ACE THE BOARDS
SURGICAL PATHOLOGY
REIMAGINED

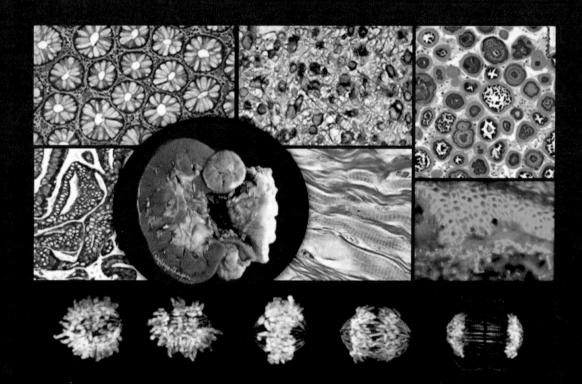

AKANKSHA GUPTA

Rajendra Singh
Terrance J. Lynn
Jared T. Ahrendsen

Kurt Schaberg
Snehal Sonawane
Upasana Joneja

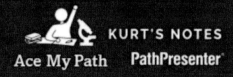
KURT'S NOTES
Ace My Path   PathPresenter®

First Edition

ISBN: 9798360734864
Copyright ©2022: Akanksha Gupta, MD
Follow us on Twitter @AceMyPath
Email: acemypath@gmail.com
Website: www.acemypath.com

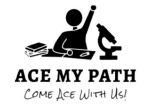

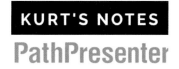

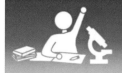 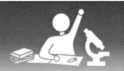
SALIENT FEATURES

- Kurt's notes, extensively revised and updated, to reflect recent advances in Surgical Pathology.
- Access to over 1000 board-relevant whole slide images, along with annotated online "high yield sections" - virtual slide collection by Path Presenter.
- More than 4000 high-resolution gross, microscopic, immunohistochemistry, and ancillary images.
- 1500 online multiple-choice question modules (work in progress).
- Videos and audio explaining the material (work in progress).

HOW YOU CAN BENEFIT MOST FROM THE BOOK

- Start reading the material from the first year of the residency.
- QR codes for virtual slides:
  - Can be scanned in the print book using electronic devices, and it is compatible with Android and IOS.
  - Most of the current mobile devices allow scanning directly via the mobile camera.
  - The other option is to download any QR code scanner application from the play store/Appstore.
  - The words "Path Presenter, Link or PP Link" are clickable on the online eBook version of the book (works on android, PC and Mac – doesn't work with some iPhones and iPads – contact us if it doesn't work).
- High Yield Sections – Virtual Microscopy Hub:
  - This high-yield board-relevant hub can be purchased at acemypath.com.
  - High-yield sections are hosted via the website acemypath.pathpresenter.com.
  - These include system-wise, compiled, and annotated 1000 virtual slides in one place.
  - As a trial, these sections are currently available on pathpresenter.net free of cost for everyone.
- Multiple Choice Questions:
  - MCQs are a work in progress currently; we plan on publishing them within a month or two.
  - These can be purchased separately at acemypath.com and can be accessed online via acemypath.pathpresenter.com.
  - MCQs will be a mix of virtual slides-based, image-based, and text-based, per the board format.
  - Around 1500 MCQs will be available for AP, including cytopathology.
- Videos / Audios:
  - Videos and Audios are a work in progress currently; we plan on publishing them within a month or two.
  - These can be purchased separately at acemypath.com and can be accessed online via acemypath.pathpresenter.com.
  - In the videos and audio, our team will discuss entities and virtual slides in the book in a system-wise format.
  - Best for people on the go or away from their book or computer screen.

ISBN: 9798360734864
Copyright ©2022: Akanksha Gupta, MD
Follow us on Twitter @AceMyPath
Email: acemypath@gmail.com
Website: www.acemypath.com

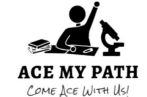

ACE MY PATH
COME ACE WITH US!

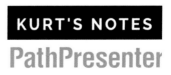

KURT'S NOTES
PathPresenter

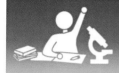
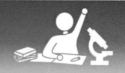
"Surgical pathology is a complex, dynamic, and ever-evolving field of medicine. This book represents **a novel contribution** to the current pathology literature. The text is **thorough, yet concise, and up to date** with the most current concepts governing the practice of surgical pathology. The book has been designed to help pathology residents preparing for board examinations; however, it will also be a useful **quick reference for practicing pathologists**.

Increasingly, the students of today want information in digital form and not in printed form. Hence book authors must cater to the needs of the new generation. The editors of this book have therefore created **a "print" book with linkage to whole slide images by scanning a QR code**. One click takes the reader to annotations. Thus, this book simulates the traditional multihead scope teaching. The only difference is that this book has an **infinite headed scope**. This unique and first of its kind simulation of teaching will help readers solidify knowledge with real life examples of surgical pathology cases. Similarly, **audio content** is also available, giving users multiple formats to customize and optimize their learning experience.

The team of authors and editors have worked tirelessly to provide a **comprehensive, user-friendly, and innovative textbook** that will be very useful for pathology residents and fellows, as well as medical students, laboratory professionals, and seasoned pathologists already in practice. **I will recommend this to our residents, fellows, and faculty.** Congratulations to the Ace My Path team for creating a novel tool for pathology education."

Vinay Kumar, MBBS, MD, FRCPath
Senior Editor/Author of Robbins Pathology textbooks
Lowell T Coggeshall Distinguished Service Professor of Pathology
Former Chairman of the Department of Pathology
Biologic Sciences Division and Pritzker School of Medicine
University of Chicago
Chicago, IL, USA

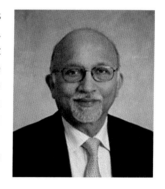

Dr Vinay Kumar is a passionate medical educator and has influenced medical education across the world for the past 35 years as the senior editor/author of **Robbins Pathology textbooks**. He is the senior editor of these books now in their 9th edition. Robbins Pathology is the most widely used medical text in the world with translations into **13 languages**. He is **the Alice Hogge and Arthur Baer Distinguished Service Professor and former Chairman** of the department of Pathology at the University of Chicago. He has made seminal contributions in the field of medical education and basic research. In 1974 **his laboratory identified Natural Killer (NK) cells** as a distinct population of lymphocytes with anti-tumor activities. Continuation of this work has led to discovery of NK cell receptors and the immunotherapeutic use of NK cells. He was elected to the American Association Advancement of Science for this "pioneering work on discovery of NK cells".
He has served on the **US National Board of medical Examiners as test writer**, and he recently coauthored a report on competency-based education commissioned by AAMC/HHMI. He has played an active role in curricular reforms globally with special interest in his native India. He believes that technology can be a powerful democratizing force in medical education and is **developing innovative ways to use technology** for educating health science professionals.

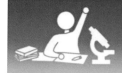 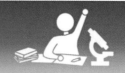
"Ace The Board: Surgical Pathology Reimagined is truly a reimagined concept to study pathology. It is designed not only for those doing residency or applying for boards, but also for all of us already practicing. This book offers more than 4000 high-resolution photomicrographs accompanied by high-yield text, which is integrated with over 1000 whole slide images. This allows a really close to "real-pathology" experience. I genuinely believe every pathologist would have loved to have this book on their side during residency and for sure will enjoy it in day-to-day practice."

VICTOR G. PRIETO, MD, PhD
Professor and Chair
Ferenc and Phyllis Gyorkey Chair for Research and Education in Pathology
Professor, Department of Dermatology
Division of Cancer Medicine
The University of Texas MD Anderson Cancer Center
Houston TX, USA

"Wow! Ace the Boards: Surgical Pathology "Reimagined" is a GAME CHANGER. Beautiful high-quality images, high yield bullet point texts, useful algorithms, and tables, and scannable QR code links to virtual microscopic slides of numerous entities. This is a high yield, efficient, modern approach to learning & studying surgical pathology. Whether you are a new pathology trainee just starting out, a senior resident studying for boards, or a pathologist who needs a high yield reference for daily practice...this book is solid gold!"

JERAD M. GARDNER, MD
Dermatopathologist/Bone and Soft Tissue Pathologist
Section Head, Bone and Soft Tissue Pathology
Co-founder, Knowledge in Knowledge out
Deputy Editor, Archives of Pathology and Laboratory medicine
Geisinger Medical Center
Danville, PA, USA

"I can undoubtedly say that "Ace the Boards: Surgical Pathology Reimagined" is a pathology review book like none other. It focuses on high-yields facts with over 3000 histologic, gross, and immunohistochemical stain images and caters to variable learning styles as audio material, virtual slides and multiple-choice questions are part of the package. It is authored by people passionate for pathology and teaching. Authors/Editors include senior pathologists and also younger generation that have gone through the stress of boards preparation themselves not too long ago. It's a book of the future with QR codes linking to annotated digital whole scanned slides to enhance learning.
Truly, a book that I wish I had while I was preparing for my boards which is SUCCINT, FOCUSED and HIGH-YIELD!!"

ANIL PARWANI, MD, PhD, MBA
Professor of Pathology and Biomedical Informatics
Vice-Chair of Anatomic Pathology
Director of Pathology Informatics
Director, Digital Pathology Shared Resources
Principal Investigator, Cooperative Human Tissue Network (CHTN) Midwestern Division
Wexner Medical Center - Department of Pathology
The Ohio State University
Columbus, OH, USA

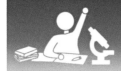 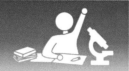
"Look forward to reading Ace the Boards: Surgical Pathology Reimagined, a new publication co-authored by Dr. Raj Singh, my co-editor of Digital Anatomic Pathology Academy (DAPA) of Digital Pathology Association (DPA). This book brings the traditional and digital board preparation material under one umbrella using over 1000 Path Presenter virtual slides. This is a much-needed supplementary resource for residents to study for the anatomic pathology board examination as well as for practicing pathologists to update their knowledge."

MARILYN BUI, MD, PhD
Co-Editor of DAPA by DPA
Scientific Director of the Analytic Microscopy Core
Professor and the Director of the Cytopathology Fellowship
University of South Florida (USF) Morsani College of Medicine
Moffitt Cancer Center & Research Institute
Tampa, FL, USA

"Ace The Boards Surgical Pathology "Reimagined" has an impressive display of surgical pathology images and descriptions that make the content comprehensive and digestible for studying. Having the option to easily access digital slides via QR codes along with a great flow of how the different branches of anatomical pathology are presented makes this a great investment for board studying and beyond."

MICHAEL WILLIAMS, MD, MSc
Neuropathology fellow
University of Alabama at Birmingham
Birmingham, AL
Founder: Diversify in Path Podcast

"I must say, the more I read, more I love the book. Why could not we have it last year at the time of our board preparation? We were lost in the sea of resources and had to juggle between them trying to find out the best so that we don't miss anything. This is such a comprehensive resource. Let it be the content or the concept of linking QR codes to the topics, it's complete! Kudos to Akanksha for thinking about this concept and kudos to the team for coming up with this beauty."

NIDHI KATARIA, MBBS
Hematopathology Fellow
Dept of Pathology and Laboratory Medicine
Donald and Barbara Zucker School of Medicine at Hofstra/Northwell
New York, NY, USA

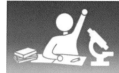

Commitment to excellence, collaborative learning, and innovation are the foundation of Ace my Path. Inspired by the overwhelmingly positive feedback on our prior books, we decided to commit to our biggest venture yet- to create a single comprehensive yet succinct surgical pathology learning resource for trainees and pathologists alike. Most of our team members are less than five years out of training; they can best see the limitations of the currently available resources and are most apt to create a new resource that is comprehensive.

During my boards preparation, I remember shuffling through my AP boards material in a hotel room in Tampa five days before the board examination. Then, two days before the exam, my co-resident came in with his much more organized handwritten anatomic pathology notes. We went through his notes within a matter of hours; truly speaking, that was a very satisfactory experience. So, the inception of the idea of creating this book happened then.

Two years later, I came across Dr. Kurt Schaberg's Pathology Notes website, an online resource that succinctly discusses innumerable pathology entities based on organ systems and is very comprehensive. I couldn't wait to reach out to him for collaboration. We are passionate about learning and teaching and imagined a surgical pathology resource with lots of histologic, gross, and immunohistochemistry correlates. Pathology is best learned by seeing slides in addition to learning the material. This concept came to fruition when we collaborated with Dr. Rajendra Singh on Path Presenter. The concept of having high-yield notes on surgical pathology entities with digital links to whole scanned slide images was innovative. We knew this would revolutionize how surgical pathology is learned. Then, we started the task of turning this idea into a reality.

It was a huge undertaking, and in January 2022, we started to look for more dedicated team members who shared our goals and enthusiasm. We formed a strong, dedicated team of forty-two pathologists that contributed to different roles: editors, authors, reviewers, and path art contributors (not counting MCQ and video/audio content generators, who are currently working on it). A special mention for the Path Twitter-verse, where pathologists from all over the world contributed images of their rare cases out of dedication as teachers. They were an indispensable part of this project. This level of project did not come without challenges- many working hours after clinical duties, day and night meetings and brainstorming sessions, work delegation and implementation, and collaborative issues, to name a few. After ten months of extensive work, numerous drafts, and multiple reviews and edits, we present to you this product that is a one-of-a-kind immersive, innovative pathology learning experience.

This book is valuable for trainees and practicing pathologists. It contains organ-based high-yield information, including advances in the field. Key gross and photomicrographs for each entity accompanied by annotated virtual slides in Path Presenter is what distinguishes this book from all others. Our readers have access to a rich repository of images and more than 1000 virtual slides at the click of a button online or by scanning a QR code in the book, creating a seamless learning experience. Meanwhile, we are working on making video and audio files discussing the entities in the book. In addition, we will go over the virtual slides in those videos/audios. This will enhance the auditory learning experience, which is best for people on the go or away from their book or computer screen. However, that is not all; multiple-choice questions with virtual slides embedded in the questions and annotated explanations for the correct answers give the learners a true boards test experience. We think this book is a must-have for trainees in their board prep, but it also undoubtedly makes a great reference resource for practicing pathologists.

This book is a collaboration between the pioneers and the leaders of Pathology teaching, "Path Presenter," "Kurt's Notes," and "Ace My Path," and we've reconceptualized ("reimagined") the way of learning. We hope that our fruit of labor is beneficial to the readers. Finally, we wish you good luck and hope to be by your side in your surgical pathology learning journey.

- **AKANKSHA GUPTA, MD**
  Founder and CEO
  Ace My Path

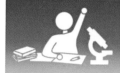
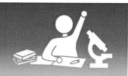

ACKNOWLEDGEMENTS

"To God, for instilling a "purpose of life" in me. To my passionate mentors, for instilling in me the passion for Pathology. To my parents, Maya Gupta and Jugalkishore Gupta for instilling my values, my character, and for living a life that I can take inspiration from. To my loving husband, Ashish Gupta, for demonstrating going after one's ambition, for encouraging me to fulfill my dreams and pushing me every day to become my best self. And lastly, to my son and best friend, Siddharth Gupta, for reminding me every day that I matter, for being my biggest fan, and for sitting on my lap / hugging me (even while sitting on the computer to write this book), making me feel the warmth of his loving heart!"

- AKANKSHA GUPTA, MD

"To my wife, Manisha, daughter Kritika and son, Satyen who have selflessly sacrificed a lot and allowed me to follow my passions. To all my friends, mentors and colleagues who have been supportive and encouraging every step of the way."

- RAJENDRA SINGH, MD

"To my family, Aiko, Ingrid, and Ben, for their love and patience. And also, to my mentors at Stanford for their inspiring teaching."

- KURT SCHABERG, MD

"To my family: MaryAnn, Scott, Jamie, and Zachariah for all their support and love. A huge thank you to my group of mentors: Dr. Yi Ding, Dr. Sara E. Monaco, Dr. Jerad Gardner, and Dr. Andrew Campbell for all their support and wisdom over the years at Geisinger."

- TERRANCE LYNN, MD

"This undertaking could not have been completed without the assistance of the Pathology Twitter verse, whose names may not be all enumerated here. Their contributions are sincerely appreciated and gratefully acknowledged. To my dearest husband, Shankar Sonawane, my beloved children Shree, Guru, and Dev, and my in-laws for their endless support, kind, and understanding spirit throughout the process of making this book. I am deeply grateful to my parents, Dr. Tulshiram and Poonam Shinde, my sister's Manswini, Trupti, my brother Ganesh, for their appreciation, encouragement, and a keen interest in my academic achievements. Above all, to the Great Almighty, the author of knowledge and wisdom, for his countless blessings."

- SNEHAL SONAWANE, MD

"To my mentors and colleagues, both past and present, for their role in my professional growth and development. Thank you to my friends and family, who have always been there for me. A special dedication to my wife and best friend, Andi, for her constant support and unwavering love."

- JARED T. AHRENDSEN, MD, PhD

"Thank you to all the collaborators! Special thanks to Akanksha Gupta for giving me this opportunity. You are inspiring!
To my wonderful family: Prabal, Mom, Dad, Akangsha, and Megha- Thank you for your unconditional love, support, and patience"

- UPASANA JONEJA, MD

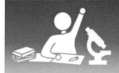 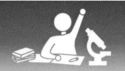
EDITORS / AUTHORS

AKANKSHA GUPTA, MD
Hematopathologist & Surgical Pathologist
Integrated Pathology Associates
Flint/Bay city/Mount Pleasant, MI

RAJENDRA SINGH, MD
Professor and Director of Dermatopathology
Associate Chair, Digital Pathology
Summit Health, New York, NY

KURT SCHABERG, MD
Pathology Residency Program Director
Associate Health Sciences Clinical Professor
UC Davis Health
Sacramento, CA

ASSOCIATE EDITORS / AUTHORS

TERRANCE J. LYNN, MD, MS, MHCI
AP/CP Residency / Cytopathology Fellowship
Geisinger Medical Center
Danville, Pennsylvania

SNEHAL SONAWANE, MD
Assistant Professor of Pathology
University of Illinois at Chicago
Chicago, IL

JARED T. AHRENDSEN, MD, PhD
Assistant Professor of Pathology
Northwestern University Feinberg School of Medicine
Chicago, IL

UPASANA JONEJA, MD
Assistant Professor
Cooper Medical School of Rowan University
Camden, NJ

MANJU AMBELIL, MD
Assistant professor
Thomas Jefferson University Hospital
Philadelphia, PA

KENECHUKWU OJUKWU, MD MPP
Bone and Soft Tissue Pathology Fellow
National Clinician Scholars Fellow
David Geffen School of Medicine
University of California, Los Angeles

NATHAN MCGRATH, MBBS
Pathology registrar
Wits Faculty of Health Sciences
Johannesburg, South Africa

AMANDEEP KAUR, MD
Molecular Genetic Fellow
University of Chicago (NorthShore)
Chicago, IL

DINESH PRADHAN, MD
Dermatopathologist & Medical Director
Sonic Healthcare USA, Jacksonville, FL

KANNAN SIVARAJ, MD, DIP RCPATH, DNB
Lab Director
Neuberg Ehrlich Laboratory
Coimbatore, India

JOSEPH CZAJA, MD
Surgical Pathologist & Cytopathologist
Integrated Pathology Associates, Flint, MI
Laboratory Director, Bay city/Mount Pleasant, MI

AUTHORS

SWATI SATTURWAR, MD
Assistant Professor,
The Ohio State University, Wexner Medical Center
Columbus, OH

SUDARSHANA ROYCHOUDHURY, MD
Breast and gynecologic pathologist
Assistant Professor, Zucker SOM at Hofstra/Northwell
Pathology and Laboratory Medicine

NAOMI HARDY, MD
Visiting Instructor
University of Maryland School of Medicine
Baltimore, MD

MARIA CECILIA D. REYES, MD
Assistant Professor
Medical University of South Carolina
Charleston, SC

BINNY KHANDAKAR, MD, DNB
Fellow, Gastrointestinal-Liver Pathology
Yale New Haven Hospital
New Haven, CT

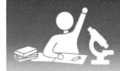 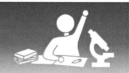

SATYAPAL CHAHAR, MD
Assistant Professor
University of Mississippi Medical Center
Jackson, MS

PUKHRAZ BASRA, MD
Assistant Professor
Case Western Reserve University
University Hospitals Cleveland Medical Center
Cleveland, OH

AMY DEEKEN, MD
Medical Examiner and President
Summit County, Ohio

DEVI JEYACHANDRAN, MD
Assistant Professor
Roswell Park Comprehensive Cancer Center
Buffalo, NY

SWATI BHARDWAJ, MBBS, MD
PGY3 AP/CP Resident
Icahn School of Medicine at Mount Sinai
New York, NY

JIAN LI, MD, PHD
PGY1 AP/CP Resident
RWJ Barnabas Health Monmouth Medical Center
New Brunswick, NJ

HANSINI LAHARWANI, MD
Breast and GYN Pathology Fellow
Washington University in St. Louis
St. Louis, MO

MANITA CHAUM, MD
PGY4 AP/CP Resident
Cedars Sinai Medical Center
Los Angeles, CA

GAGANDEEP KAUR , MD
Oncologic Surgical Pathology Fellow
Memorial Sloan Kettering Cancer Center
New York, NY

NIDHI KATARIA, MBBS
Hematopathology Fellow
Dept of Pathology and Laboratory Medicine
Donald and Barbara Zucker School of Medicine at
Hofstra/Northwell, NY

NUPUR SHARMA, MD
Hematopathology fellow
University of North Carolina
Chapel Hill, NC

KRISTY WAITE, MD
Deputy Medical Examiner
Summit County, Ohio

MAYURI SHENDE, MBBS, DCP, FCPS, DNB, SH(ASCP)^{CM}
Specialist in Hematology
Hematopathology fellowship training
Loyola University Medical Center, Maywood IL
Current AP/CP Resident
University of Tennessee Health Science Center, TN

KRUTIKA PATEL, MBBS, MD
Assistant Professor
Department of Pathology
Vanderbilt University Medical Center
Nashville, TN

AASTHA CHAUHAN, MD
Assistant Professor
University of Minnesota Medical Center
Minneapolis, MN

VISHU PASHAM, MD
AP/CP Resident
Medical University of South Carolina
Charleston, SC

REVIEWERS

SNEHAL SONAWANE, MD
Assistant Professor of Pathology
University of Illinois at Chicago
Chicago, IL

JARED T. AHRENDSEN, MD, PhD
Assistant Professor of Pathology
Northwestern University Feinberg School of Medicine
Chicago, IL

UPASANA JONEJA, MD
Assistant Professor
Cooper Medical School of Rowan University
Camden, NJ

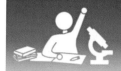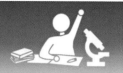
KSHITIJA KALE, MD
Ph.D. Graduate Student
Experimental Pathology
University of Iowa, Iowa City, IA

NIDHI KATARIA, MBBS
Hematopathology Fellow
Dept of Pathology and Laboratory Medicine
Donald and Barbara Zucker School of Medicine at
Hofstra/Northwell, NY

HARINI VENKATRAMAN RAVISANKAR, MBBS, MD
MD Pathology
Rajiv Gandhi University of Health Sciences
Karnataka, India

BINNY KHANDAKAR, MD, DNB
Fellow, Gastrointestinal-Liver Pathology
Yale New Haven Hospital, New Haven, CT

SWATI BHARDWAJ, MBBS, MD
PGY3 AP/CP Resident
Icahn School of Medicine at Mount Sinai
New York, NY

DEEPA ANANTHA LAXMI N.V, MBBS, MD
Consultant Pathologist & Lab Head,
Healthians Labs, Telangana, India

RAMA DEVI, MD
Oncopathology DM Resident
Gujarat Cancer Research Institute
BJ Medical College, Ahmedabad, India

HANSINI LAHARWANI, MD
Breast and GYN Pathology Fellow
Washington University in St. Louis
St. Louis, MO

ABHILASHA BORKAR, MD
Cytopathology Fellow
Loyola University Medical Center, IL

NEHA SETH, MD
Hematopathology fellow 2024-25
Donald and Barbara Zucker School of Medicine
at Hofstra/Northwell, Greenvale, NY
Former Practicing Hematopathologist
CMC Vellore, TN India
Sehgal Path Lab, Mumbai, India

OTHER CONTRIBUTORS

PRIYA SKARIA, MD
(Helped in designing the book concept)
Hematopathologist and Surgical Pathologist
Yuma Regional Medical Center
Yuma, AZ

PATHART CONTRIBUTORS

ZIAD EL-ZAATARI, MD
Surgical Pathologist
Methodist Hospital
Houston, TX

ANDY MOORE, PhD
Cell biologist
Arlington, VA

SUSAN PRENDEVELLE, MD
GU Pathologist
University Health Network
Toronto, Canada

AMY ENGEVIK, PhD
Epithelial Cell Biologist and Physiologist
Charleston, SC

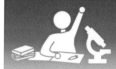

OUTLINE

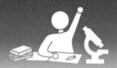

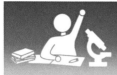 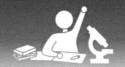

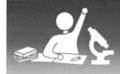
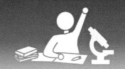

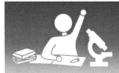
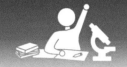

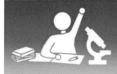

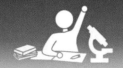

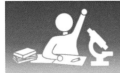 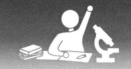

DETAILED INDEX (VOL 1)
(PREPARED BY HARINI V RAVISANKAR, MD)

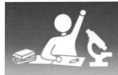
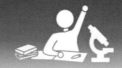

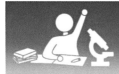
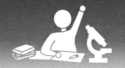

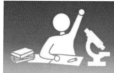
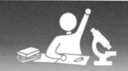

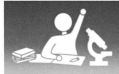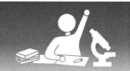

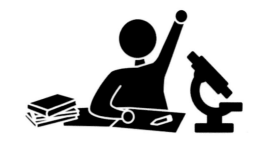

ACE MY PATH
Come Ace With Us!

CHAPTER 1: APPROACH TO THE UNITED
STATES AP/CP BOARD EXAMS

Nupur Sharma, MD
Hansini Laharwani, MD
Nidhi Kataria, MD
Akanksha Gupta, MD

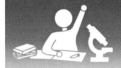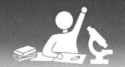
INTRODUCTION

This chapter will cover the following topics:
- Approach to AP/CP board exams
- Pre-exam requirements
- Preparation timeline and resources
- Post exam follow-up

PRE-EXAM REQUIREMENTS:

- Combined Anatomic Pathology and Clinical Pathology (AP/CP) Certification
- The applicant must have 48 months of full-time training in an accredited AP/CP program. Training must include at least 18 months each of structured AP and CP training. The remaining 12 months are flexible and may include AP and/or CP rotations
- Training may include up to 6 months of research during the pathology training program with the approval of the program director
- The applicant must have completed at least 30 autopsies by the time the application for certification is submitted.
- A list of completed autopsies must be uploaded with the application (see Appendix A: Autopsy Requirements)
- Candidates for combined AP/CP certification will not be certified by the ABPath until both the AP and the CP examinations are passed, and all requirements are met

APPLICATION:

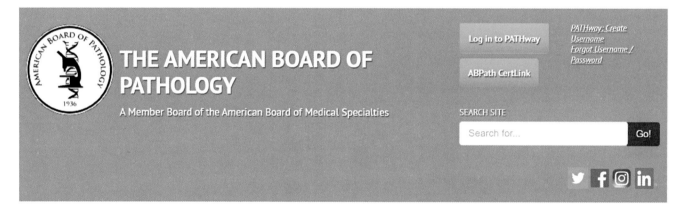

- Link: https://wds.dataharborsolutions.com/ABPathOrg/Default.aspx
- You will receive an email from ABPath about Board registration at the end of August
- Please keep your personal information up to date
- 2022 exam details:
  - ➢ Application Start   9/15/2021
  - ➢ Application Deadline   1/15/2022
  - ➢ Application Fee $2600 for AP/CP combined
  - ➢ Late submission deadline mid-February (costs additional $1050 (AP or CP only) or $1300 (combined AP/CP)
  - ➢ The window for scheduling exam: 3/9 – 5/2/2022
  - ➢ Exams will be administered : **5/16 – 6/3/2022**
- Schedule your exam date in March
- You will receive an email from ABPath for details

AUTOPSY LOG:

- Enter at least 30 cases with brief main diagnosis (cause of death)
- Link: https://apps.acgme.org/connect/login?returnUrl=https%3A%2F%2Fapps.acgme.org%2Fads%2F&redirect=True
- Export the Autopsy Log as PDF format
- The end product that goes in your application look like this

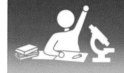
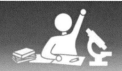
ROTATION LOG:

- Breakdown of weeks on AP & CP rotations

Anatomic Pathology	No. of Months
Autopsy Pathology	2
Surgical Pathology	14
Cytopathology	4
Pediatric Pathology	0.5
Forensic Pathology	2
Neuropathology	0.5
Informatics	1
Laboratory Management	0
Molecular Pathology	1
Research	0
Other	5
Other (specify; excluding vacation)	4 tumor board, 1medical renal/lung
Subtotal for Anatomic Pathology	30

Clinical Pathology	No. of Months
Chemical Pathology	3
Hematopathology	4
Blood Banking/Transfusion Medicine	3
Microbiology	3
Medical Microscopy	0
Informatics	1
Laboratory Management	1
Molecular Pathology	1
Research	0
Other	2
Other (specify; excluding vacation)	Introduction test utilization
Subtotal for Clinical Pathology	18
Total	48

CASE NUMBERS OF SURGICAL PATHOLOGY, CYTOPATHOLOGY, AND CLINICAL CONSULTATION
Clinical consultation includes Chemistry, Hematopathology, Blood bank, Tumor board, and CP on-call

	4 year total
Number of surgical specimens examined by you	2112
Number of cytopathologic specimens examined by you	1512
Number of bone marrows performed by you	0
Number of FNAs performed by you	1
Clinical pathology consultations participated in by you. A clinical consultation is defined by the ABPath as any interaction (formal or informal) between you and another health care professional regarding handling of specimens and/or interpretation of data. These consultations may be oral or written and do not have to be billable. **Do not include written anatomic pathology reports.**	1450

- Program Director must sign off that you have satisfactorily completed residency requirements
- After you submit your application, you will hear nothing for months. Be patient!

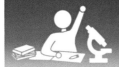

- You need following things in order to get your results: Remember to finish your full and unrestricted licensing!

2022 Spring PRIMARY Exam Application Tracking.

- ☑ Application and payment have been received.
- ☑ Medical license reviewed.
  - ☑ Approved.
  - ☐ Expired. **Withhold Results
  - ☐ Not approved (training or restricted license).
  - ☐ Applied for. **Withhold Results
    - Step 3 score or equivalent.

  Medical school diploma.
  - ☑ Approved.
- ☑ Application to Program Director for review.
  - ☑ Completed.
- ☑ Evaluation 1 received (Vidant Medical Center/East Carolina University Program).
  Application to Credentials Committee.
    Approved.
    Not Approved.

SCHEDULE:
2022 AP BOARD EXAM SCHEDULE

One Day (10.1 hours)			
Time	**Section**	**Number of Items**	**Comments**
(20 min)	Tutorial/Honor Code		
(72 min)	Combined Section A	72	1 min per item
(15 min)	*Break*		
(81 min)	Virtual Microscopy I	27	3 min per item
(15 min)	*Break*		
(72 min)	Combined Section B	72	1 min per item
(60 min)	*Long Break*		
(81 min)	Virtual Microscopy II	27	3 min per item
(15 min)	*Break*		
(71 min)	Combined Section C	71	1 min per item
(15 min)	*Break*		
(78 min)	Virtual Microscopy III	26	3 min per item
(10 min)	Exam Survey		

- 3 multiple choice question sections, 215 questions (1 min/question)
- 3 virtual microscope sections, 80 questions (3 min/question)

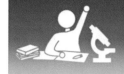 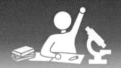

2022 CP BOARD EXAM SCHEDULE

One Day (9.1 hours)			
Time	**Section**	**Number of Items**	**Comments**
(20 min)	Tutorial/Honor Code		
(66 min)	Combined Section A	55	1.2 min per item
(15 min)	*Break*		
(66 min)	Combined Section B	55	1.2 min per item
(15 min)	*Break*		
(66 min)	Combined Section C	55	1.2 min per item
(60 min)	*Long Break*		
(66 min)	Combined Section D	55	1.2 min per item
(15 min)	*Break*		
(66 min)	Combined Section E	55	1.2 min per item
(15 min)	*Break*		
(66 min)	Combined Section F	55	1.2 min per item
(10 min)	Exam Survey		

- 6 multiple choice question sections (1.2 min/question)
- 330 questions

EXAMINATION BLUEPRINT

Anatomic Pathology Exam Blueprint	Approximate %	
	Written/Practical	**Virtual Microscopy**
AP Management & General Pathology Principles	2	0
Breast	7	10
Male Genital	4	8
Cardiovascular	2	1
Lymph Nodes and Spleen	4	6
Bone Marrow	4	3
Head and Neck	4	8
Alimentary Canal, Pancreas, Liver, Extrahepatic Biliary Tree, Gall Bladder	10	13
Endocrine	5	6
Female Genital, Placenta, Peritoneum	8	8
Urinary/Renal	7	6
Respiratory, Pleura, Mediastinum	6	8
Central and Peripheral Nervous System	3	6
Soft Tissue and Bone	5	6
Skin	6	8
Molecular	1	0
Forensic	2	0
Cytopathology	18	3
Laboratory Management-General	2	0
Total Percentage	**100**	**100**
Total Number of Questions in Each Section	**215**	**80**
Total Hours Allotted for Each Section	**3 Hrs 35 Mins**	**4 Hrs**

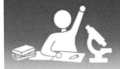
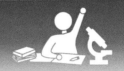
Updated for 2022

Clinical Pathology Exam Blueprint	Approximate % Written/Practical
Blood Banking/Transfusion Medicine	23
Chemical Pathology	20
Hematology	25
Management and Informatics	9
Medical Microbiology	23
Total Percentage	100
Total Number of Questions in Each Section	330
Total Hours Allotted for Each Section	6 Hrs 36 Mins

LICENSURE:
(Disclaimer: You don't have to get PA license, many residents in the past have gotten it, since it's easier and convenient; but feel free to choose a state license that is convenient as per your needs and future plans)

Full and Unrestricted Medical License Application
(**Pennsylvania** State)

- Fingerprints (FD-1164) $40
- Criminal record investigation (FBI) $18
- https://www.edo.cjis.gov/#/
- **Apply online, Pay online.** Mail fingerprint card
- You will receive an email link in a week
- Criminal record investigation (NC) $14
- https://ncsbi.gov/Services/SBI-Forms/SBIRight-to-Review__FILLABLE-2021.aspx
- Mail application, fingerprint card and money order together
- You will receive a letter in 2-3 weeks
- Go to the **Pennsylvania Licensing System (PALS)**
- (PALS.pa.gov) and create your account

Welcome to the Pennsylvania Licensing System (PALS)

PALS can help you apply for, renew, and check your professional license.

How do I get started?

A good starting point is to use our application checklist to see all of the requirements and needed documents to apply for your license.

If this is your first time using PALS, create an account or if you are a returning user, log in to your account. Once you are logged in, your dashboard will provide you with clear next steps.

- Start application and pay $85 online
- Upload the following documents

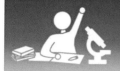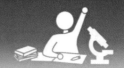
CheckList Name	Instructions
Application	All applications are processed in order of submission. If this application is not completed **within six months**, updates of certain sections and/or supporting documents will be required. If the application has not been completed within one year from the date it was received, applicants will be required to submit a new application (**another application processing fee**) and supporting documents, as necessary.
Application Fee	**NON REFUNDABLE FEE** in the amount of **$85.00**, made payable by credit/debit card. If the application has not been completed within one year from the date it was received, applicants will be required to submit a new application (**another application processing fee**) and supporting documents, as necessary.
Child Abuse CE	All health-related licensees/certificate holders and funeral directors are considered "mandatory reporters" under section 6311 of the Child Protective Services Law (23 P.S. § 6311). Therefore, all persons applying for issuance of an initial license or certificate from any of the health-related boards (except the State Board of Veterinary Medicine) or from the State Board of Funeral Directors are required to complete, as a condition of licensure, 3 hours of approved training by the Department of Human Services (DHS) on the topic of child abuse recognition and reporting. After you have completed the required course, the approved provider will electronically submit your name, date of attendance, etc. to the Bureau. For that reason, it is imperative that you register for the course using the information provided on your application for licensure/certification. A list of DHS-approved child abuse education providers can be found on the Department of State Website.
Criminal History Check	Provide a recent Criminal History Records Check (CHRC) from the state police or other state agency **that is the official repository for criminal history record information** for every state in which you have lived, worked, or completed professional training/studies for the past ten (10) years. The report(s) must be dated within 90 days of the date the application is submitted. For applicants living, working, or completing training/studies in Pennsylvania, your CHRC request will be automatically submitted to the Pennsylvania State Police upon submission of this application. The PATCH fee will be included at checkout. Your PA CHRC will be sent directly to the Board/Commission. You will be notified if additional action is required. For individuals living, working, or completing training/studies outside of Pennsylvania during the past ten (10) years, in lieu of obtaining individual state background checks, you may elect to provide BOTH a state CHRC from the state in which you currently reside, AND your FBI Identity History Summary Check, available at https://www.fbi.gov/services/cjis/identity-history-summary-checks. Please note: For applicants currently living, working, or completing training/studies in California, Arizona, or Ohio: Due to the laws of these states, the Board is not an eligible recipient of CHRC's or your CHRC will not be issued to you for upload to the Board. Please obtain your Federal Bureau of Investigation (FBI) Identity History Summary Check, available at the link noted above.

Databank Report	Provide an official notification of information (Self Query) from the National Practitioner Data Bank. Please refer to the NPDB website for additional information. When you receive the "Response to your Self Query," you will need to upload it to your online application. The report will need to be uploaded, where prompted, in order to submit your application.
Diploma	Request that your school provide a certified copy of your diploma. **NOTE: All documents must be in ENGLISH or an official translation must be submitted to the Board from an official translation agency or professor of the language.**
Education Verification	Complete Section 1 of the Verification of Medical Education form and forward to your medical school for completion of Section 2. **The school must return the completed verification directly to the Board. The form will be available for download and printing when the application is submitted.**
Educational Transcripts	Request that your school provide an official transcript. If the official transcript does not provide detailed information regarding the courses attended from which the applicant's eligibility is determined, the Board retains the right to request a copy of the medical school curriculum.
Exam Results	Submit proof of obtaining a passing score on one of the examinations acceptable to the Board by contacting the appropriate agency and **request scores be sent directly to the Board**
Graduate Training	Complete Section 1 of the Verification of ACGME Approved Graduate Medical Training form and send to the U.S./Canadian hospital(s) where you completed your PGY 1, PGY 2, and PGY 3 postgraduate training. Section 2 should be completed by the training hospital(s). For applicants still in PGY 3, the program director **may not sign and date the form more than thirty (30) days prior to the completion of the approved training. Forms postmarked or signed prior to the thirty days will not be accepted. The hospital(s) must return the completed form directly to the Board. The form will be available for download and printing when the application is submitted.**

- If you have current ECFMG certification, you DO NOT need to request the record of graduation, educational transcript, and diploma from your medical schools

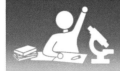
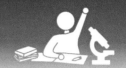
International Education Verification	Request verification of your ECFMG Certification directly from ECFMG. Your certification must be current and valid. **The name of the State Medical Board that the Status Report should be sent to is Pennsylvania State Board of Medicine–State Code: 039.** If you completed an approved Fifth Pathway Program, submit a notarized copy of the Fifth Pathway Certificate.
Letter of Good Standing (LOGS)	Contact the licensing authorities of the states, territories or countries where you hold or have ever held a license, certificate, permit, registration or other authorization to practice a health-related profession (whether active, inactive, expired or current) and request letters of good standing/verification of licensure in that state or jurisdiction. The letter must include the following: license issue and expiration date, license status (current or expired) and disciplinary standing. **The letter(s) of good standing must be sent directly to the Board.**
Opioid CE	Section 9.1(a) of ABC-MAP* requires that all prescribers or dispensers, as defined in Section 3 of ABC-MAP, applying for licensure/approval complete at least 4 hours of Board-approved education consisting of 2 hours in pain management or the identification of addiction and 2 hours in the practices of prescribing or dispensing of opioids. Applicants seeking licensure/approval on or after July 1, 2017, must document, within one year from issuance of the licensure/ approval, that they completed this education either as part of an initial education program, a stand-alone course from a Board-approved course provider, or a continuing education course from an approved continuing education provider. The 4 hours of Board-approved education needs to be completed only once. See the Board's website for the Opioid Education Forms and additional information. *The Achieving Better Care by Monitoring All Prescriptions Program Act (ABC-MAP) (Act 191 of 2014, as amended) is available on the Legislature's website at: http://www.legis.state.pa.us/cfdocs/Legis/LI/uconsCheck. cfm?txtType=HTM&yr=2014&sessInd=0&smthLwInd=0 &act=191. The Board's Regulations are available on the Board's website.
Resume/Curriculum Vitae	You will need to upload, where prompted, a current Curriculum Vitae listing **all** periods of employment or unemployment (i.e., child rearing, research, etc.) from graduation from medical school to present. The list must be in chronological order, include the month and year, and indicate the state/territory in which the employment occurred. The resume/curriculum vitae will need to be uploaded, in order to submit your application.

- FSMB (transcript directly to PA medical board) $70
- https://www.fsmb.org/transcripts/

ECFMG CERTIFICATION VERIFICATION SERVICE (CVS) ON-LINE $60
- https://secure2.ecfmg.org

OPIOID CE: https://www.train.org/pa/welcome

CHILD ABUSE CE: https://www.dos.pa.gov/ProfessionalLicensing/BoardsCommissions/Pages/Act-31.aspx

REGISTRATION:
- https://www.reportabusepa.pitt.edu//Login.aspx
- The online course will take four hours to finish
- Upload the certificate to PALS

RESOURCES AND TIMELINE:
Timeline for preparation:
- Start reading this book from the first year. This will go a long way!!
- Initial reading for boards: Approximately 2-3 hours of questions and text and 1 hour of group study per day starting in September
- January onwards: (6-7 hours per day), gradually increasing as time permits
- Recognize your strength and weakness early in 4th year
- Divide your time between reading text, doing questions and virtual slides each day to break the monotony
- Group study helps tremendously with understanding concepts and building recall ability. Ace My Path has developed many WhatsApp based groups for Pathologists and creates each year separate group for exam going residents. Contact us to be included in the groups

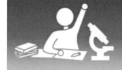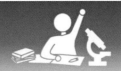
- Use flashcards for things like mutations in soft-tissue tumors
- Go through cases in your rotations and try to understand the etio-pathogenesis of diseases

Resources:
- AP: Kurt's notes, Board review courses, Path presenter high yield section with virtual images, one or more popular question banks (e.g., Pathdojo, PathPrimer, ASCP Question Banks etc.)
- What we have to offer:
  ➢ Ace the boards: Surgical Pathology will give you a combined experience of question banks, notes, virtual slides, and videos all in one space
  ➢ Contact us for buying a boards relevant annotated virtual slide hub, which has >1000 boards relevant virtual slides
  ➢ In addition, videos/audios are available, which will go over our text and explain virtual slides
  ➢ Multiple choice question module by Ace My Path consists of over 1500 board style questions, including questions with virtual microscopic slides
  ➢ MCQs and videos will be rolled out within few months of release of this book. For more information, visit www.acemypath.com
- CP: CP compendium, CDC (microbiology images), selective reading- Henry's, popular question banks (e.g., Spitalnik, Pathdojo)
- Our other boards relevant resources include:
  ➢ Ace the boards: Neoplastic Hematopathology
  ➢ Ace the boards: Non-Neoplastic Hematopathology and Coagulation
  ➢ Ace the boards: Cytopathology

EXAM DAY:
- The day: Try to stay relaxed!!!! (Easier said than done 😊)
- The exam is currently being conducted at Pearson-VUE exams center, and information is available on the ABPath website as well as on the link below
- Reach the center well before time and bring 2 identity proofs with you. Get light snacks (e.g., Banana, yogurt, chocolate, peanut sandwich, coffee, water bottle, coke etc. Bring lunch if you can, it will save your time and you can relax more in your lunch break). Sometimes, the exam center buildings have cafeteria, but it is good to have some snacks for the small breaks
- For the exam, first and foremost in the tutorial session make sure virtual slides and images are working well. If not, please contact the proctor ASAP
- Preferably, follow the exam format as provided by ABPath, taking all the breaks to refresh your minds in between different sessions
- Try to stay focused and relaxed, getting through last 2 sessions can become challenging
- Use your system from Med School/Steps – flag questions, use scratch paper, choose an answer and don't look back
- Instructions and test interface are super straightforward; REALLY, NO ONE IS TRYING TO TRICK YOU
- Time allotted is adequate
- You may come across diagnoses you've never heard of – and that's okay, happens to the best of us!
- Odd clinical factoids you don't know about common entities can be encountered
- Best way to prepare for this is to stay engaged during residency
- Senior year is a good time to go over weak areas (sit in on sign outs and pay attention!)
- Focus on Hematology and Coagulation, as they are high yield as well. Do lots of morphology for heme
- Follow ABPath's blueprint for system wise distribution of questions and their weightage. Our book is created keeping the blueprint in mind
- As per their website, board passing rate is >90% for both AP and CP. So, work hard and smart and stay relaxed

Test center information:
American Board of Pathology (abpath.org)

POST-EXAM FOLLOW UP:
- Results are available usually in 8 weeks, so look out for the email from ABPath. Again, keep your email updated on ABPath website to receive your results
- Most important: Don't give away this book to juniors after boards, you will benefit hugely with it while starting to practice as well!

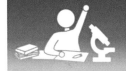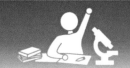

Disclaimer: While the authors believe that the information stated in this chapter is correct and current for 2022 to the best of their knowledge, applicants are requested to verify all information before use. The authors claim no responsibility for any change/update in the above-mentioned data.

ALL THE BEST FOR YOUR BOARDS AND PATHOLOGY CAREER!! COME ACE WITH US!!

ACE MY PATH TEAM

References:
- Abpath.org
- PALS.pa.gov

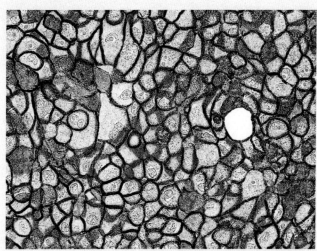

HER-2 Immunostain, invasive ductal carcinoma of the breast. Image courtesy: Takashi Fujisawa, MD, Ph.D. (@Patholwalker)

CHAPTER 2: BREAST PATHOLOGY

Terrance Lynn, MD
Aastha Chauhan, MD
Pukhraz Basra, MD
Akanksha Gupta, MD
Jian Li, MD

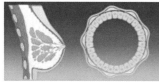 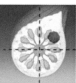

NORMAL ANATOMY

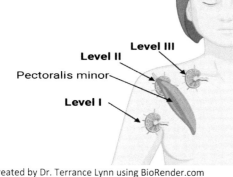

Lobules with acini | Duct

NORMAL BREAST PARENCHYMA
STRUCTURE
- Breast parenchyma is composed of terminal duct lobular units (TDLU)
- Variable amounts of adipose present, as age increases → adipose increases
- Each TDLU is composed of acini, dense connective tissue, loose connective tissue, and Cooper's ligament
- Milk originates in lobules and travels to the mammary ducts →lactiferous sinuses → lactiferous ducts, and is excreted out of the nipple
- Acini and duct network → Composed of outer myoepithelial cells and inner cuboidal-columnar epithelial cells

OTHER HIGH YIELD POINTS
- Myoepithelial cells IHC: Positive for **calponin, p63, CK5/6, S100**, actin
- Ductal epithelium IHC: **Cytokeratin**

Level III
Level II
Pectoralis minor
Level I

Created by Dr. Terrance Lynn using BioRender.com

Breast Lymph Node Levels	
Level I	Located at the **lateral border of pectoralis minor** Has an anterior (pectoral axillary), posterior (subscapular axillary), and lateral (humeral) groups
Level II	Centrally located and are **deep to pectoralis minor** Central axillary and some apical axillary lymph nodes
Level III	**Medial to pectoralis minor** Composed of interpectoral lymph nodes (Rotter's Nodes) and the majority of apical axillary nodes

REACTIVE AND BENIGN EPITHELIAL LESIONS

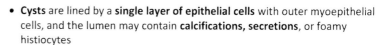

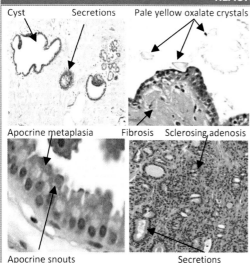

Cyst | Secretions | Pale yellow oxalate crystals

Apocrine metaplasia | Fibrosis | Sclerosing adenosis

Apocrine snouts | Secretions

Columnar cell change | Grossly visible cystic spaces

NON-PROLIFERATIVE CHANGES (FIBROCYSTIC CHANGES)
MORPHOLOGY
- **Cysts** are lined by a **single layer of epithelial cells** with outer myoepithelial cells, and the lumen may contain **calcifications, secretions**, or foamy histiocytes
- **Stromal fibrosis** commonly **surrounds the cyst wall** and can be exaggerated upon repeated cyst ruptures, inflammation, and lead to scarring
- **Apocrine metaplasia** shows eosinophilic ductal epithelial cells with **apical snouts, round nuclei with conspicuous nucleoli**; cysts may contain oxalate crystals but are challenging to see on H&E due to being pale yellow or colorless
- **Columnar cell change** shows cells that are **perpendicularly oriented** to the basement membrane and **round nuclei** and occasionally conspicuous nucleoli, and pale eosinophilic to amphophilic cytoplasm
- **Increased acini per lobule define adenosis**, and they are often columnar and seen in **pregnant women**; they may have stromal fibrosis, especially after rupture

OTHER HIGH YIELD POINTS
- **Most common non-proliferative lesion** of the breast
- **No significant** increased **risk** of cancer
- Pathogenesis: Excess hormone secretion
- **Risk factors:** Late age menopause (**prolonged estrogen exposure**), hormonal replacement therapy, **nulliparity**, and **low BMI**

Path Presenter

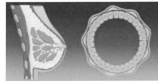
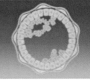

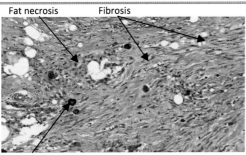

Fat necrosis   Fibrosis

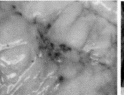
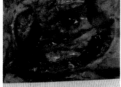

Giant cells

Core Biopsy Site   Excisional Biopsy Cavity

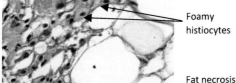

Foamy histiocytes

Fat necrosis

BIOPSY SITE CHANGE
MORPHOLOGY
- **Organizing hemorrhage** (with hemosiderin-laden macrophages and blood)
- **Fat necrosis** (with foamy macrophages)
- Foreign body **giant cells** and/or foreign material, **granulation tissue, fibrosis**
- Acute and chronic **inflammation**
- **Squamous metaplasia**
- "**Epithelial displacement**" of ductal epithelium

OTHER HIGH YIELD POINTS
- **Pitfall warnings:**
  - Post-biopsy, there can be "**epithelial displacement**" where epithelium (benign or atypical) can be found within the stroma or vascular spaces
  - Epithelial displacement is **more common in papillary lesions,** which can result in an **erroneous diagnosis of invasive carcinoma**
  - When the epithelial fragments are **confined to the biopsy site**, a diagnosis of epithelial displacement should be favored
  - A diagnosis of **invasive carcinoma** should only be made if epithelium is found in the stroma **away from the biopsy site**

Path Presenter

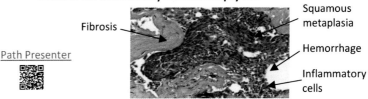

Squamous metaplasia

Fibrosis

Hemorrhage

Inflammatory cells

Histiocytes   Adipose tissue   Chronic inflammation

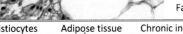

FAT NECROSIS
MORPHOLOGY
- **Necrotic adipose tissue** characterized by cystic spaces surrounded by lipid-laden ("**foamy**") macrophages
- **Variable** acute and chronic **inflammation**
- **Early** stage → **hemorrhage** and **histiocyte** reaction
- **Late** stage → **fibroblastic proliferation** and **collagen** deposition

OTHER HIGH YIELD POINTS
- Can **mimic malignancy** clinically and/or radiographically
- Occurs secondary to **injury** following surgery, biopsy, or **trauma**
- IHC: **CD68** positive histiocytes

Path Presenter

Empty spaces   Histiocytes

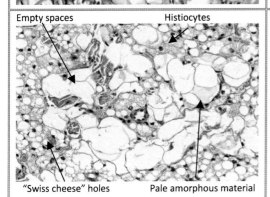

"Swiss cheese" holes   Pale amorphous material

REACTIONS TO FOREIGN MATERIAL
SILICONE GRANULOMA
MORPHOLOGY
- Many **oval** and **empty spaces** ("**Swiss cheese**") may or may not contain pale **amorphous material**
- Adjacent **histiocytes/giant** cells reacting to the polydimethylsiloxane

OTHER HIGH YIELD POINTS
- Silicone leakage can be **seen even without frank** implant **rupture**
- Newer silicone implants have **liquid** silicone (at body temperature), which can **migrate locally and distantly**

Path Presenter

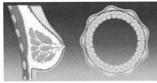 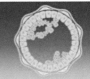

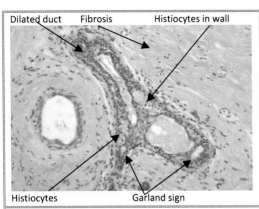

Labels: Dilated duct | Fibrosis | Histiocytes in wall | Histiocytes | Garland sign

DUCT ECTASIA
MORPHOLOGY
- Varying amounts of **periductal chronic inflammation**, **fibrosis**, and duct **dilation**
- Inspissated **lipid-rich material**, with **foamy macrophages** that often infiltrate the wall
- May have **squamous metaplasia** or **"Garland" sign** (obliterated duct lumen with recanalization around the periphery of ducts by small tubules)

OTHER HIGH YIELD POINTS
- Primarily **perimenopausal and post-menopausal** women
- Can present with pain, discharge, mass, or calcification

Path Presenter

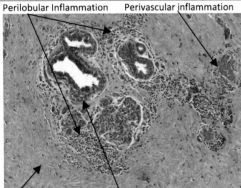

Labels: Perilobular Inflammation | Perivascular inflammation | Fibrosis | Myofibroblasts

DIABETIC MASTOPATHY
MORPHOLOGY
- Dense, **keloid-like fibrosis** with **epithelioid myofibroblasts** in stroma
- Periductal, perivascular, and perilobular **lymphocytic infiltrates** containing predominantly **B-cells**

OTHER HIGH YIELD POINTS
- **Fibroinflammatory** breast lesion, which presents as a **dense breast mass** and is **often bilateral**
- Characteristically presents in **premenopausal women** with long-standing **type 1 diabetes mellitus** and can be recurrent
- It can be **seen with other autoimmune** disorders (Grave's, Hashimoto, Pernicious anemia, SLE, RA, etc.) and in men
- IHC: **CD20 (+) B-Cells**   *Path Presenter*

Labels: Dense lymphoplasmacytic inflammation | Fibrotic stroma | Obliterative phlebitis

IgG4 RELATED MASTITIS
MORPHOLOGY
- Dense **lymphoplasmacytic infiltrate** in a fibrotic stroma with **storiform pattern** and **obliterative phlebitis**
- The absence of neutrophils, granulomas, and giant cells is essential

OTHER HIGH YIELD POINTS
- Can have **bilateral involvement** of the breast and **lymphadenopathy**
- Occurs in middle-aged females; ~50% have **hypocomplementemia**
- May have substantial **weight loss** or **peripheral eosinophilia**
- Other organs are often involved at the time of diagnosis
- IHC: Increased **IgG4 positive plasma cells (>40% IgG4/IgG ratio)**

Path Presenter

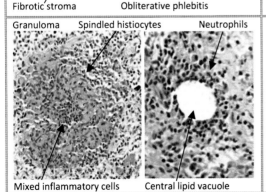

Labels: Granuloma | Spindled histiocytes | Neutrophils | Mixed inflammatory cells | Central lipid vacuole

GRANULOMATOUS MASTITIS
MORPHOLOGY
- Nonspecific **lobulocentric** granulomatous inflammation with epithelioid and spindled histiocytes, multinucleated **giant cells**, and a **central lipid vacuole**
- Often will have neutrophils, lymphocytes, plasma cells, and eosinophils

OTHER HIGH YIELD POINTS
- It can be seen in certain **Corynebacterium infections**
- Other considerations: **Sarcoidosis**, prior procedure site changes, infection, and idiopathic

Path Presenter

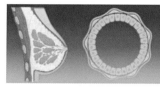

BENIGN EPITHELIAL LESIONS AND PRECURSOR LESIONS

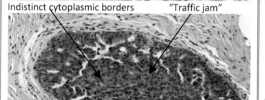
Slit-like spaces   Pseudoinclusions   Irregular nuclei

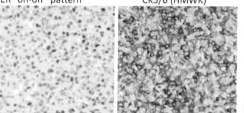
Indistinct cytoplasmic borders   "Traffic jam"

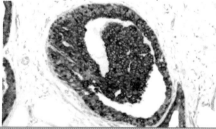
ER "on-off" pattern   CK5/6 (HMWK)

BNC-5 showing polyclonal keratin expression

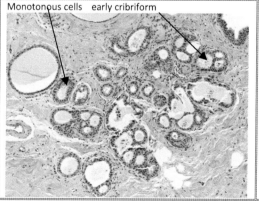
Monotonous cells   early cribriform

USUAL DUCT HYPERPLASIA (UDH)
MORPHOLOGY

- A **cohesive proliferation** of epithelial cells arranged in **a haphazard architecture** with irregular, **slit-like spaces**, often peripherally located
- **Epithelial cells** are variably sized cells with **indistinct borders**, **overlapping nuclei** with frequent **nuclear grooves**, and some **pseudoinclusions**
- **Any bridges are thin** and stretched with **"traffic jam"** type pattern
- **Any micropapillae** have broad bases and **narrow tips** with small pyknotic nuclei

OTHER HIGH YIELD POINTS

- Epithelial cells stain with a **mixture of low molecular-weight** (e.g., CK7) and **high-molecular weight cytokeratins** (e.g., CK5/6)
- **BNC-5 stain** will show brown staining for p63 (nuclear) and brown cytoplasmic CK903, and cytoplasmic red CK7 and CK8/18 staining
- **Heterogeneous ER staining** pattern: **Some are "on," others are "off"**
- Confers approximately a **2-fold increased risk for breast cancer**

UDH	DCIS
Think: Polyclonal	**Think: Monoclonal**
Irregular, slit-like lumina, often peripheral	Regular, punched out lumina, often central
Streaming architecture	**Prominent polarization** around lumina
Variation in cell size/shape	Monomorphic cells/shape
Indistinct cell margins	**Distinct cell margins**
Admixture of cell types (epithelial, myoepithelial and/or apocrine): Stain with high and low-molecular weight cytokeratins	Proliferating cells are epithelial. Myoepithelial cells are against the basement membrane: Epithelium stains with low-molecular weight cytokeratins only
Heterogenous ER staining (think: "some on, some off")	Strong, diffuse ER staining (think: "all on")
CK5/6 positive	CK5/6 negative

Path Presenter
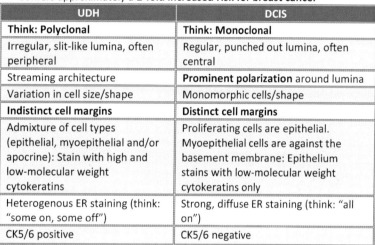

ATYPICAL DUCT HYPERPLASIA (ADH)
MORPHOLOGY

- **Neoplastic proliferation of evenly spaced epithelial cells** with round nuclei, dense chromatin, arranged in **cribriform architecture**, **bridging** or **micropapillae**

OTHER HIGH YIELD POINTS

- Confers a **4 to 5-fold relative risk for breast cancer**
- Size: **≤2mm and <2 duct spaces**; otherwise, it is DCIS
- Findings that **increase the likelihood of malignancy: multiple foci** of ADH, **marked nuclear atypia**, or **micropapillary** architecture
- Treatment: On biopsy → surgical excision to exclude DCIS/invasive; Found on excision → no additional treatment
- IHC: High ER (+) expression   Path Presenter

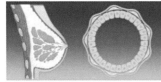

LOW-GRADE DCIS

Micropapillary

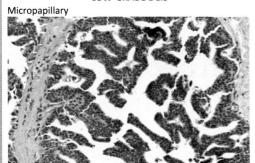

Polarization | Cribriform pattern

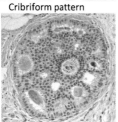

Cancerization of lobules by DCIS

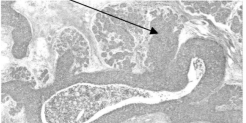

Picture courtesy: Lorand Kis, MD

HIGH-GRADE DCIS

Comedo necrosis | Pleomorphism

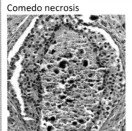
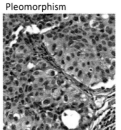

IMMUNOHISTOCHEMISTRY

ER "Clonal pattern" | CK5/6 Negative

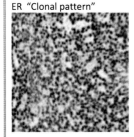
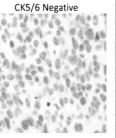

DUCTAL CARCINOMA IN SITU

MORPHOLOGY

- Neoplastic proliferation of epithelial cells of **ductal origin**
- **Morphologic** appearance **defines the grade** (not architecture)
- Nuclei can be round to oval, have regular or irregular nuclear contours, and conspicuous or inconspicuous nucleoli

OTHER HIGH YIELD POINTS

- Often limited to one duct system but can involve the lobules and is specifically called "**cancerization of lobules**"
- No specific size requirement is needed (unlike ADH)
- Majority are non-palpable and thus usually detected on mammography with associated with **linear calcifications** which are microcalcifications
- **Relative risk** of **invasive cancer** in ipsilateral breast is **~10 X**
- Approximately 40% of low-grade lesions progress to invasive carcinoma if left untreated
- High-grade lesions often associated with stromal reaction with fibrosis, sclerosis, or infiltrative lymphocytes
- **Graded** based **on nuclear morphology**
  - ➤ **Low grade:** Think "**small bland**" monomorphic cells
  - ➤ **Intermediate grade:** Features between low and high-grade
  - ➤ **High-grade:** Think "**ugly and pleomorphic**" cells
- Treatment: Excision with "wide" negative margins; +/- radiation therapy and/or hormone therapy
- IHC: Dependent on grade, but **ER/PR is positive** in a **clonal** pattern, HER2 is variable (HER2 not performed on in situ), negative for CK5/6; myoepithelial cells are positive for p40, p63, CK5/6. E-Cadherin retained (Lost in LCIS)
- Molecular: **PIK3CA** (~25%), **TP53** (10-15%), **GATA3** (~10%) mutations
- Cytogenetics:
  - ➤ **Low grade:** Chromosomal **losses** in **16q, 17p**, and **gains** at **1p**
  - ➤ **High grade:** Chromosomal **losses** at **8p, 11q, 13q, 14q**, and **gains** at **5p, 8q, 17q**

Low-grade DCIS	High-grade DCIS
Small monomorphic cells 1.5-2x size of RBCs Regular nuclear contours Even chromatin Small to inconspicuous nucleoli	**Large, pleomorphic cells** >2.5x size of RBC Irregular nuclear contours Coarse chromatin Prominent nucleoli
Usually **cribriform** or **micropapillary** growth	Usually **solid** growth, but may have any architectural pattern
Polarization around lumina	**No polarization** around lumina
Necrosis **uncommon**	Necrosis **common**, especially comedo
Must be >2mm and **involve more than 2** complete spaces	**No size** requirement
ER and PR **positive** (frequently)	ER and PR **negative** (more frequently)
HER2 is **negative** (frequently)	HER2 is **positive** (frequently)
Few mitoses	**Many** mitoses
Low-grade associated cancers	High-grade associated cancers

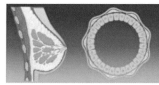

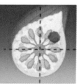
BNC-5 stain demonstrating retained myeoepithelial cells (nuclear p63, cytoplasmic CK5/6; brown stain) and clonal luminal cytokeratin expression (CK8/18)

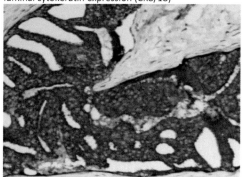

Figure: Comparison of multicentric versus multifocal DCIS created by Dr. Terrance Lynn, MD using BioRender.com

Multicentric	Multifocal
(>5 cm apart and in different quadrants)	(<5 cm apart and in same quadrant)

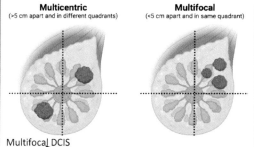

Multifocal DCIS

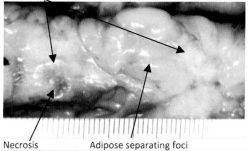

Necrosis   Adipose separating foci

Monotonous cells   discohesive

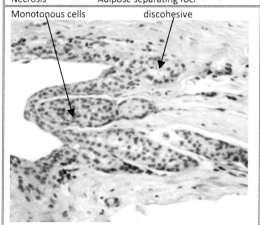

	UDH	Low-grade DCIS
CK5/6		
ER		

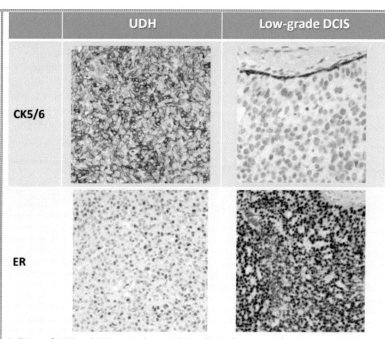

Collision of DCIS and LCIS, sorted out with E-cadherin (courtesy: Rhard Owings, MD)

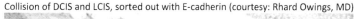

LCIS
E-Cad (-)

DCIS
E-Cad (+)

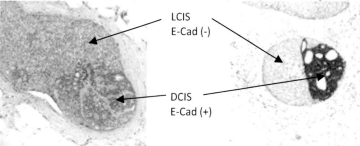

Path Presenter

ATYPICAL LOBULAR HYPERPLASIA (ALH)

MORPHOLOGY

- A small proliferation of **discohesive**, **monomorphic** epithelial cells low to moderate grade nuclei
- It may have **pagetoid spread** through the ductal spaces

OTHER HIGH YIELD POINTS

- Cytologically **similar to LCIS** but **limited to <1/2 of duct** involvement
- **Non-obligate precursor lesion**, common in premenopausal women
- Confers a **4 to 5-fold relative risk** for breast **cancer**
- The **lifetime risk of invasive carcinoma is about 15%,** and approximately **67% of carcinoma occurs in the ipsilateral breast** and 33% in the contralateral breast

Path Presenter

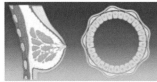

Monomorphic discohesive cells

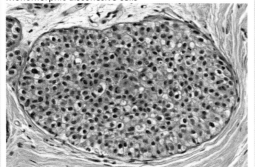

Florid LCIS expanding lobules

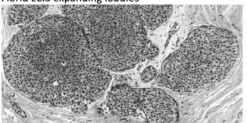

"Pagetoid" spread of LCIS in a duct

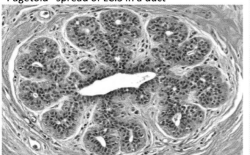

Pleomorphic LCIS (courtesy Mark Ong, MD)
x20

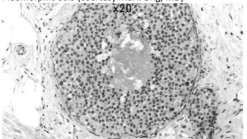

Cytoplasmic p120   Loss of E-cadherin on IHC

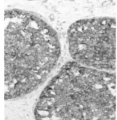

Credits: @tissuepathology

LOBULAR CARCINOMA IN SITU

MORPHOLOGY

- **Classic LCIS**
  - ➢ **Discohesive, monomorphic** epithelial cells low to moderate grade nuclei that originate from the TDLU, **>50% of the acini are filled and expanded, often >8 cells thick**
  - ➢ It may have pagetoid spread through the duct space
- **Pleomorphic LCIS subtype:**
  - ➢ **Large epithelial cells** (>4x lymphocyte) with **marked** nuclear **pleomorphism** and may have **nucleoli** and **mitoses, intracytoplasmic vacuoles**
- **Florid LCIS Subtype:**
  - ➢ Classic LCIS cells but form a **confluent, mass-like lesion** with **little** or no **intervening stroma** between the distended TDLU (often ~50 cells in diameter)

OTHER HIGH YIELD POINTS

- More than 50% of acini are filled/expanded by the neoplastic cells
- **Non-obligate precursor lesion** to invasive carcinoma that is most common in premenopausal women
- Confers an **8-10-fold relative risk for invasive breast cancer**
- The **lifetime risk** of invasive carcinoma is about **15%**, and approximately 67% of carcinoma occurs in the ipsilateral and 33% in the contralateral breast
- If **classic LCIS is present on core biopsy, there is no need to excise**; on surgical excision, no need to have clear margins
- Most often is **not associated with mammographic findings**
- If pleomorphic or florid LCIS, **excise with negative margins** due to their increased genomic instability and more aggressive behavior
- Increased incidence in women who are post-menopausal on HRT
- Possible treatment includes chemoprevention which reduces the subsequent risk of ER (+) cancer ➔ **Tamoxifen reduces risk by ~50%**
- Special stains: Intracytoplasmic vacuole is **mucicarmine positive**

IHC STAIN	NORMAL EPITHELIUM	LOBULAR NEOPLASIA	DCIS
E-Cadherin	Membrane +	Negative	Membrane +
p120	Membrane +	Cytoplasmic	Membrane +
β-Catenin	Membrane +	Membrane stain lost	Membrane +

Feature	LCIS	DCIS
Loss of cohesion	Present	Absent
Intracytoplasmic vacuoles	More common	Less common
Pagetoid ductal involvement	More common	Less common
Microacini	Absent	Present
Polarization at duct periphery	Absent	Present

Path Presenter

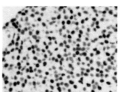

Pleomorphic LCIS: ER   Pleomorphic LCIS: BNC-5

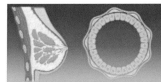 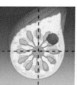
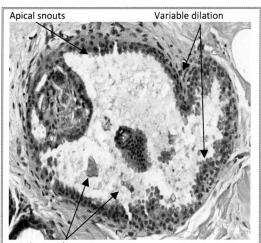

Apical snouts | Variable dilation

Calcification/Secretions

COLUMNAR CELL CHANGE
MORPHOLOGY
- Characterized by enlarged, **variably dilated acini** lined by **columnar epithelial cells** arranged **perpendicular to the basement membrane** and are 1-2 cells in thickness
- Cells are **uniform** and have **ovoid nuclei with regular chromatin** distribution, **inconspicuous nucleoli**, and have **apical cytoplasmic** blebs
- Apical snouts and **calcifications/secretions** are often present
OTHER HIGH YIELD POINTS
- The **earliest step in the low-grade** carcinoma **pathway**
- If > 2 cell layers thick → columnar cell hyperplasia
- **Infrequently associated with ADH, low-grade DCIS,** or invasive carcinoma
- **Risk of developing** a subsequent **carcinoma is negligible** (1.5x relative risk)
- IHC: Strongly ER (+), CK8/18 (+); CK5/6 (-)

Path Presenter

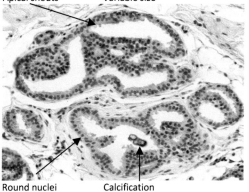

Apical snouts | Variable size

Round nuclei | Calcification

Path Presenter

FLAT EPITHELIAL ATYPIA
MORPHOLOGY
- **Monomorphic cuboidal to columnar cells** with nuclei that are round with minimal nuclear contour irregularities, and are **polarized**
- It can be arranged in **complex architecture**
- May have **calcifications**, secretions, and apical snouts
OTHER HIGH YIELD POINTS
- The **relative risk for cancer is 1.5-fold**, and the **lifetime risk of 5%**
- If FEA is found in the targeted lesion, less than 5% of cases will have associated cancer but is an indication for excision to exclude worse lesion in close proximity
- **Same cells as in ADH/DCIS**
- If complex architecture present it is not FEA but rather ADH or DCIS
- IHC: **ER will be strongly and diffusely positive** throughout the lesion
- Molecular: Often has loss of 16q

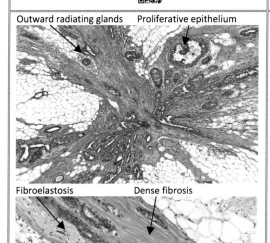

Outward radiating glands | Proliferative epithelium

Fibroelastosis | Dense fibrosis

RADIAL SCLEROSING LESION (RADIAL SCAR)
MORPHOLOGY
- **Stellate**, dense **fibroelastosis** with **entrapped glandular structures** in a **radiating outward** configuration
- **Two cell layers** maintained throughout lesion
- It may have associated proliferative epithelial lesions (e.g., UDH/ADH/DCIS)
OTHER HIGH YIELD POINTS
- **Radiographically** is a **spiculated lesion** & may have associated calcifications
- **Radial scar** → Smaller with a stellate configuration
- **Complex sclerosing lesion** → Larger and more disorganized than radial scar
- Approximately **2/3rd will have a PIK3CA mutation**
- Myoepithelial IHC helps exclude invasive carcinoma
- Confers **approximately a 1.5-to-2-fold increase in the risk of invasive carcinoma**, and the **lifetime risk of carcinoma is 5-7%** in either breast regardless of which had the radial sclerosing lesion

Path Presenter

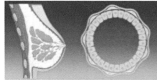 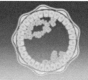

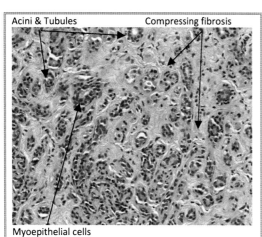
Acini & Tubules | Compressing fibrosis
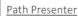
Myoepithelial cells

SCLEROSING ADENOSIS
MORPHOLOGY
- **Lobulocentric proliferation** of **acini and tubules** accompanied by **compressing fibrosis**
- **Epithelial cells** are often **cuboidal, small,** and cytologically **bland**
- **Myoepithelial cells** have spindled, hyperchromatic nuclei and inconspicuous to prominent clear cytoplasm
- **Microcalcifications** are common

OTHER HIGH YIELD POINTS
- Can be involved by epithelial proliferations (UDH, etc.)
- **Easily confused** with **carcinoma**
- Useful IHC stains: **Myoepithelial markers** (p63, CK5/6). S100 (-); BNC-5 polyclonal cytokeratin expression and retained **myoepithelial** cells

Path Presenter

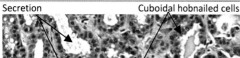
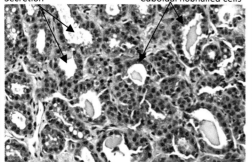
Secretion | Cuboidal hobnailed cells

Densely pack glands

LACTATING ADENOMA
MORPHOLOGY
- **Well-circumscribed** proliferation of closely packed **hyperplastic secretory lobules** separated by **delicate connective tissue**
- **Cuboidal to hobnailed** epithelial cells are **bland** with **vacuolated to granular cytoplasm** and small, uniform, pinpoint nucleoli

OTHER HIGH YIELD POINTS
- Benign nodules are usually **diagnosed during pregnancy/breastfeeding**
- **Spontaneously regresses** after completion of lactation
- **No** known **progression to carcinoma**
- Can be **present anywhere along the mammary line**

Path Presenter

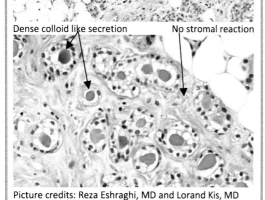
Haphazard tubular glands | Cytologically bland cells
Dense colloid like secretion | No stromal reaction
Picture credits: Reza Eshraghi, MD and Lorand Kis, MD

MICROGLANDULAR ADENOSIS
MORPHOLOGY
- A **haphazard proliferation** of small, round, uniform, **tubular glands** composed of a **single layer of epithelium** (without associated myoepithelial cells) that have **bland nuclei** and **amphophilic cytoplasm**
- Luminal spaces are open and often have **eosinophilic colloid-like secretion**

OTHER HIGH YIELD POINTS
- About **25% of cases** are **associated** with **invasive carcinoma**
- Hypothesized to be **non-obligate precursor of basal-type** breast **cancer**
- IHC: **(+) Cytokeratin**, s100; (-)for ER, PR, HER2, and **myoepithelial markers**
- Molecular findings include **copy number alterations**, *TP53* mutations, *PIK3CA*, and *BRCA1* mutations

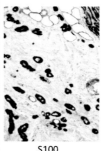 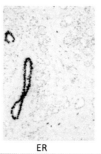 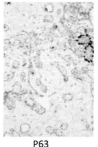

Path Presenter

S100 | ER | P63

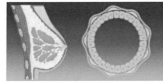

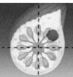

Well circumscribed

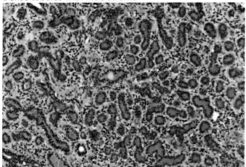

Dense tubules with little stroma

Picture credits: Reza Eshraghi, MD

TUBULAR ADENOMA
MORPHOLOGY
- Well-circumscribed, sharply demarcated, and dense proliferation of closely approximated round to oval tubular structures with little background stroma
- Glands have the usual two layers: Epithelium and myoepithelium

OTHER HIGH YIELD POINTS
- Uncommon, usually in younger women in the upper outer quadrant
- Lack a *MED12* mutation (seen in fibroepithelial lesions)

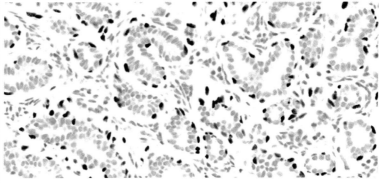

Path Presenter

P63 immunostain

Eosinophilic cytoplasm   Secretions

Round nuclei

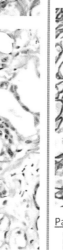

Courtesy: Amal Asar, FRCpath.

APOCRINE ADENOSIS
MORPHOLOGY
- **Lobulocentric proliferation** of benign **glandular** structures composed of epithelial cells with **abundant granular cytoplasm**
- Apocrine cells have **round nuclei** and **prominent nucleoli**

OTHER HIGH YIELD POINTS
- Think **apocrine metaplasia + sclerosing adenosis = apocrine adenosis**
- If significant cytologic **atypia → Atypical Apocrine Adenosis**
- If **complex architecture** (cribriform, marked pleomorphism): **Apocrine DCIS**
- IHC : **(+)** myoepithelial cells; epithelial cells are ER**(-)** but AR and GCDFP-15**(+)**

Path Presenter

SMM immunostain

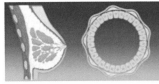

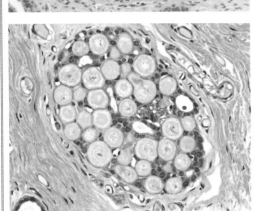

Amorphous deposits   Myoepithelial cells

Courtesy: Ari Abdullah, MD

COLLAGENOUS SPHERULOSIS
MORPHOLOGY
- **Intraductal deposits** of **basement membrane** which are **amorphous** and **eosinophilic**, acellular or fibro papillary spherules
- **Myoepithelial cells surround the lumina** and are often compressed and spindle-shaped
- May or may not have calcifications

OTHER HIGH YIELD POINTS
- **Commonly seen** with **papilloma, UDH,** or **sclerosing lesions**
- Easily **confused for DCIS** or **adenoid cystic carcinoma**
- The matrix material is **PAS-positive** and **Alcian Blue positive**

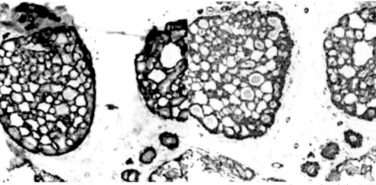

Calponin and SMA immunostains   Courtesy: Mohamed Kahila, MD

Path Presenter

No acini, branching ducts, loose periductal stroma

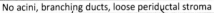

Pyramid-shaped micropapillae   epithelial hyperplasia

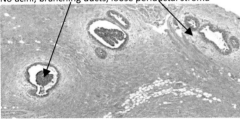

Pseudoangiomatous stromal hyperplasia

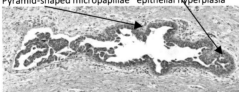

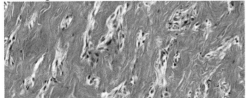

GYNECOMASTIA
MORPHOLOGY
- Contains **fibrous stroma** and **branching ducts**, and terminal ductules, but extremely few (if any) acini
- **Early stage** → Loose **periductal stroma** and **mixed chronic inflammatory infiltrate**, extensive epithelial **hyperplasia**, tapering tufts (**pyramid-shaped micropapillae**)
- **Late stage** → Fibrosis and **hyalinization** of periductal stroma and **epithelial atrophy**
- May have **pseudoangiomatous hyperplasia (PASH)**
- Absence of lobules

OTHER HIGH YIELD POINTS
- **Benign lesion** of the male breast and is **often bilateral**
- Caused by **androgen/estrogen imbalance** and is **physiologic in children** but often **pathologic in adults**
- Can be seen during **puberty**, taking **dopaminergic medications**, hormone therapy, **Klinefelter syndrome, cirrhosis,** or **obesity**
- **Not associated with** any risk of **cancer**

Path Presenter

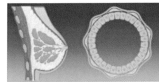 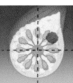

FIBROEPITHELIAL LESIONS

FIBROADENOMA

MORPHOLOGY

- **Circumscribed, benign neoplasm** of the Terminal Duct Lobular Unit (TDLU) with a **biphasic proliferation** of **epithelial** and **stromal** cells
- **Intracanalicular pattern:**
  - ➢ Expansion of stroma compresses ducts into slit-like spaces
- **Pericanalicular pattern:**
  - ➢ Stroma grows around open ducts
- **Absence of stromal overgrowth**, cytologic **atypia**, significant **mitotic activity**, or **well-developed fronds**

OTHER HIGH YIELD POINTS

- The **most common benign** solid breast **mass in young women**
- Most are **slow growing** and **painless**, and **unilateral**
- Most fibroadenomas **do not recur** after complete surgical excision
- **Juvenile Fibroadenoma:** Usually large and have rapid growth and predominantly have pericanalicular growth
- Immunohistochemistry:
  - ➢ **Stromal cells: (+)** for CD34, PR, ER-beta, Beta catenin (nuclear)
  - ➢ **Epithelial cells: (+)** for CK7, CKAE1/AE3, ER-alpha
- **About 60-65% will have a *MED12* mutation** (stromal cells) but the **myxoid fibroadenoma will lack** this mutation

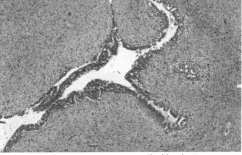

Stromal expansion

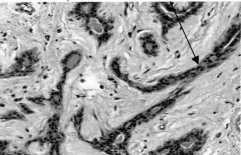

Pericanalicular pattern: Open duct

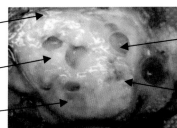

Well-circumscribed — Cystic change

Fibrotic appearance — Slit-like space

Mucoid appearance

Intracanalicular pattern   Slit-like ducts

Path Presenter

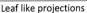

PHYLLODES TUMOR

MORPHOLOGY

- **Biphasic tumor** composed of spindled stromal cells and benign epithelial cells
- **Stromal cellularity is variable** and ranges from paucicellular to hypercellular
- Prominent intracanalicular growth pattern
- Exaggerated intracanalicular growth→ **"Leaf-like" projections** into variably dilated lumina

OTHER HIGH YIELD POINTS

- **Increased incidence** in patients **with Li-Fraumeni syndrome**
- Presents as a **palpable painless breast mass**
- Can have **heterologous elements that are malignant**
- **Molecular:** MED12 and RARA mutations seen in benign phyllodes; TERT promoter, ERBB4, TP53, EGFR, PIK3CA, **RB1 seen in borderline and malignant** phyllodes tumors

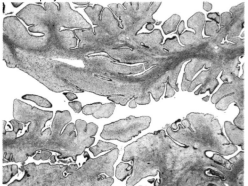

Leaf like projections

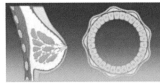 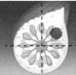

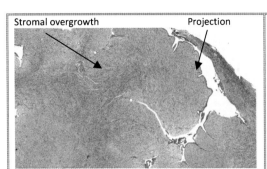

Stromal overgrowth — Projection

Benign Phyllodes tumor

Minimal atypia — Cellular stroma

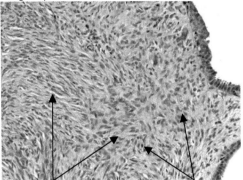

- Treatment: wide local excision
- **Singapore nomogram** used for predicting **recurrence**
  - ➤ **Atypia** in stroma
  - ➤ **Mitoses**
  - ➤ **Overgrowth**
  - ➤ Surgical **margin**

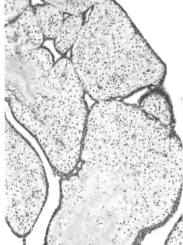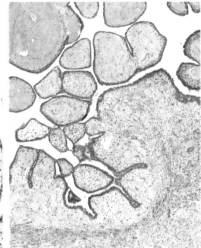

<u>Path Presenter</u>

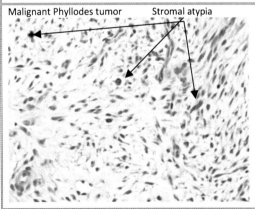

Malignant Phyllodes tumor — Stromal atypia

CLASSIFICATION OF PHYLLODES TUMORS			
	BENIGN	**BORDERLINE**	**MALIGNANT**
Stromal Atypia	Mild	Moderate	Marked
Stromal Cellularity	Minimal to mild	Moderate	Marked and diffuse
Stromal Overgrowth	Not present	Not present or very focal	Present
Mitoses	<5/10 HPF	5-9/10HPF	≥10/10 HPF
Border	Well defined	Well defined	Infiltrative
Malignant Heterologous elements	Not present	Not present	If present, upgrades to malignant

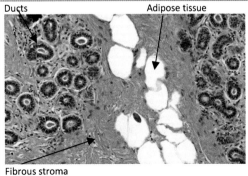

Ducts — Adipose tissue

Fibrous stroma

HAMARTOMA
MORPHOLOGY
- Composed of **normal ducts, lobules, fibrous tissue, and adipose tissue** in varying proportions (normal components)
- **Well circumscribed**
OTHER HIGH YIELD POINTS
- Sometimes called "adenolipoma"
- Clinical presentation is a **painless breast mass**
- Requires clinical &/or imaging correlation to distinguish from normal breast
<u>Path Presenter</u>

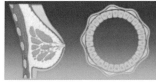
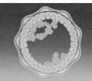

SPINDLE CELL LESIONS

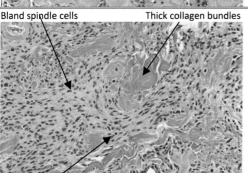

Myofibroblasts   Slit-like spaces   Keloid – like stroma

PSEUDOANGIOMATOUS STROMAL HYPERPLASIA (PASH)

MORPHOLOGY

- **Keloid-like stroma** with **complex anastomotic spaces** that are often empty and have **peripherally placed myofibroblasts**

OTHER HIGH YIELD POINTS

- Benign breast lesion with **aberrant stromal response** to hormone
- Presents as an **incidental mass-forming lesion**
- IHC: Spindle cells **(+)** for CD34, PR, and ER; **(-)** for cytokeratins and CD31

Path Presenter

Bland spindle cells   Thick collagen bundles

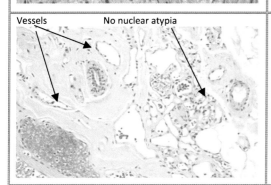

Haphazard intersecting fascicles

MYOFIBROBLASTOMA

MORPHOLOGY

- **Bland**, **spindled cells** composed of **fibroblasts** and **myofibroblasts** that are arranged in short, **haphazardly intersecting fascicles**
- Interspersed **thick collagen bundles**, **minimal** mitoses, and **atypia**

OTHER HIGH YIELD POINTS

- Often presents as a **slow-growing, painless mass**
- **Well-circumscribed** and **unencapsulated**
- IHC: Shows **loss of RB1**; spindle cells are **(+)** for desmin, CD34, ER, PR, AR
- FISH: 13q14 deletions
- **Treatment**: Cured by **local excision**

Path Presenter

Spindle cells

DESMOID FIBROMATOSIS

MORPHOLOGY

- **Broad, sweeping fascicles** of uniform **spindled cells** with small, pale nuclei with pinpoint nucleoli
- **Moderate amounts** of **collagen** and may be slightly myxoid
- **Microhemorrhages** and scattered **chronic inflammation** are common

OTHER HIGH YIELD POINTS

- Benign (**never metastasize**), but **infiltrative** with a strong **tendency to recur** (>25%), microscopic **margins do NOT predict recurrence**
- Often have infiltrative growth into surrounding structures
- IHC: **(+)** Nuclear β-catenin, **(+/-)** Actin
- Molecular: FAP (if syndromic); CTNNB1   Path Presenter

Vessels   No nuclear atypia

HEMANGIOMA

MORPHOLOGY

- Benign **proliferation of mature** blood **vessels without** nuclear **atypia** (hyperchromasia or pleomorphism), **mitoses, or multi-layering**

OTHER HIGH YIELD POINTS

- Usually found incidentally and most common in middle-aged females
- If superficial, it can show red-purple coloring on the skin
- IHC: **(+) for CD31, CD34, and ERG**

Path Presenter

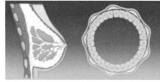

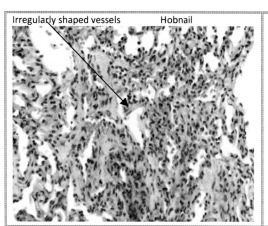

Irregularly shaped vessels   Hobnail

ATYPICAL VASCULAR LESION
MORPHOLOGY

- **Irregularly shaped**, thin-walled **vessels** with **branching** and anastomotic growth
- Lumen is lined by a **single layer of endothelial cells** with some **hobnail** and **hyperchromatic** features
- **No** endothelial cell **multilayering** or true cytologic **atypia**

OTHER HIGH YIELD POINTS

- **Benign** condition, often occurs in irradiated skin of breast
- **Multiple lesions** may be present
- If superficial, it can show red-purple coloring on the skin
- IHC: **(+)** for CD31, CD34, ERG; **no MYC overexpression/amplification**

Path Presenter

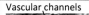

Vascular channels   Epithelioid cells

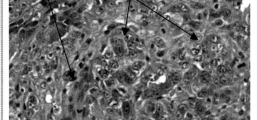

Plump endothelial cells   Vascular channels

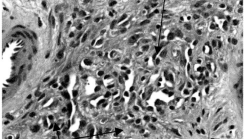

Extravasated red cells

ANGIOSARCOMA
MORPHOLOGY

- **Spindled** to **plump epithelioid cells** line vascular channels
- Vascular spaces are pinpoint or dilated and have **exuberant anastomosis**
- The **nuclei** of these cells often contain **a "bullet" shaped nucleolus**
- May have **hemosiderin, necrosis, atypical mitoses**, and **high-grade foci**

OTHER HIGH YIELD POINTS

- Usually found **incidentally** and most common in **middle-aged females**
- If superficial, it can show **red-purple coloring on the skin**
- **Post-radiation angiosarcoma** occurs approximately **5 years post-radiation**
- IHC: **(+)** for CD31, CD34, **ERG, high ki-67** proliferation index; **(+) MYC** in **post-radiation** angiosarcoma

Atypical mitosis

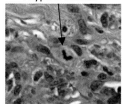

Irregular anastomosing spaces with atypical endothelial cells

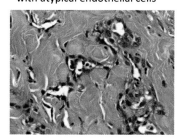

Path Presenter

Ductal cells   Myoepithelial cells

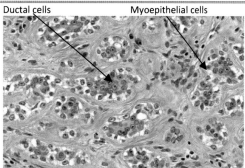

ADENOMYOEPITHELIOMA
MORPHOLOGY

- **Biphasic proliferation** of **inner ductal** cells and **outer myoepithelial** cells
- May have **various patterns**, but can be **papillary** or **tubular** with prominent myoepithelial cells with clear cytoplasm or can be more spindled
- **Well circumscribed** and can be encapsulated
- May have **sebaceous, squamous, or apocrine metaplasia**
- May have **mild to moderate** nuclear **atypia** but **no mitosis or necrosis**

OTHER HIGH YIELD POINTS

- Usually found **in older females** with a **palpable breast mass**
- **Peripheral location** more often seen than central or areolar

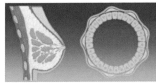

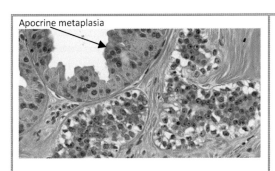

Apocrine metaplasia

- **Can de-differentiate** into **carcinoma (any type)** or **malignant transformation**
  - ➤ High mitotic count, infiltrative borders, severe atypia in either myoepithelial or ductal cells
- Immunohistochemistry:
  - ➤ **Epithelial component: (+)** CKAE1/AE3, CK7, EMA, Cam5.2, ER
  - ➤ **Myoepithelial component: (+)** p63, S100, SMMHC, SMA
- Molecular: Frequent mutations in PIC3CA or AKT1 (in ER positive) and HRAS Q61R (in ER negative)

Path Presenter

BREAST SPINDLE CELL NEOPLASM ALGORITHM FOR SELECTING IHC PANEL

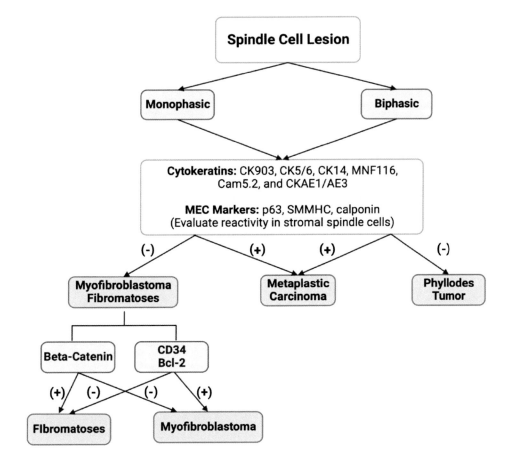

Tip: For spindle cell lesions, always consider **metaplastic carcinoma** and/or **stromal overgrowth in a Phyllodes Tumor.** Sample the lesion well, looking for an epithelial component and stain it with multiple epithelial markers. Given the limitations of sampling, be particularly careful (and perhaps more descriptive) on core biopsies! **Always** be very weary diagnosing a primary sarcoma in the breast! MEC: Myoepithelial component.

Created by Dr. Terrance Lynn using BioRender.com. Adapted from Liu. H. Application of immunohistochemistry in breast pathology: a review and update. Arch Pathol Lab Med. 2014 Dec;138(12):1629-42.

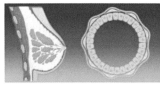

STEP-WISE ALGORITHM OF BENIGN AND INSITU BREAST NEOPLASMS

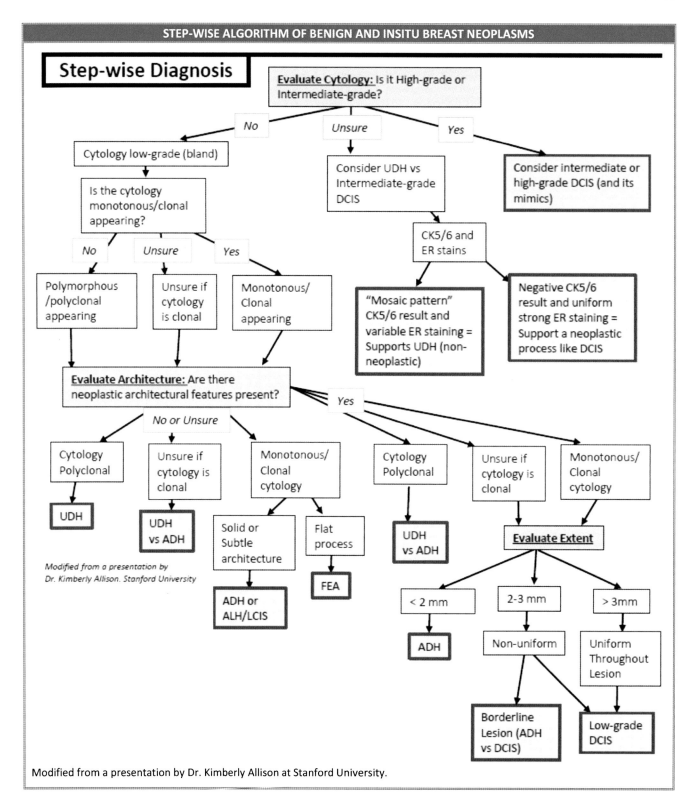

Modified from a presentation by Dr. Kimberly Allison at Stanford University.

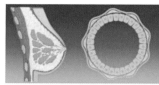

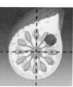

PAPILLARY LESIONS

Intraductal papillary proliferation

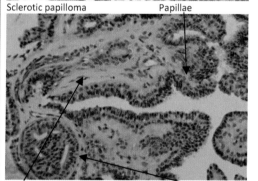

Epithelial layer   Myoepithelial layer

Sclerotic papilloma   Papillae

Sclerotic stroma   Usual Duct Hyperplasia

BNC-5 stain showing retained myoepithelial cells and polyclonal keratin expression

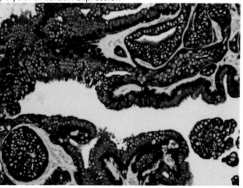

INTRADUCTAL PAPILLOMA
MORPHOLOGY
- **Benign intraductal proliferation** composed of **papillary projections** with fibrovascular cores, covered by **epithelial** and **myoepithelial** cell **layers**
- May have **superimposed proliferative changes** such as UDH, apocrine metaplasia, sclerosing adenosis, or duct ectasia
- Can be **sclerotic** or undergo **infarction**, especially **after biopsy**

OTHER HIGH YIELD POINTS
- Can be broken into **two categories** based on their location within the ducts
- **Small duct papilloma (SDP):**
  - **Peripherally located** within TDLU and **usually** there are **multiple**
  - The relative **risk of carcinoma** is approximately a **3-fold increase**
  - Usually is mass that is < 1cm and not readily palpable on exam
- **Large duct papilloma:**
  - **Centrally located** within lactiferous duct and usually solitary
  - The relative **risk of carcinoma** is approximately a **2-fold increase**
  - Standard treatment is to **surgically excise**
- Often present with **serosanguinous nipple discharge**
- **Risk factors for carcinoma** on excision include: >1 cm in size, **old age**, and palpable **mass** or **discharge**
- **Gross examination**: Usually tan-pink bosselated or papillary nodule that is protruding into dilated duct space; may have serosanguinous fluid
- Immunohistochemistry:
  - **Myoepithelial markers: (+) p63, SMA**
  - **Epithelial markers: (+) CK5/6 (heterogenous), ER (heterogenous),** and a **BNC-5** showing a **polyclonal keratin** expression
- **Molecular: PIK3CA (about 40%), AKT1 (about 30%) activating point mutations** and about **50% of all papillomas** will **have** either **mutation**

Path Presenter

Section showing Sclerotic IDP

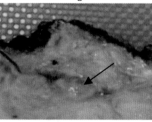

Section of large duct papilloma

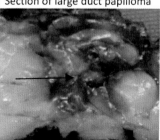

Ultrasound of IDP

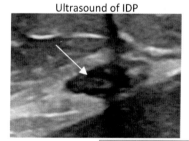

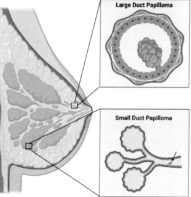

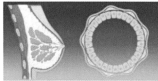

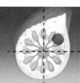

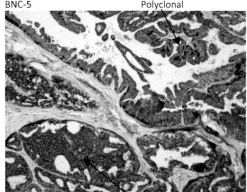

Polarization — Monotonous cells

BNC-5 — Polyclonal

Size > 3 mm — Clonal

PAPILLOMA INVOLVED BY DUCT CARCINOMA IN SITU
MORPHOLOGY
- **Foci of DCIS (or ADH)** superimposed **in** an intraductal **papilloma**
- Focal population of **monotonous cells** with **cytologic** and **architectural** atypia showing low-grade neoplastic ductal process
- **Monotonous cells** will demonstrate **polarization** around lumina

OTHER HIGH YIELD POINTS
- **Size criteria** for ADH versus DCIS is utilized **except for** lesions in which there is **intermediate** or **high-grade cytology** as these **automatically** are DCIS
- For low-grade lesions:
  ➢ **Lesions <3 mm** are classified as **atypical duct hyperplasia (ADH)**
  ➢ **Lesions ≥ 3 mm** are best classified as **Ductal carcinoma in situ (DCIS)**
- Immunohistochemistry:
  ➢ **DCIS component:** BNC-5 will show clonal cytokeratin expression and ER will be **diffuse and strong**
  ➢ **Papilloma component:** BNC-5 will show polyclonal cytokeratin expression and ER will be **heterogenous**

Diffuse ER in DCIS component   Variable ER in the papilloma

Path Presenter

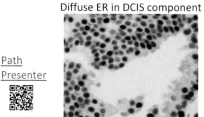
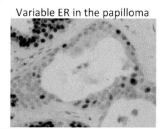

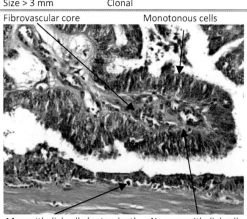

Fibrovascular core — Monotonous cells

Myoepithelial cells (outer duct)   No myoepithelial cells

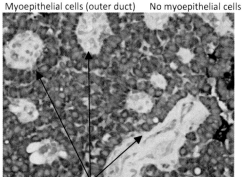

Papillae with no myoepithelial cells (no nuclear p63)

PAPILLARY DUCTAL CARCINOMA IN SITU
MORPHOLOGY
- **Monotonous clonal ductal** epithelial **cells** lining **arborizing filiform fibrovascular cores** that are **devoid** of **myoepithelial cells**
- **Nuclei can be variable** based on grade and are round to oval, have regular or irregular nuclear contours, and conspicuous or inconspicuous nucleoli
- The **duct containing** the **neoplasm** has **preserved myoepithelial cells** (which is different than the papillary fronds that lack myoepithelial cells)
- Neoplasm **may be deceptively bland** with stratified spindled cells, compact columnar cells, or clear cells

OTHER HIGH YIELD POINTS
- The **comedo pattern** is the **only clinically relevant pattern**
- Neoplasm is **graded based** on the **nuclear** cytologic **features**
- **Graded** based **on nuclear morphology**
  ➢ **Low grade:** Think "small bland" monomorphic cells
  ➢ **Intermediate grade:** Features between low and high-grade DCIS
  ➢ **High-grade:** Think "ugly and pleomorphic" cells
- Immunohistochemistry
  ➢ Myoepithelial cells: **(+)** for p40, **p63, CK5/6, calponin**, SMH
  ➢ Ductal cells: **(+)** for **CK7/18 (luminal)**, p120 (strong membranous), E-cadherin; **(-)** for **CK903** (34βE12), CK5/6, CK14
  ➢ Prognostic markers: ER and PR must be performed

Path Presenter

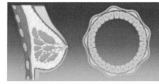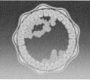

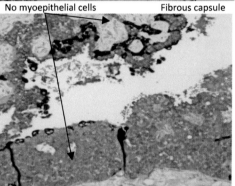

Papillae — No mypoepithelial cells

No myoepithelial cells — Fibrous capsule

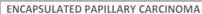

BNC-5 stain showing (+) CK7/18, (-) p63 and (+/-)CK5/6

ENCAPSULATED PAPILLARY CARCINOMA
MORPHOLOGY
- Carcinoma composed of **fine fibrovascular (papillary) fronds** covered by **neoplastic** epithelial **cells** of **low to intermediate** nuclear **grade**
- Carcinoma is most often in a **cystic space** with surrounding **fibrous capsule**
- **No myoepithelial cells** are present **in the fibrovascular fronds** or at the **periphery of cystic space**

OTHER HIGH YIELD POINTS
- WHO recommend **classification as a Tis lesion** (similar to DCIS) **but** is **lacking** the **myoepithelial cells**
- If there is **invasion past the capsule**, then **use** area of **invasion for T classification**
- **Very low risk of metastasis** and a very **favorable prognosis** (>95%, 10-year)
- No need to sample lymph nodes if stromal invasion absent
- Pitfall: If there are **isolated tumor cells**, consider **displaced epithelial cells** from biopsy procedure **rather than true invasion** unless absolutely sure
- Most **frequently seen** in **older post-menopausal females** and presents as a **centrally located**, well-circumscribed **palpable mass** (+/- nipple discharge)
- Immunohistochemistry
    - Myoepithelial cells: **(-)** for **p63** (most useful)
    - Ductal cells: **(+)** for **CK7/18**; **(-)** for CK5/6 (except high-grade lesions)
    - Prognostic markers: Nearly all positive for ER and PR; HER-2 negative
- Molecular: **PIK3CA hotspot mutations** seen in about **20% of cases**

Path Presenter

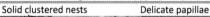

Solid clustered nests — Delicate papillae

Circumscribed

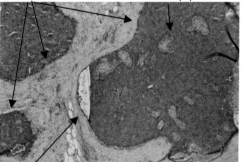

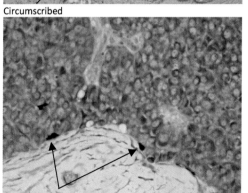

Sparce myoepithelial cells

SOLID PAPILLARY CARCINOMA
MORPHOLOGY
- **Heterogenous** or **monotonous round to spindled-shaped** epithelial **cells** with mild to moderate nuclear atypia, and eosinophilic, granular cytoplasm lining delicate papillae
- Arranged in **multiple clustered** and **circumscribed solid nests**
- **Myoepithelial** cells may be **sparse** but are present
- Mitoses are seen and there is **variable mucin** within cytoplasm or lumens
- May have **neuroendocrine differentiation** in approximately **45% of cases**

OTHER HIGH YIELD POINTS
- **Uncommon** and composes <1% of all breast carcinomas
- Typically, it is seen in **older females** with a palpable **multinodular mass**
- Associated with a **good prognosis**
- If **entirely well-circumscribed nodules** (even in absence of myoepithelial cells) are present and no invasion is present
    - Solid papillary carcinoma in situ
    - Utilize the **AJCC Tis classification** (similar to DCIS)
- If **infiltrating strands** or **ragged borders** are present
    - **Solid papillary carcinoma with invasion** or **invasive solid papillary carcinoma**
    - Utilize the AJCC T classification for the area of invasion
- Immunohistochemistry
    - Myoepithelial cells: **(+)** for **p63**, p40, calponin, SMH
    - Ductal cells: **(+)** for **CK7/18**; **Negative** for CK5/6; **variable** neuroendocrine expression (synaptophysin, INSM-1, chromogranin)
    - Prognostic markers: Almost **all (+)** for **ER/PR**; **(-) Her-2**

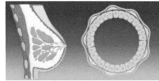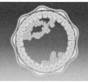

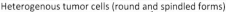

Heterogenous tumor cells (round and spindled forms)

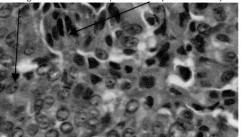

- Molecular findings
  - ➢ **PIK3CA** hotspot mutations seen in approximately **25-35% of cases**
  - ➢ **Copy number changes**: Gains in 1p and 16q, losses in 16q

Path Presenter

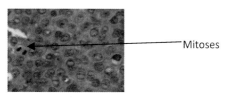

Mitoses

Fibrovascular cores   Monotonous cells

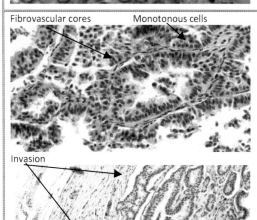

Invasion

INVASIVE PAPILLARY CARCINOMA
MORPHOLOGY
- **Monotonous** neoplastic epithelial cells with **low to intermediate grade nuclei** that are **round** to **oval** with **variable chromatin** distribution, **occasionally** conspicuous **nucleoli** arranged on **fibrovascular cores** with **delicate vessels**
- Usually are **poorly circumscribed** and have an **infiltrative growth** pattern
- **Absence** of myoepithelial cells
- **Stromal desmoplastic response** where infiltration occurs at periphery

OTHER HIGH YIELD POINTS
- **Extremely rare** breast carcinoma (<1% of all breast carcinomas)
- Most common in **post-menopausal women** but can be seen in **men**
- **Differential diagnosis** includes **metastasis** (**lung, ovary, thyroid**), solid papillary carcinoma, invasive solid papillary carcinoma, encapsulated papillary carcinoma, and invasive micropapillary carcinoma
- Immunohistochemistry
  - ➢ Prognostic markers: Majority are **(+)** for **ER/PR**; **(-)** for **HER2**

Path Presenter

ALGORITHM TO APPROACH PAPILLARY LESIONS OF THE BREAST

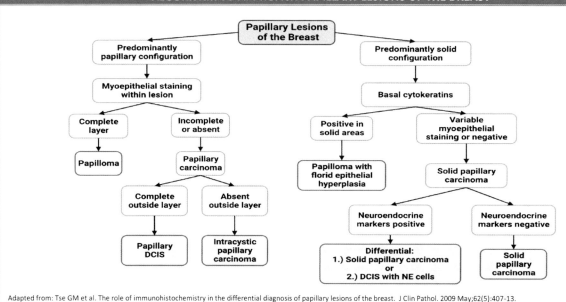

Adapted from: Tse GM et al. The role of immunohistochemistry in the differential diagnosis of papillary lesions of the breast. J Clin Pathol. 2009 May;62(5):407-13.

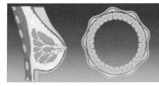

SUMMARY OF PAPILLARY LESIONS OF THE BREAST						
	Intraductal papilloma	Papilloma with DCIS	Papillary DCIS	Encapsulated Papillary Carcinoma	Solid Papillary Carcinoma	Invasive Papillary Carcinoma
Papillary Architecture	• Broad, blunt fronds	• Broad, blunt fronds	• Slender fronds, sometimes branching	• Numerous slender fronds, sometimes branching • Typically, well developed and peripheral; fibrous capsule	• Solid with inconspicuous fibrous septa	• Infiltrative carcinoma with papillary morphology, including fibrovascular cores
Epithelial cells	• Heterogeneous non-neoplastic cells. • Sometimes proliferative lesions (UDH…)	• Focal areas with cytologic features of DCIS (usually Low-grade)	• Entirely occupied by a cell population with features of DCIS (often low-grade)	• Entirely occupied by a cell population with features of DCIS (Often low grade) • Cribriform, micropapillary, and solid patterns may be present, with fusion of papillae	• Entire lesion occupied by a population of cells with low to intermediate grade nuclei • Often spindled or neuro - endocrine morphology.	• Low, intermediate, or, rarely, high grade nuclei
Myoepithelial cells in papillae	• Present	• Present in papilloma but may be scant in DCIS component	• Absent	• Absent	• Absent or Present	• Absent
Myoepithelial cells at periphery	• Present	• Present	• Present	• Absent (usually)	• Absent or Present	• Absent
CK5/6	• Positive in myoepithelial cells and UDH	• Positive in myoepithelial and UDH; Negative in DCIS	• Positive in peripheral myoepithelial • Negative in lesion	• Negative	• Negative	• Negative
ER & PR	• Positive, but heterogeneous	• Strong and diffuse in DCIS	• Strong diffuse	• Strong diffuse	• Strong diffuse	• Positive
Other Stains	• None	• None	• None	• None	• Frequent synaptophysin and chromogranin expression	• None

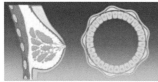

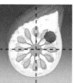
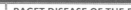

DISEASES OF THE NIPPLE

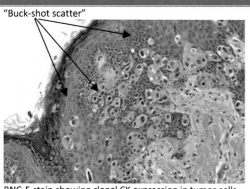

"Buck-shot scatter"

BNC-5 stain showing clonal CK expression in tumor cells

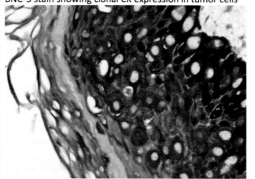

HER-2 IHC highlighting "Buckshot scatter" of tumor cells

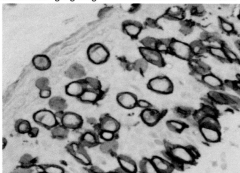

ER negative tumor cells   PR negative tumor cells

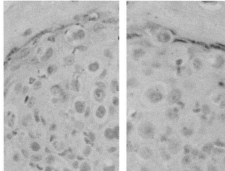

Path Presenter

PAGET DISEASE OF THE BREAST (MAMMARY PAGET DISEASE)

MORPHOLOGY

- **Intraepidermal proliferation** of malignant glandular **epithelial** cells with a "**buckshot scatter**" (transepidermal distribution) appearance
- Malignant cells have **large nuclei, prominent** conspicuous **nucleoli**, and abundant **pale eosinophilic cytoplasm**
- Malignant cells can be in **clusters** or **singly**
- May **form glandular structures** and **may contain mucin**
- Often has an associated **lichenoid lymphocytic infiltrate** in papillary dermis

OTHER HIGH YIELD POINTS

- **Uncommon presentation** of breast cancer and is seen in **women and men**
- Presents as a **pruritic scaling skin crust** with **erythema** (majority of cases), but **can be** a **dark hyperpigmented macule**, and/or it can be **ulcerated**
- Patient may complain of a **moist or wet-breast** due to **extravasation of fluid** from **disrupted tight junctions**
- As many as **50% of patients have no mammographic findings**
- Most cases are a **cutaneous extension of DCIS** or **invasive carcinoma**
  - ➤ Many cases involve lactiferous sinuses of the nipple
  - ➤ If not present, **may be derived** from **Toker cells** or other **adnexal-derived cell** type
- May secondarily invade the dermis in more aggressive cases
- Approximately **50% of cases are associated** with **invasive carcinoma**
- **Prognosis** is **determined** by the **presence of invasive** cancer
  - ➤ Skin **ulceration/erosion**, **dermal invasion**, and **hemorrhage** are **not sufficient** for a AJCC **T4b classification**
  - ➤ Any **tumor cells in the superficial dermis** are **not associated with** any **increased risk** of **metastasis**
  - ➤ Paget disease with DCIS only has a **survival of >95% at 20-years**
- Immunohistochemistry & special stains
  - ➤ Majority are **(+)** for **CK7**, Cam5.2, **HER2**, **GATA3** (80%)
  - ➤ **(-)** for **S100** (75% of cases), CK5/6, **MelanA**, **HMB45**, ER, and PR
  - ➤ May be **(+) for PASD** or **mucin stains** (shows glandular origin)
- Differential diagnoses: Squamous cell carcinoma in situ (Bowen Disease), Melanoma, Toker cell hyperplasia, clear cell change in keratinocytes, sebaceous carcinoma, or carcinoma directly involving the skin

HMB45 negative tumor cells

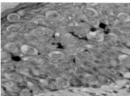

Gross excision showing scaling and crusts involving nipple and areola

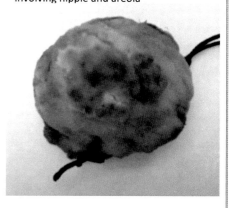

S100 negative tumor cells

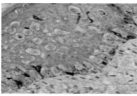

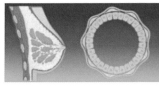

USEFUL SMALL IHC PANEL FOR PAGET DISEASE AND MIMICS					
	Paget Disease of Beast	**Toker cell hyperplasia**	**SCC in situ (Bowen Disease)**	**Melanoma**	**Sebaceous carcinoma**
CK7 or Cam5.2	**Positive**	Positive	**Negative**	**Negative**	Variably positive
CK5/6	Negative	Negative	**Positive**	Negative	Positive
p63	Negative	Negative	**Positive**	Negative	Positive
S100	Negative	Negative	Negative	**Positive**	Negative
MelanA/MART1	Negative	Negative	Negative	**Positive**	Negative
HMB45	Negative	Negative	Negative	**Positive**	Negative
ER	**Usually negative**	**Positive**	Negative	Negative	Variably positive (30%)
Her2	**Strong positive**	Strong positive	Negative	Negative	Variably positive (35%)
Adipophilin	Negative	Negative	Negative	Negative	**Positive**

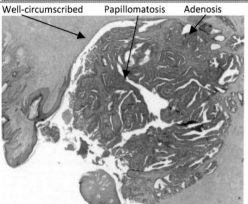

Well-circumscribed   Papillomatosis   Adenosis

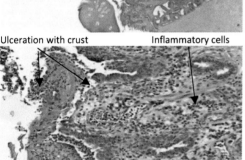

Ulceration with crust   Inflammatory cells

NIPPLE ADENOMA
MORPHOLOGY
- **Benign, epithelial proliferation composed** of any or a **mixture of**:
  - ➤ Simple **ducts**
  - ➤ **Papillomatosis** or sclerosing papillomatosis
  - ➤ **Adenosis**
  - ➤ **Usual duct hyperplasia** or florid hyperplasia
- Epidermis **may have Toker cell hyperplasia** or **hyperkeratosis**
- **Myoepithelial** cells **surround** all the **ducts**
- May have **epidermal erosion** and/**or hemorrhage**, or **focal necrosis**
- Often **well-circumscribed** lesion, but **stromal fibrosis may entrap ducts** in a pattern that **can resemble invasive carcinoma**

OTHER HIGH YIELD POINTS
- **Uncommon** breast lesion that is most often seen in **middle-aged females**
- Patients present with an **irregular or lobulated palpable breast mass** and can have **nipple discharge** and/or be **tender**
- Clinically it **can mimic Paget's disease** due to the erythema, hyperkeratosis and crusts, and erosion/ulceration
- Benign lesion but **can reoccur without complete excision** of the lesion
- Molecular: **PIK3CA present** in **half of all cases**
- Main significance is not to confuse it with invasive carcinoma

Path Presenter

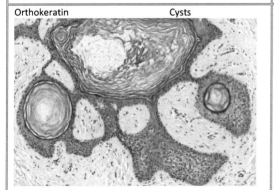

Orthokeratin   Cysts

SYRINGOMATOUS TUMOR
MORPHOLOGY
- **Benign infiltrative neoplasm** composed of **tubules**, solid **nests**, and **cysts**
- The tubules are **composed of more than one cell layer** that usually are cuboidal (glandular) or flattened (squamous)
- The **tubules often display branching** and have **eosinophilic luminal secretions**
- **Squamous metaplasia** can be solid or cystic and are frequently **"tadpole"** or **"comma" shaped**
- **Cystic spaces** are **filled with orthokeratin**
- Tumor frequently **infiltrates around bundles of smooth muscle, lactiferous sinuses** and may have **perineural invasion**
- **No necrosis** and **mitoses are extremely rare** (if any)

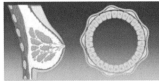
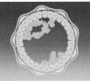

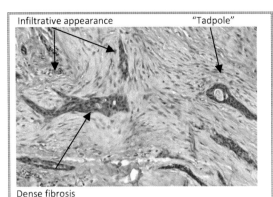

Infiltrative appearance   "Tadpole"

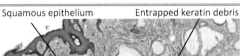

Dense fibrosis

- **Stroma is variable** and can be myxoid, hyaline, fibrous, or loosely cellular and is denser around the tumor nests
- May have **pseudoepitheliomatous hyperplasia** or **lymphocytic infiltrate**

OTHER HIGH YIELD POINTS
- **Very rare tumor** occurring almost exclusively in middle-aged females
- Presents as a **palpable firm mass** in the dermis of the **nipple/areola**
- **Recurrence occurs in 30%** of cases that have a positive margin
- Immunohistochemistry:
  - ➤ Glandular: **(+)** for CK8/18
  - ➤ Squamous: **(+)** for p63, CK10
  - ➤ Myoepithelial-like cells: **(+)** for p63
  - ➤ **(-)** for ER, PR, and HER2

Path Presenter

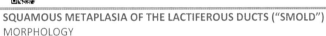

Squamous epithelium   Entrapped keratin debris

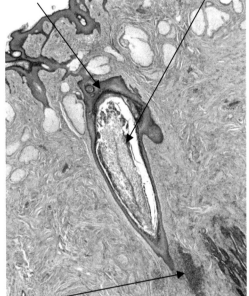

Chronic inflammation
Image credit: Dr. Patrick J. McIntire, MD

Inverted nipple

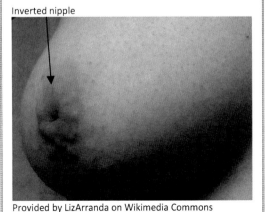

Provided by LizArranda on Wikimedia Commons

SQUAMOUS METAPLASIA OF THE LACTIFEROUS DUCTS ("SMOLD")
MORPHOLOGY
- Duct epithelium with **squamous metaplasia** and **entrapped keratin**
- Often has **acute** and **chronic inflammation** surrounding nests
- **Giant cells may be present adjacent to the duct space and is** more common when keratin debris is present in the stroma
- Chronic **fibrosis** may be seen from prolonged **chronic inflammation**
- **Bacteria can be present** if there is a **secondary infectious** etiology

OTHER HIGH YIELD POINTS
- **Occurs at any age >20 years** and is seen in **females and males**
- This entity is essentially a **special form** of **duct ectasia**
- Presents as a **very painful** and **erythematous subareolar mass** that is sterile (no organisms)
- **Highly associated with tobacco use** and **inverted nipples** as nearly all patients have history of both
- Proposed **hypothesis** for the findings are:
  - ➤ **Squamous metaplasia** is caused by the **toxins from** the **tobacco and** mediating a **vitamin A deficiency** and thus **causing the metaplasia**
  - ➤ **Inverted nipples** are caused by the **recurrent inflammation** and **fibrosis** surrounding the duct
- Surgical intervention (wedge resection) is the main treatment but may cause fistula track near the areolar perimeter

Pathogenesis of SMOLD

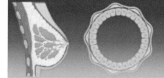 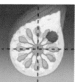

2. BREAST PATHOLOGY

INVASIVE BREAST CARCINOMA	

GENERAL BACKGROUND	• **Most common cancer in women** and **leading cause of** female **cancer death** worldwide
	• Presenting signs and symptoms:
	  ➢ **Unscreened populations:** Mass, skin erythema and edema due to cancer in dermal lymphatics
	  ➢ **Screened populations:** Spiculated mass, architectural distortion, MRI enhancement
	• **Three pillars of diagnosis:** Physical exam, imaging, needle biopsy/cytology
	  ➢ **When** these are **concordant**, the **risk of missing breast cancer is extremely low** but requires careful correlation
	• **General risk factors:** Increased estrogen, seen with early menarche, fewer children, less lactation, and obesity, increased alcohol consumption

PATHOGENESIS AND MOLECULAR BASIS	• **Two main pathways** separated by Estrogen Receptor (ER) status:
	  ➢ **ER-positive (ER+, HER2-):** Diploid with specific chromosomal gains/losses (e.g., gain 1q, loss of 16q) and are usually low to intermediate-grade cancers
	  ➢ **ER-Negative (ER-, HER2+/-):** Aneuploid with complex karyotypes, frequent TP53 mutations, and are most frequently high-grade tumors with high proliferation rate
	• Both pathways show **PIK3CA mutations**, but it is **more common in ER-positive** tumors
	• **Non-obligate precursors to ER (+) cancers:** FEA, ADH, and low-grade DCIS
	• **Non-obligate precursors ER (-) cancers:** Microglandular adenosis and high-grade DCIS

MOLECULAR CLASSIFICATION (BASED ON HIERARCHICAL CLUSTER ANALYSIS OF GENE EXPRESSION)

	Luminal A	Luminal B	HER2-Positive	Basal type
Percent of all tumors	50%	20%	15%	15%
Classic ER/HER2 status	ER+, HER2-	ER+, HER2-	ER-, HER2+	ER-, HER2-
Ki-67	Low	Intermediate	High	High
Actual ER/HER2	ER+		HER2+	Triple negative
Grade	Low			High
Recurrence Risk	Low, but long term		High, but short term	
Therapies used	Hormone Rx		HER2 Rx	Chemotherapy

* Note: Other molecular classifications exist and include additional/alternate groupings; this is just the most well established frequently utilized classification

GRADING	• Grade using the **Nottingham system** based on 3 characteristics:
	  ➢ **Tubule formation:** Only structures with central lumina surrounded by polarized cells are counted
	  ➢ **Nuclear pleomorphism:** Assessed in the area showing the worst cytologic atypia
	  ➢ **Mitotic count:** Assessed in mitotic hot spot. Remember to factor in your field area

Tubule Formation	Score	Nuclear Pleomorphism	Score	Mitosis	Score
Majority of tumor (>75%)	1	**Small, regular, uniform** (<1.5x the size of normal nucleus)	1	<3/mm²	1
Moderate degree (10-75%)	2	**Moderate increase in size/variability** (1.5-2x cell size)	2	4-7/mm²	2
Little or none (<10%)	3	**Marked variation** (>2x cell size), vesicular chromatin, prominent nucleoli	3	≥8/mm²	3

Total Nottingham Score	Grade
3-5	1
6 or 7	2
8 or 9	3

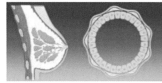 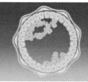 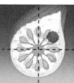

NOTTINGHAM GRADING EXAMPLES	NUCLEAR PLEOMORPHISM		
	NORMAL / SCORE 1	SCORE 2	SCORE 3
	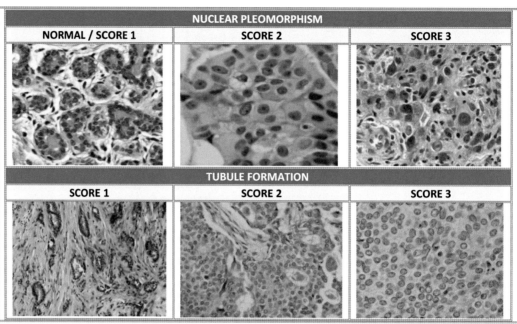		
	TUBULE FORMATION		
	SCORE 1	SCORE 2	SCORE 3

GENERAL IHC

- **Invasive cancers** usually **stain with LMWCK** (including CK7 and CK19), EMA, and **GATA3**
- Some cancers (often the **well-differentiated** ones) **stain** with **GCDFP-15(BRST2)** and **mammaglobin**
- Higher-grade **triple-negative cases stain** with **basal markers** including **HMWCK** (CK5/6)
- A subset of cancers (often **metaplastic** and/or triple negative) express **S100, SOX10,** and/or **p63**
- **TRPS1 will stain all breast cancers except apocrine** adenocarcinoma

MYOEPITHELIAL CELL MARKERS			
Marker	Clone	Staining pattern	Comment
p63	4A4	Nuclear	• One of the **most sensitive** and **specific** markers • Normal ducts show **continuous dot-like pattern** • **In situ** carcinomas are **focally discontinuous** • Attenuated or **non-reactive in invasive** & papillary carcinoma
SMMHC	SMMS-1	Cytoplasmic	• **More sensitive than p63** • Some **cross-reactivity with vascular smooth muscle cells** and **stromal myofibroblasts** (but less than calponin) • Linear cytoplasmic pattern with **gaps in the in-situ carcinoma**
Calponin	EP798Y	Cytoplasmic	• Linear cytoplasmic pattern with **gaps in the in-situ carcinoma** • **Higher frequency** of **cross-reactivity** to vascular **smooth muscle cells** and stromal **myofibroblasts** • **Reactive to** small proportion of **tumor cells**
SMA	1A4	Cytoplasmic	• **Sensitive** but **not a specific marker** due to the **marked cross-reactivity** to **vascular smooth muscle cells** and **myofibroblasts**
Maspin	G167-70	Nuclear, cytoplasmic	• **Very sensitive marker** and **lacks the cross-reactivity** to vascular smooth muscle cells and stromal myofibroblasts • **Reacts to tumor cells**, which **limits the utility** of this marker
CD10	56C6	Cytoplasmic, membranous	• **Somewhat sensitive marker** but has **cross-reactivity** to **stromal myofibroblasts, non-specific reactivity** to **epithelial cells**, but **no reactivity to vascular smooth muscle cells**

Adapted from: Liu H. Application of Immunohistochemistry in Breast Pathology: A Review and Update. Archives of Pathology & Laboratory Medicine: December 2014, Vol. 138, No. 12, pp. 1629 1642.

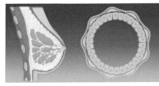 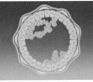
IS IT INVASIVE OR A MIMIC?	<ul><li>**Invasive** breast is **defined by** the **absence of** peripheral **myoepithelial cells**</li><li>Stains for myoepithelial cells should be employed as part of a panel or cocktail with at least one nuclear and one cytoplasmic stain</li><li>**Do not rely** solely **on negative myoepithelial stains** to diagnose invasion, H&E findings must be concordant</li><li>Nests of **in situ carcinoma may** be **surrounded by reduced numbers** or **weak staining of myoepithelial cells**</li></ul>

MORPHOLOGIC FEATURES OF CANCER VERSUS MIMICS

Feature	Invasive cancer	Complex Sclerosing lesions	DCIS involving sclerosing adenosis
Stroma	Desmoplastic	Dense	Dense
Cytology	Atypical	Bland	Atypical
Gland profile	Angulated	Compressed	Solid/Cribriform
Architecture	Infiltrative	Lobulated	Lobulated
Myoepithelial cells	Absent	Present	Present

Modified From: Peng et al. Update on Immunohistochemical Analysis in Breast Lesions. Archives of Pathology & Laboratory Medicine: August 2017, Vol. 141, No. 8, pp. 1033-1051.

SUBTYPES OF INVASIVE CARCINOMA

NO SPECIAL TYPE (NST)	CARCINOMAS OF SPECIAL TYPE	
	Non-salivary gland type tumors	**Salivary gland-type tumors**
Invasive ductal carcinoma Medullary pattern Osteoclastic-like giant cell pattern Neuroendocrine differentiation pattern Pleomorphic pattern Choriocarcinomatous pattern Melanotic pattern Oncocytic pattern Lipid-rich pattern Glycogen-rich clear cell pattern Sebaceous pattern	Microinvasive carcinoma Invasive lobular carcinoma Tubular & cribriform carcinoma Mucinous (colloid) carcinoma Mucinous cystadenocarcinoma Invasive papillary carcinoma Invasive micropapillary carcinoma Metaplastic carcinoma Low-grade Adenosquamous carcinoma Triple-negative and Basal-like carcinoma Inflammatory carcinoma Invasive apocrine carcinoma Neuroendocrine tumor (NET) and carcinoma	Acinic cell carcinoma Adenoid cystic carcinoma Secretory carcinoma Mucoepidermoid carcinoma Polymorphous adenocarcinoma

Note: Tumors showing a special histologic pattern in ≥ 90% of the tumor are designated as pure special tumor. If less than 90%, they are designated as "No Special Type" (NST), which accounts for the majority of breast cancer cases. If a special type composes 10-90% of the carcinoma, it is reported as a "Mixed invasive breast carcinoma of no special type and special subtype".

INVASIVE CARCINOMA OF NO SPECIAL TYPE

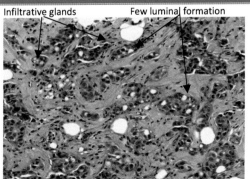
Infiltrative glands   Few luminal formation

INVASIVE "DUCTAL" CARCINOMA
GENERAL MORPHOLOGY
- Composed of infiltrative **malignant epithelial cells** that can be in **irregular and stellate glands, cribriform** pattern, **solid**, or **small clusters**
- **Morphology is variable** based on if there are any morphologic patterns
- **No myoepithelial cells** surround any of the tumor cells
- **May infiltrate lymphovascular** channels **or** have **perineural invasion**
- Often has a **desmoplastic stromal response** to the infiltration of tumor cells
- **Necrosis and calcifications** may or **may not be present** in the lesion
- May have biopsy site changes (granulation tissue etc.)

OTHER HIGH YIELD POINTS
- **Represents** approximately **75% of invasive** breast **carcinomas**

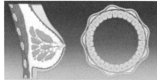

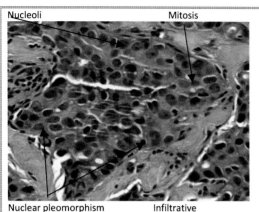

Nucleoli   Mitosis

Nuclear pleomorphism   Infiltrative

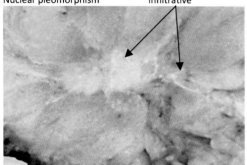

- The **grade** of carcinoma is **based on the Nottingham** grading **scale**
- Can present as a hard lump within the breast if it is at least 2cm in size
- **Nearly 90% of all palpable cancers are identified by the patient** themselves with the remainder detected by examination
- Patients are **usually middle-aged females** and **only 1% of cases** occur in **males**
- **Immunohistochemistry is dependent on the specific subtype** but those with no morphologic patterns show:
  - ➤ **Ductal cells: (+)** for LMWCK (CK8/18, CKAE1/AE3, CK7), p120, e-cadherin, TRPS1, GATA3 (variable on HR status), variable positivity for HMWCK (CK5/6, CK14, CK17), SOX10 (variable)
- **Prognostic markers** should be **performed on all invasive carcinomas**
  - ➤ **Report the % of tumor cells positive and the intensity** of staining
- Molecular:
  - ➤ **ER-positive:** Gains of 1q and loss of 16q
  - ➤ **ER-negative:** Gain of 11q13, loss of of 13q, amplification of 17q12
  - ➤ **HER2-amplification** is seen in **approximately 15% of cases** but allows for targeted therapy albeit toxic
  - ➤ **PIK3CA and ESR1** mutations are **associated with endocrine therapy resistance**
- **Gene expression profiles:** Helpful to classify if they are luminal A, luminal B, HER2-enriched, triple-negative/basal-like
  - ➤ Majority of **low-grade NST** cases are **luminal A subtype**

Path Presenter

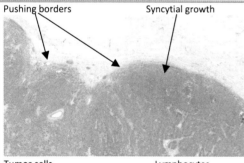

Pushing borders   Syncytial growth

Tumor cells   Lymphocytes

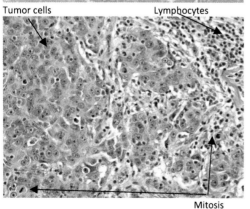

Mitosis

INVASIVE CARCINOMA OF NST WITH MEDULLARY PATTERN
GENERAL MORPHOLOGY

- **Well-circumscribed**, high-grade carcinoma with "**pushing margins**"
- Tumor cells have **high-grade nuclei** have a **syncytial** (sheet-like) **architecture** with **no glandular formation** in any part of the tumor
- **Prominent** tumor **infiltrating lymphocytes** between the tumor cells and at the periphery of the tumor
- **Mitoses can be seen** throughout the tumor
- **Dense fibrous tissue surrounds the tumor** & desmoplasia may be present

OTHER HIGH YIELD POINTS

- Presents in **younger females** (usually age 50) as a **soft, palpable circumscribed mass**
- May have **palpable lymph nodes but** it is **from hyperplasia**
  - ➤ **Nodal metastasis** is **not common**
- **Better outcome** than other stage-matched high-grade cancers
  - ➤ Hypothesized to be due to the tumor infiltrating lymphocytes
- IHC: **Epithelial cells are (+)** for **CK5/6, CK14, EGFR, p53**, and **PDL1** expression (more than 80% of cases)
- **Prognostic markers**: Majority are **triple negative** (basal-like)
- **Molecular**: About **15% of patients are BRCA1** mutation **carriers**
- **Differential diagnoses**: Metastatic high-grade carcinoma from other organs and lymphoma

Path Presenter

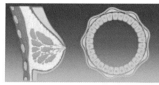

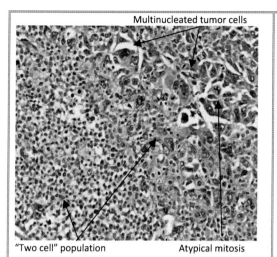

Multinucleated tumor cells

"Two cell" population   Atypical mitosis

INVASIVE CARCINOMA OF NST WITH CHORIOCARCINOMATOUS FEATURES
GENERAL MORPHOLOGY
- **Markedly pleomorphic tumor cells** that appear as **two different populations**
- **Large, pleomorphic, and multinucleated tumor cells** have **smudged nuclei, eosinophilic cytoplasm** with **occasional vacuoles**, and **irregular cytoplasmic projections**
- Second tumor cell population is **monocytoid in appearance**
- Scattered, **highly atypical mitoses** are seen throughout

OTHER HIGH YIELD POINTS
- **Extremely rare** morphologic pattern of invasive carcinoma with NST
- May have an **elevated β-hCG**, but **nearly 60% of patients with IC-NST also have this**, so this is a **non-specific finding**
- All cases have been seen in women and are **middle-aged** to **elderly**
- IHC: Often **(+) for hPL** and **β-hCG; (-)** for **ER** and **PR**

Path Presenter

Osteoclast-like giant cell pattern
Benign osteoclast-like giant cells

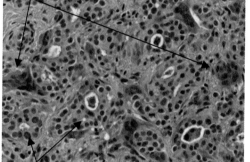

Invasive carcinoma

Neuroendocrine pattern

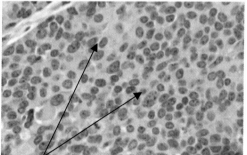

Salt and pepper chromatin

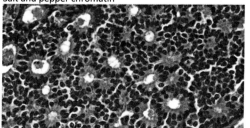

OTHER RARE MORPHOLOGIC ENTITIES OF INVASIVE CARCINOMA OF NST
- **IC-NST with osteoclast-like giant cells** – Giant cells are **similar to histiocytes** and **osteoclasts** and **are benign**, lesion is associated with hypervascular stroma with surrounding hemosiderin and hemorrhage; associated with **any histologic type of carcinoma**

- **Neuroendocrine differentiation pattern** – Any carcinoma with **salt and pepper chromatin,** variable conspicuous nucleoli, eosinophilic cytoplasm, for which **lacks the features** to be called **a neuroendocrine carcinoma;** **stains with** some **neuroendocrine markers** (synaptophysin, chromogranin, INSM-1); frequently are **ER-positive** and **HER2-negative**

- **Oncocytic pattern** – Carcinoma cells have **increased** numbers of **mitochondria** which make the **cytoplasm granular and eosinophilic**

- **Melanotic pattern** – The carcinoma cells are reminiscent of melanoma; can be cohesive, epithelioid, spindled, binucleated, conspicuous nucleoli, have dusty eosinophilic cytoplasm, produce melanin pigment

- **Pleomorphic pattern** – The tumor cells have marked pleomorphism, often have multinucleation

- **Lipid-rich pattern** – The tumor cells have **abundant intracytoplasmic lipid** which are positive for **Oil Red O** or **Sudan** (both **require fresh tissue**, FFPE eliminates the lipid); commonly are **grade 3** carcinomas which are **ER-negative, PR-negative,** and **HER2-positive**

- **Glycogen-rich pattern** – The tumor cells have abundant intracytoplasmic glycogen stores which are **PAS-positive** and **diastase resistant**

- **Sebaceous pattern** – The tumor cells can be oval to round and have vacuolated, clear cytoplasm, and have nuclei that are irregularly-shaped; intracytoplasmic lipid is **positive** for **Oil Red O**

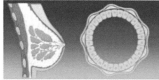
INVASIVE CARCINOMA OF SPECIAL TYPE (NON-SALIVARY GLAND TYPE)

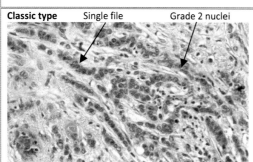

In situ carcinoma / Microinvasion / Desmoplastic stromal response

MICROINVASIVE CARCINOMA

MORPHOLOGY

- **Invasive carcinoma ≤ 1mm in size**, often **adjacent to high-grade DCIS**
- **Earliest recognizable forms** of **invasive** carcinoma that presents as:
  - ➢ **Invasion beyond myoepithelium**
  - ➢ **Small, angulated clusters** of tumor cells infiltrating stroma
  - ➢ Associated with **desmoplastic stromal** changes

OTHER HIGH YIELD POINTS

- **Better prognosis than larger invasive** tumors
- **Often multifocal** and if any single **invasive focus is > 1mm then** it is called **invasive carcinoma** (not microinvasive)
- Be **wary diagnosing** this **on a biopsy** as more **invasion may be on excision**
- Best practice is to **get levels** to **exclude any larger focus** of invasive carcinoma

Path Presenter

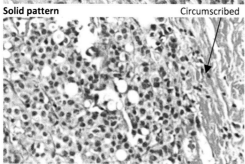

Classic type / Single file / Grade 2 nuclei

Solid pattern / Circumscribed

Pleomorphic

INVASIVE LOBULAR CARCINOMA

MORPHOLOGY

- Malignant epithelial cells with **variable cytologic features**
- **Classic type** – Tumor cells are discohesive and have **nuclei grade 1 or 2, round** nuclear **contours**, and have **scant to moderate cytoplasm**
- **Signet ring cell type** – Tumor cells are **discohesive** and have **eccentrically** located **nuclei** that are **compressed** from the **intracytoplasmic mucin vacuole**
- **Pleomorphic type** – Tumor cells are **discohesive** and **are > 4x that of a lymphocyte** and have **nuclei that are markedly irregular**, conspicuous **nucleoli**, and **variable chromatin**, and **variable cytoplasm**

OTHER HIGH YIELD POINTS

- Accounts for nearly **15% of all invasive** breast **carcinomas**
- Presents in women that are **usually middle aged** and **may not be palpable** or is **poorly defined**; may be **seen in males that have BRCA2 mutations**
- Often **little host stromal reaction** or disturbance of background architecture
- Nearly **90% of classic type are Grade 2 tumor cells**
- **Lymphovascular invasion is very rare** due to the dispersion of single cells
- Growth patterns are variable and can be any of the following:
  - ➢ **Classic pattern (most common)** – Single file rows of tumor cells that dissect collagen fibers
  - ➢ **Alveolar pattern (~10%)** – Tumor cells are in round aggregates and are separated by a fibrous band and may resemble LCIS
  - ➢ **Solid pattern (~5-10%)** – Tumor cells form large, circumscribed nests, mimic lymphoma, and often have the classic pattern at the edges of the nests
  - ➢ **Tubulolobular pattern (<1~)** – Tumors have mixtures of classic type and few scattered, miniature round tubules of tumor cells with grade 1 nuclei
  - ➢ **Mucinous pattern (rare)** – Tumor cells with signet ring cell morphology and are suspended in extracellular mucin
- IHC: **(+)** for **cytokeratins, GATA3, p120 (cytoplasmic)** AR, ER, PR, MUC1, GCDFP15, and **(-)** for HER2, e-cadherin, CDX-2
- **Special stains:** Intracytoplasmic mucin is **mucicarmine positive**

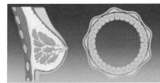
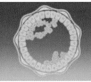

Signet Ring cell type   Eccentric nuclei

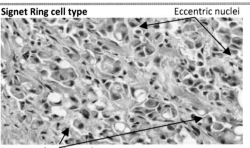

Intracytoplasmic mucin

Tubulo-lobular pattern   Small tubules

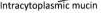
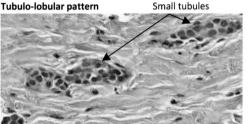

- **Molecular classification:** Majority are **luminal A type**, and second most common is luminal B type
- **Molecular mutations: CDH1** and **PIK3CA** mutations
- **Cytogenetic abnormalities:** Gain of 1q and 16p, and loss of 16q

IHC Stain	Normal Epithelium	Lobular Carcinoma	No Special Type
E-Cadherin	Membrane staining	Negative	Membrane staining
P120	Membrane staining	Cytoplasmic	Membrane staining
β-Catenin	Membrane staining	Absence of membrane staining	Membrane Staining

Path Presenter

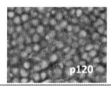
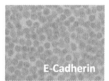

p120   E-Cadherin

Well-formed tubules

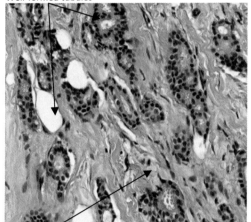

Stromal desmoplastic response

TUBULAR CARCINOMA
MORPHOLOGY

- **Haphazard proliferation** of **infiltrative tumor cells** that are arranged in **well formed tubules** with **angled** and **tapered edges** (90% of tumor must have)
- Tumor cells have **low-grade nuclei** with **uniform chromatin distribution**, small **single conspicuous nucleoli**, and **cytoplasm with occasional snouts**
- **Stromal desmoplastic response** is present
- **No myoepithelial cells** surround the tubules

OTHER HIGH YIELD POINTS

- An **uncommon low-grade** invasive **carcinoma** with a **good prognosis**
- Often **associated with a low-grade DCIS component**, CCH, ALH, and FEA
- Often **mimics sclerosing adenosis, DCIS,** and **Microglandular adenosis**
- IHC: **(+)** for **ER** and **PR** and **negative for HER2; (-)** for myoepithelial markers

Path Presenter

Nests of cribriform tumor

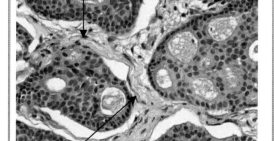

Stromal desmoplasia

CRIBRIFORM CARCINOMA
MORPHOLOGY

- **Haphazard fenestrated proliferation** of infiltrative **cribriform nests** and compose **> 90% of tumor**
- Tumor cells have **low-grade, polarized nuclei** with **uniform chromatin** distribution, small **single conspicuous nucleoli**, and **eosinophilic cytoplasm**
- **Stromal desmoplastic response** is present
- **No myoepithelial cells** surround the tubules (tumor cells get crushed and appear like myoepithelial cells)

OTHER HIGH YIELD POINTS

- **Rare** and **uncommon low-grade carcinoma** with a **good prognosis**
- IHC: **(+)** for **ER** and **PR** and **negative for HER2; (-)** for myoepithelial markers

Path Presenter

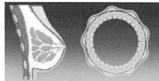

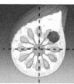
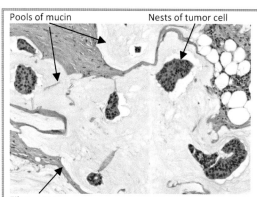

Pools of mucin   Nests of tumor cell

Fibrous septa
Well-circumscribed

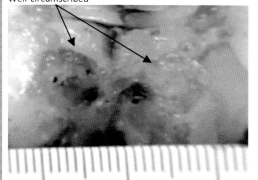

Gelatinous appearance of core biopsy

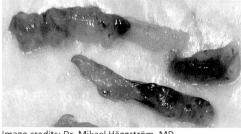

Image credits: Dr. Mikael Häggström, MD

MUCINOUS CARCINOMA

MORPHOLOGY

- **Scattered groups** and **nests** of **invasive carcinoma** floating **in pools of extracellular mucin**
- **Delicate fibrous septae** separate the pools of extracellular mucin
- The tumor cells are composed of **low to intermediate-grade nuclei** that are **round to oval**, have **regular chromatin** distribution, and **variable eosinophilic cytoplasm**
- Lesion is **well-circumscribed**

OTHER HIGH YIELD POINTS

- **Uncommon** invasive carcinoma occurring in **elderly women** and presents as a **soft, palpable mass** that mimics a **benign process**
- Has **three main histologic patterns:**
  - ➢ **Pure mucinous carcinoma** – composed of two subtypes, **type A is paucicellular** and **type B is more cellular** and **less mucin**; has a **favorable prognosis**; **type B frequently** has **neuroendocrine differentiation**
  - ➢ **Mixed mucinous carcinoma** – has both a **mucinous component** and an **invasive component** which **lacks the mucin component** (>10% of tumor); has an **intermediate prognosis**
  - ➢ **Micropapillary mucinous carcinoma** – micropapillary architecture & often has an **inverted appearance** in which the **cytoplasm points towards the outside** of the spherules; has a **worse prognosis** when compared to the other patterns of mucinous carcinoma
- **Prognostic markers**: Majority are **(+)** for **ER** and **PR**; **(-)** for **HER2**
- **IHC**: **(+)** for **WT1, EMA**; **variable** neuroendocrine expression (synaptophysin, chromogranin, CD56, INSM1)
- **Molecular**: Mutations in **GATA3** (~25%), **KMT2C** (20%), **MAP3K1** (~15%), **PIK3CA** (~10%), and **fusion of OAZ1-CSNK1G2** (<5%, recurrent but not pathognomonic)
- **Differential includes** a rare entity called **mucinous cystadenocarcinoma**:
  - ➢ Invasive breast cancer characterized by cystic structures lined by tall columnar cells with intracytoplasmic and intracystic mucin, like pancreatic IPMNs or ovarian mucinous carcinoma

Path Presenter

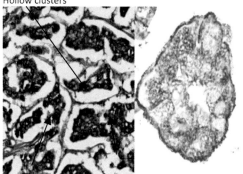

Hollow clusters

Delicate stroma

EMA, image credits :
Takashi Fujisawa M.D.,
Ph.D. (@Patholwalker)

INVASIVE MICROPAPILLARY CARCINOMA

MORPHOLOGY

- The tumor cells can be **cuboidal to columnar** and have **intermediate** to **high-grade nuclei**, with **granular eosinophilic cytoplasm**
- Tumor cells are **arranged in small, hollow**, or **morula-like clusters** with an **inside out-growth pattern** and are **surrounded by spaces** with **intercellular fluid** and a **delicate stromal network**
- **No fibrovascular cores** (as is the case with all micropapillary tumors)
- Tumor cells have **reverse polarity** (apical cytoplasm faces outwards)

OTHER HIGH YIELD POINTS

- **Very rare** and often occurs in **younger patients** and **affect both sexes**
- **Nearly 67%** of cases **have lymph node metastasis at presentation**
- Despite having tubules, they are **graded as a Nottingham score 3**
- **Survival is not significantly worse** than stage-matched IC-NST
- **IHC**: **(+)** for **MUC1, e-cadherin** (basolateral), and **p120** (basolateral)
- **Prognostic markers**: **(+)** for **ER** and **PR**, and **50%** are **(+)** for **HER2**

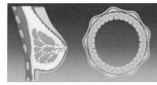

Low-grade adenosquamous carcinoma

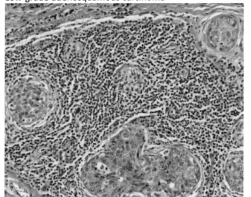

Fibromatosis-like metaplastic carcinoma

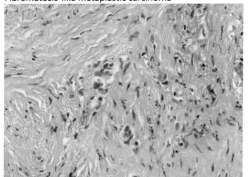

Spindle cell carcinoma

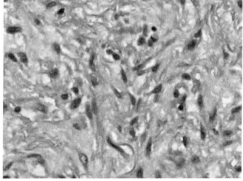

Squamous cell carcinoma

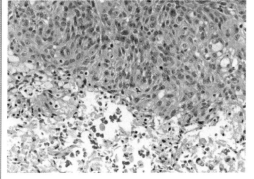

METAPLASTIC CARCINOMA
MORPHOLOGY
- **Invasive carcinoma** with a **wide spectrum of differentiation** of the epithelium towards squamous or mesenchymal-like elements
- **Several distinct patterns** (with some overlap, often mixed)
  - **Low-grade adenosquamous carcinoma** – Well-developed, rounded glands and tubules associated with solid squamous nests infiltrating through desmoplastic stroma; sometimes associated "cannon ball" lymphoid aggregates; associated with a **good prognosis**
  - **Fibromatosis-like metaplastic carcinoma** – Bland spindled cells with pale eosinophilic cytoplasm and slender nuclei with mild atypia (or may be plump and epithelioid) in stroma with variable collagen and often arranged in fascicles; associated with a **good prognosis**
  - **Spindle cell carcinoma** – Atypical spindle cells with a variety of architectural patterns (fascicles, herringbone) and have elongated to plump spindled cells with moderate to high-grade cytologic atypia; there is often associated inflammation; this category includes a spectrum of tumors from sarcomatoid SCC to myoepithelial carcinoma; associated with a **worse prognosis**
  - **Squamous cell carcinoma** – Pure squamous cell carcinoma and is often cystic; most important thing is to exclude a metastasis; associated with a **worse prognosis**
  - **Metaplastic carcinoma with heterologous mesenchymal differentiation** – Is essentially a carcinosarcoma and the heterologous elements may include chondroid, osseous, or rhabdoid components; epithelial and mesenchymal components can have variable atypia; extensive sampling is often necessary to find the epithelial component and exclude a primary sarcoma of the breast

OTHER HIGH YIELD POINTS
- **Rare type** of cancer that **composes <1% of all breast cancers**
- Usually presents as a **large palpable mass**
- **Prognostic markers:** Negative for ER, PR, and HER2 **(triple negative)**
- IHC: **(+) for TRPS1, p63, HMWCKs**(CK5/6), **CKAE1/AE3, SOX10** (~50%); **(-) for CK7, CD34**; variable SMA, CD10, desmin, and β-catenin
- **Molecular:** Mutations in **TP53** (~65%), **PIK3CA** (~60%), **TERT promoter** (~45%) **PTEN** (~15%), NF1 (~!5%), PIK3R1 (~10%), and AKT (~5%), Wnt, and RB1

Path Presenter

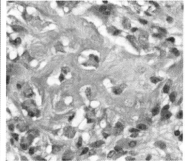

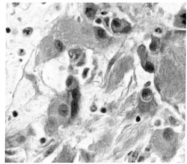

Osseous component   Rhabdoid component

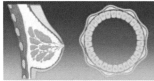

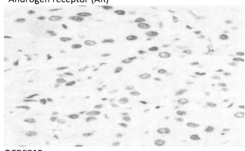

Apocrine carcinoma (Metastasis to bone)   Nucleoli

Large nuclei   Granular cytoplasm

Androgen receptor (AR)

GCDFP15

AR and GCDFP15 , image credits : Takashi Fujisawa M.D., Ph.D. (@Patholwalker)

INVASIVE APOCRINE CARCINOMA
MORPHOLOGY
- The tumor cells have **large nuclei** with **prominent conspicuous nucleoli**, **vesicular chromatin**, and have **abundant granular eosinophilic cytoplasm**
- Must have **>90% of tumor cells and must have** apocrine **morphology**
- May be arranged in **well-formed tubules**, **solid** or **sheet-like**, or **single cell** "**lobular**" **pattern**
- **Type A cells:** Intensely staining, abundant granular eosinophilic cytoplasm and round nuclei with prominent conspicuous nucleoli
- **Type B cells:** Abundant, finely vacuolated cytoplasm (resemble histiocytes) and have round nuclei with prominent conspicuous nucleoli

OTHER HIGH YIELD POINTS
- **Rare** breast carcinoma seen in older women
- **Favorable prognosis**
- IHC: **(+)** for **cytokeratins, AR, GCDFP15; (-)** for **TRPS1, GATA3**
- **Special stains:** Intracytoplasmic granules are **PAS positive**
- **Prognostic markers:** Negative for ER, PR, HER2 (~50%) (**triple-negative**)
- **Molecular**: Mutations in **PIK3CA** (>80%), **TP53** (~30%), **PTEN** (~30%)
- **Electron microscopy: Prominent mitochondria** with occasional **abnormal cristae**; and membrane bound **vesicles** that are **400-600 nm** and have **dense secretory granules**
- **Cytogenetics:** Loss of heterozygosity of 17p13 (TP53), 3p25 (VHL), 16p13 (PKD1/TSC2), and 1p35-36 (NB), and abnormalities of 7q (encodes GCDFP15)

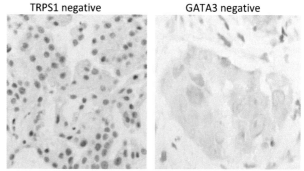

TRPS1 negative   GATA3 negative

Image credits: Dr. Terrance Lynn, MD

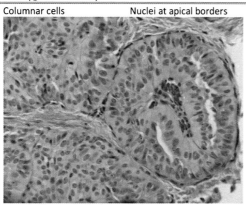

Columnar cells   Nuclei at apical borders

Provided by Dr. Kimberly Heightchew, MD

TALL CELL CARCINOMA WITH REVERSE POLARITY
MORPHOLOGY
- **Tall columnar cells** with **reverse nuclear polarity** (nuclei at apical border)
- Nuclei are round to oval and have mild contour irregularities, conspicuous nucleoli, variable chromatin, and eosinophilic cytoplasm
- Tumor cells are arranged in **solid** and **solid papillary patterns**
- Scattered calcifications can be seen in the papillary areas

OTHER HIGH YIELD POINTS
- **Rare** and **indolent** invasive carcinoma that resembles papillary thyroid carcinoma but nuclei are not basally located
- IHC: **(+)** for **HMWCK** and **LMWCK** (CK5/6, CK7), and **calretinin**
- Prognostic markers: **(-)** for ER, PR, and HER2 **(triple negative)**
- **Molecular: IDH2 R172 hotspot mutation** (>80% of cases), **PIK3CA** (~67%)

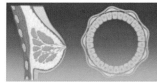

INVASIVE CARCINOMA OF SALIVARY-GLAND TYPE

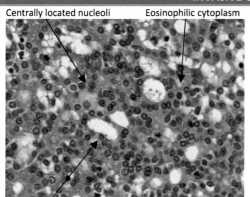

Centrally located nucleoli / Eosinophilic cytoplasm

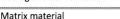

Microglandular formation

ACINIC CELL CARCINOMA
MORPHOLOGY
- Invasive carcinoma composed of tumor cells that have **centrally located, round nuclei, prominent** conspicuous **nucleoli**, and **finely granular pale eosinophilic** to **clear vacuolated cytoplasm**
- May have **dark staining granules** in cells which **may resemble Paneth cells**
- Often has a **microglandular formation**
- Frequently has **easily seen mitosis** scattered throughout

OTHER HIGH YIELD POINTS
- **Very rare** carcinoma of the breast with <20 known cases
- In the rare cases, many were **female in their 30s-40s**
- Grossly tumor is **well-circumscribed** with a pink hemorrhagic cut surface
- IHC: **(+) for CK7**, E-cadherin, EMA; **(-) for GCDFP15**, MUC2, SMA,
- **Prognostic markers: (-)** for ER, PR, and HER2 **(triple negative)**

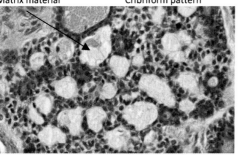

Matrix material / Cribriform pattern

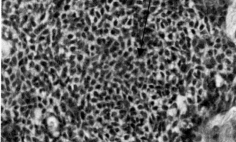

Solid pattern / Epithelial/myoepithelial cells

ADENOID CYSTIC CARCINOMA
MORPHOLOGY
- Malignant **epithelial cells and myoepithelial cells** that are arranged in **tubules, cribriform,** and **solid patterns** with an associated **basophilic matrix** and **basement membrane material**

OTHER HIGH YIELD POINTS
- **Very rare** and majority occur in **middle-aged females**
- Presents as a **palpable lobulated** or **circumscribed mass below** the **nipple**
- **Prognosis is good,** >90% survival at 10 years
- **Distant metastasis is uncommon; solid-basaloid pattern** more **likely to metastasize** and has a **poorer prognosis** than classic pattern
- IHC: Epithelial cells **(+)** for **MYB, LMWCK, EMA**, CEA, and **CD117**
- **Myoepithelial cells (+)** for p63, SMA, calponin, naspin, CK14, CK17
- **Prognostic markers: (-)** for ER, PR, and HER2 **(triple negative)**
- **Molecular: Translocation of t(6;9)(q22-23;p23-24)** resulting in a **MYB-NFIB fusion**
- Treatment is surgical with complete excision and negative margins

Path Presenter

 (Round nuclei / small nucleoli)

Round nuclei / small nucleoli

Secretory material
Path Presenter

SECRETORY CARCINOMA
MORPHOLOGY
- Malignant **epithelial cells with uniformly round nuclei** with **no significant pleomorphism, small nucleoli, vacuolated eosinophilic cytoplasm** containing **secretory material**
- Lumina contains **dense eosinophilic secretions**
- May be in a **solid, tubular,** or **microcystic** pattern

OTHER HIGH YIELD POINTS
- Special stains: **Secretory material is PASD positive**
- IHC: **(+)** for **GATA3, CEA, S100,** cytokeratins, e-cadherin, **C-kit, Pan-TRK,** p63, **SOX10, MUC4**
- **Prognostic markers: (-)** for ER, PR, and HER2 **(triple negative)**
- **Molecular: Balanced translocation of t(12;15)(p13;q25) → ETV6-NTRK3**
- FISH: Break apart probes for ETV6

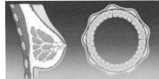

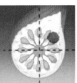
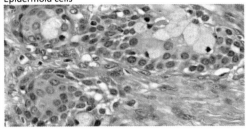

Mucinous cells   Intermediate cells

Epidermoid cells

MUCOEPIDERMOID CARCINOMA
MORPHOLOGY
- Malignant epithelial carcinoma that is **composed of mucinous cells, intermediate cells,** and **epidermoid (squamous) cells**
- The tumor cells are usually arranged in a **solid or cystic pattern**
- **Mucinous and intermediate cells** are most often **seen lining the cystic spaces or** within the **epidermoid areas**
- The background **stroma may be sclerotic** and there may be **foci of mucin**
- **High-grade** tumors often have **scattered mitosis, necrosis,** and **pleomorphism**

OTHER HIGH YIELD POINTS
- **Very rare** carcinoma of the breast and resembles salivary counterpart
- **Very good prognosis if low-grade**
- IHC: **(+)** for **HMWCK, p63, EMA**, CEA
- **Prognostic markers: (-)** for ER, PR, and HER2 **(triple negative)**
- **Molecular: MAML2 fusions;** MAML2 is located on **chromosome 11q**
  - Most common is **t(11;19)(q14-21;p12-13)** → **CRTS1(MECT1)-MAML2**
- FISH: Break apart probe for MAML2

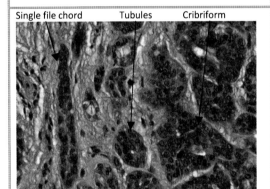

Single file chord   Tubules   Cribriform

POLYMORPHOUS ADENOCARCINOMA
MORPHOLOGY
- Monotonous **neoplastic cells** with **round to ovoid nuclei, vesicular chromatin,** and **eosinophilic cytoplasm**
- Tumor cells are **arranged in** a variety of patterns including **large nests, tubules, trabeculae, cribriform, alveolar,** or **single file chord patterns**
- **Mitosis are easily seen** and usually there is **no necrosis**

OTHER HIGH YIELD POINTS
- **Very rare** carcinoma of the breast
- IHC: **(+)** for **CK7 (weak), BCL2** (strong), **CK5/6, GFAP** (focal); **(-)** for EMA and CD117
- **Prognostic markers: (-)** for ER, PR, and HER2 **(triple negative)**

BRCA & SYNDROMIC-RELATED BREAST CANCERS

BREAST CANCER GENE 1 AND 2 (BRCA1, BRCA2)
- BRCA-genes are **tumor suppressors** involved in the **homologous recombination repair pathway**
- **Highest risk** is for breast and **ovarian cancer**
- Accounts for nearly **3.5% of all breast cancers;** more common in certain populations, like **Ashkenazi Jews**
- **Treatment:** patients may opt for **prophylactic bilateral mastectomy** and **salpingo-oophorectomy** before **40 years of age**
  - Must submit entire fallopian tube and ovary looking for **serous tubal intraepithelial carcinoma (STIC) lesions**
- Carcinomas can be **treated** with **poly-ADP ribose polymerase (PARP) inhibitors**
  - When a single stranded DNA break occurs, PARP binds to the DNA, then undergoes confirmational change and begins synthesis of polymeric adenosine diphosphate ribose, which acts as a signal for other repair enzymes
  - Addition of **PARP inhibitor in conjunction with BRCA mutations,** the **cancer cells cannot repair and DNA** strand breaks

Characteristic	BRCA1	BRCA2
Risk of breast cancer	40-90%	45-85%
Risk of ovarian /fallopian tube high grade serous carcinoma	40-50%	10-20%
Male breast cancer risk	Lower	Higher
Other cancer risk	Possibly pancreatic and colon	Pancreatic cancer, prostate cancer
Morphology	Circumscribed growth pattern with pushing borders, lymphocytic infiltrate, high-grade	Variable morphology and grade
Molecular cancer type	Basal-like(triple-negative)	Luminal A (ER/PR+; HER2-)

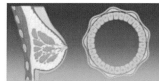

LI FRAUMENI SYNDROME 1 (TP53-ASSOCIATED)
- Inheritance pattern: **Autosomal dominant**
- Gene affected: **TP53** (prominent tumor suppressor gene)
- Defect causes early onset of a **broad spectrum of cancers**, of which the **most common is breast (>90% lifetime risk)** but also soft tissue sarcomas, osteosarcomas, brain (esp. choroid plexus carcinoma), adrenal cortical carcinoma, acute leukemia, melanoma, Wilms' tumor, gastroesophageal, colorectal, pancreas, and gonadal cancers

LI FRAUMENI SYNDROME 2 (TP53-UNASSOCIATED; CHK2-ASSOCIATED)
- **Heterozygous germline mutation with low to moderate penetrance**
- Gene affected: **CHEK2 (tumor suppressor gene)**
- Mutation: **CHEK2 1100delC**
- Risk of cancer: There is a **30% lifetime risk of breast cancer** and there is an **increased risk of** a variety of **other cancers**
- Normal gene function: **CHEK2 is activated by double strand DNA breaks** (upstream of TP53 and BRCA1)
  - ➢ **Mutations disrupt DNA repair** which allows for more errors and leads to carcinogenesis.

PEUTZ-JEGHERS SYNDROME
- Inheritance pattern: **Autosomal dominant**
- Gene affected: **STK11 (tumor suppressor gene)**
- Characteristic **hamartomatous polyps** in **>95% of patients** (often small bowel), **mucocutaneous melanin pigmentation**
- **Increased risk of many cancers** including **breast**, colon, stomach, pancreas, ovary (SCATs), etc.

CDH1-ASSOCIATED DIFFUSE GASTRIC AND LOBULAR BREAST CANCER SYNDROME
- Inheritance pattern: **Autosomal dominant**
- Gene affected: **CDH1 inactivating mutations** (cell adhesion and tumor suppression gene) on **chromosome 16q22**
- **Lifetime risk of cancer** in carrier individuals is **>80%**; **Nearly 60% of all female carriers develop lobular carcinoma** of the breast
- Cancers present as a characteristic **single file, discohesive, signet ring cells** and **pagetoid spread**
- **Cancers in the stomach are signet ring cell adenocarcinoma** and usually **affects the submucosa** and is **not seen endoscopically**
- **Somatic mutations in CDH1 are also seen** in individuals **with sporadic** lobular carcinoma and diffuse gastric cancer

ATAXIA-TELANGIECTASIA
- Inheritance pattern: **Autosomal recessive**
- Gene affected: **ATM gene** (tumor suppressor that phosphorylates p53 and BRCA1 when dsDNA breaks occur)
- **Carriers** (heterozygous: one normal and one mutant allele) **have an increased risk of breast cancer at a young age** but **do not have syndrome** because they maintain a normal copy of the gene
- Patients present with **progressive cerebellar ataxia, oculocutaneous telangiectasia, variable immunodeficiency**, sterility, and **recurrent sinopulmonary infections**
- **High risk of malignancy** and patients are very **sensitive to ionizing radiation** (including X-rays for medical purposes)

COWDEN SYNDROME (MULTIPLE HAMARTOMA SYNDROME)
- Inheritance pattern: **Autosomal dominant**
- Gene affected: **PTEN gene** (tumor suppressor gene)
- Affected patients usually have **macrocephaly, facial trichilemmomas, acral keratoses, papillomatous papules, lipomas,** esophageal **glycogen acanthosis**, multiple **stomach polyps resembling hyperplastic polyps**, colon polyps with cystically dilated glands, **colon with adipocytes in lamina propria** (unique), and **ganglioneuromatous polyps**
- Mutation **predisposes patients to breast cancer (highest risk), multiple hamartomas** (mouth, GI tract), **follicular thyroid carcinoma** (most often), and **endometrial cancer**
- Other PTEN syndromes include: **Bannayan-Riley-SMITH-Myhre-Ruvalcaba syndrome,** and **Lhermitte-Duclos disease**

PROGNOSTIC MARKER TESTING

ESTROGEN RECEPTOR (ER)
- **Step 1: Preanalytical quality control check and appropriateness of prognostic marker testing**
  - ➢ Is the **cold-ischemia time** (time from tissue removed to placement in fixative) documented?
    - ○ Cold ischemia time is **preferred to be less than 1 hour** as **prolongation results in antigen degradation**
  - ➢ **What fixative is used?** Do these meet the latest ASCO/CAP guidelines?
  - ➢ Is the **fixation time at least 6 hours or more?** Does it meet the latest ASCO/CAP guidelines?
  - ➢ Has the **tissue been altered** in any way that could **affect immunogenicity (decalcification)**?

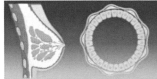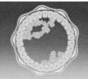

- o **ER is degraded in acidic fixatives**; such fixatives include Bouin's and B-5
- o **Buffered formalin** is the recommended and should have a **pH between 7.0 and 7.4**
- o **Prolonged fixation** can also **result in loss of immunogenicity**
- o Each lab should have their validated acceptable fixation time window
- ➤ **If the information is not available**, then a **statement regarding the absence of certain information** should be **added to report** and results should be **interpreted with caution**

- • Step 2: Analytical quality control check
  - ➤ Is the **sample adequate for testing** (sufficient tumor for testing)?
  - ➤ Are the **correct antibody clones** being used? Are they FDA approved or are they a laboratory developed test?
  - ➤ What is the **status of the internal control** (normal epithelial cells that are positive)?
    - o If there is no normal internal control, this should be mentioned in the report
  - ➤ What is the **status of the external control** (cancer cell lines that are positive, etc)?
    - o If this is negative, repeat staining (if enough tissue exists)
    - o If positive control failed, a negative result cannot be confirmed

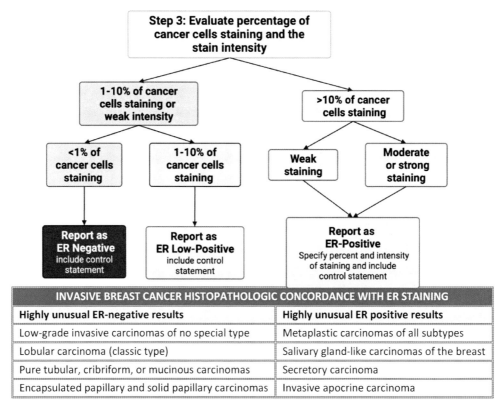

INVASIVE BREAST CANCER HISTOPATHOLOGIC CONCORDANCE WITH ER STAINING	
Highly unusual ER-negative results	**Highly unusual ER positive results**
Low-grade invasive carcinomas of no special type	Metaplastic carcinomas of all subtypes
Lobular carcinoma (classic type)	Salivary gland-like carcinomas of the breast
Pure tubular, cribriform, or mucinous carcinomas	Secretory carcinoma
Encapsulated papillary and solid papillary carcinomas	Invasive apocrine carcinoma

- • Step 4: Post-analytic control check prior to reporting results
  - ➤ If a **result** is considered **highly unusual/discordant**, **additional steps should be taken prior** to report sign-out
  - ➤ Perform a **review of the preanalytical** and **analytic testing factors**
  - ➤ Check the **accuracy of the histologic type and grade**, if matches, proceed to an **independent, second review**
  - ➤ Perform an **independent second review** (by another pathologist) and **repeating testing**
  - ➤ If all **results appear valid** on independent second review and repeat testing matches, the **result can be reported**
    - o Add a comment noting that the findings are highly unusual, and repeat testing was concordant, document second pathologist reviewed results, and add that testing of additional samples may be of value to confirm the findings

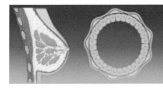 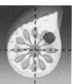
HUMAN EPIDERMAL GROWTH FACTOR RECEPTOR 2 (HER2)

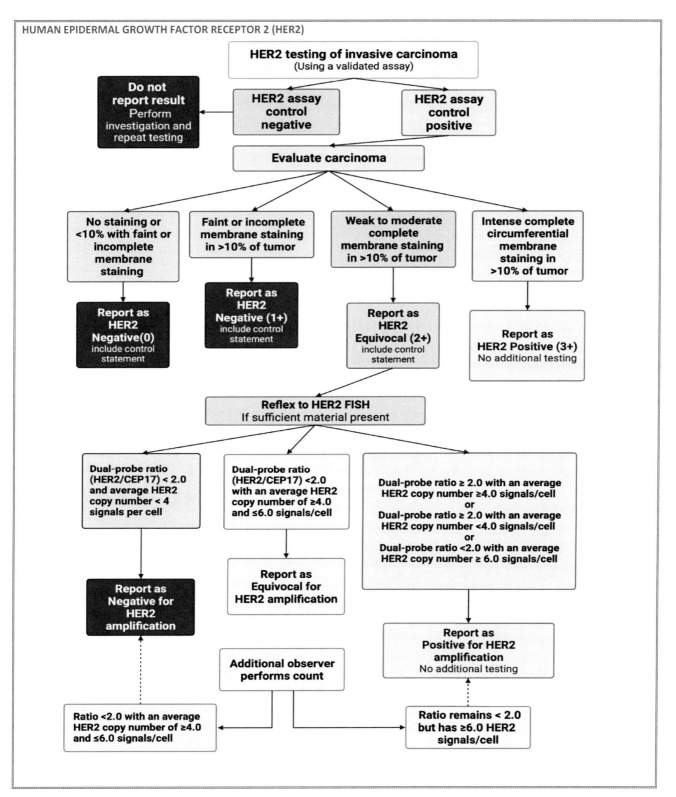

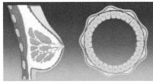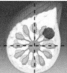

IMMUNOHISTOCHEMISTRY GRADING OF HER2 IN INVASIVE CARCINOMA OF THE BREAST				
Score	Interpretation	Staining pattern	Thickness	IHC Image
0	Negative	**No staining** is observed, **or membrane staining** is observed in **<10% of tumor** cells	Essentially **nothing**, like an eraser	
1+	Negative	A **faint/barely perceptible membrane staining** is detected **in >10% of tumor** cells; the cells exhibit incomplete membrane staining	Slight **pencil tracing**	
2+	Equivocal (order FISH)	A **weak to moderate complete, circumferential membrane staining** is observed in **>10% of tumor cells**	**Ballpoint** pen	
3+	Positive	A **strong complete membrane staining** is observed in **>10% of tumor** cells	**Sharpie** marker	

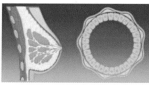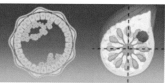
HER2 FLUORESCENCE IN SITU HYBRIDIZATION IN INVASIVE BREAST CANCER

Enumeration Probe Set
Utilizing Locus-Specific & Centromeric Probe for Chromosome 17

Normal Diploid	Monosomy	Deletion	Triploidy	Amplification

Chromosome Appearance	HER2/ CEP17 Ratio	HER2 signals per cell	FISH Appearance
Classic Amplified	≥ 2.0	≥ 6.0	
Classic Non-amplified	< 2.0	<4.0	
Equivocal	< 2.0	4.0-6.0	

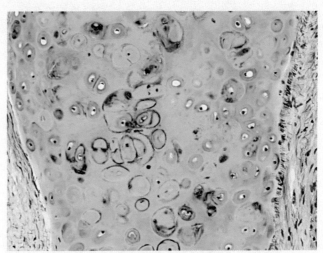

Movat Pentachrome stain in Bronchial cartilage.
Image courtesy: Sanjay Mukhopadhyay, MD

CHAPTER 3: PULMONARY PATHOLOGY

Jian Li, MD
Jared T. Ahrendsen, MD, PhD
Akanksha Gupta, MD

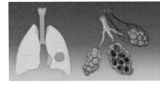
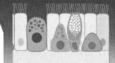
HISTOLOGIC FINDINGS OF IDIOPATHIC INTERSTITIAL PNEUMONIA						
	Nonspecific Interstitial Pneumonia (NSIP)	Usual Interstitial Pneumonia (UIP)	Desquamative Interstitial Pneumonia (DIP)	Acute Interstitial Pneumonia (AIP)	Lymphoid Interstitial Pneumonia (LIP)	Cryptogenic Organizing Pneumonia (COP)
Temporal appearance	Uniform	**Varied**	Uniform	Uniform	Uniform	Uniform
Interstitial inflammation	**Prominent**	Scant	Scant	Scant	**Prominent**	Scant
Interstitial collagen	Variable, diffuse	Patchy	Variable, diffuse	No	Some cases	No
Interstitial fibrosis	Rare, diffuse	No	No	**Yes, diffuse**	No	No
Organizing pneumonia pattern	Occasional, focal	Occasional, focal	No	Occasional, focal	No	**Prominent**
Fibroblastic foci	Occasional, focal	**Typical**	No	No	No	No
Honeycombing	Rare	**Typical**	No	No	Occasional	No
Intra-alveolar macrophages	Occasional, patchy	Occasional, focal	**Yes, diffuse**	No	Occasional, patchy	No
Hyaline membranes	No	No	No	**Yes**	No	No
Granulomas	No	No	No	No	No	No

DISEASES WITH BRONCHOGENIC GRANULOMAS	
Aspiration	Degenerating **food particles**; history of stroke, epilepsy, GERD, dementia, etc.
Sarcoidosis	Tightly formed, non-necrotizing granulomas; also, along pleura and septa
Infection	Positive cultures or special stains
Hypersensitivity Pneumonitis	**Peribronchiolar** inflammation, chronic bronchiolitis, peribronchiolar metaplasia ("Lambertosis"), relevant exposure history (birds, molds, occupational, etc.)
Allergic Bronchopulmonary Aspergillosis (ABPA)	Allergic mucin (Charcot-Leyden crystals and eosinophils), eosinophilic pneumonia, asthma/asthmatic airway changes, rare fungal elements
Granulomatosis with Polyangiitis	**Vasculitis**, capillaritis, diffuse alveolar hemorrhage, positive ANCA, relevant history/clinical findings
Middle Lobe Syndrome	Limited to the middle lobe
Rheumatoid Arthritis	Rheumatoid nodules, relevant clinical history (arthritis, +RF, etc.)

MEDICAL LUNG DISEASE - FIBROSIS

Distorted cystic spaces (honeycombing)

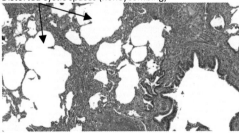

Fibroblastic focus

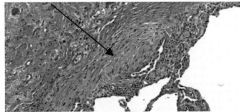

USUAL INTERSTITIAL PNEUMONIA(UIP)/IDIOPATHIC PULMONARY FIBROSIS
MORPHOLOGY
- **Temporally and spatially heterogeneous**: The disease is patchy, with some advanced areas and other early areas
- Minimal inflammation
- **Fibroblastic foci**: Immature fibroblastic areas
- **Honeycombing**: Architecturally distorted cystic spaces with respiratory epithelium and surrounding fibrosis
- Fibrosis is worst in **lower lobes** adjacent to pleura and septa (cannot diagnose on transbronchial biopsy)

OTHER HIGH YIELD POINTS
- **UIP is a histologic pattern**; it can be seen with connective tissue diseases, chronic hypersensitivity pneumonitis, drug reactions, or idiopathic
- Typical presentation: Older male with gradually increasing shortness of breath; eventually fatal

Path Presenter

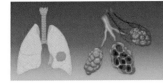
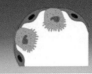
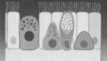
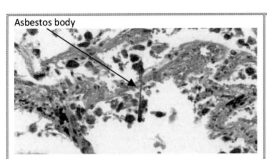
Asbestos body

ASBESTOSIS
MORPHOLOGY
- **Interstitial fibrosis** with minimal associated inflammation; fibroblastic foci absent
- **Asbestos bodies**: Dumbbell-shaped iron deposits
- **Pleural plaques** visible grossly

OTHER HIGH YIELD POINTS
- Caused by **inhalation of silicate mineral fibers** (not just asbestos)
- Often due to **occupational** exposure (miner, construction, shipyards, etc.)
- Increased risk of lung cancer and mesothelioma

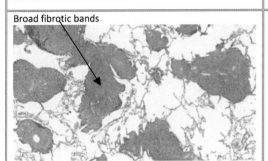
Giant cells

HARD METAL PNEUMOCONIOSIS
MORPHOLOGY
- **Giant cell interstitial pneumonia**
- Intra-alveolar **giant cells** and **fibrosis** with variable inflammation
- Frequent emperipolesis

OTHER HIGH YIELD POINTS
- Caused by **inhalation of hard metals**, usually **cobalt**
- Other metals: tungsten, titanium
- Occupational exposure: manufacturing, drilling, sawing

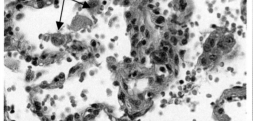
Broad fibrotic bands

Foamy macrophages

ERDHEIM-CHESTER DISEASE
MORPHOLOGY
- **Broad fibrotic bands** with intermixed foamy to pink **histiocytes**
- Scattered **touton-type giant cells**

OTHER HIGH YIELD POINTS
- **Multisystem histiocytosis** that can involve any organ (it frequently involves long bones)
- IHC: Macrophages stain **(+)** for CD68, Factor XIIIa; **(+/-)** S100
- Some show BRAF V600E gene mutations

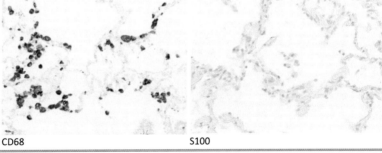
CD68   S100

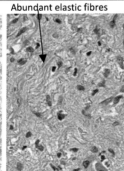
Subpleural fibrosis   Abundant elastic fibres

PLEUROPARENCHYMAL FIBROELASTOSIS
MORPHOLOGY
- **Upper lobe predominant subpleural fibrosis with abundant elastic fibers** (highlight with elastin stain), which are smaller and more lightly colored than collagen
- Minimal to no inflammation, granulomas, or fibroblastic foci

OTHER HIGH YIELD POINTS
- Rare, diffuse interstitial disease
- Idiopathic or associated with stem cell transplant, medications, exposure, etc.
- If localized apical mass lesion, consider "apical cap"

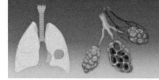
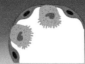
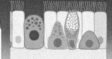
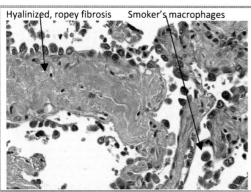

Hyalinized, ropey fibrosis   Smoker's macrophages

OTHER FIBROTIC DISEASES
- SMOKING-RELATED INTERSTITIAL FIBROSIS (SRIF)
  - **Hyalinized, ropey fibrosis**; respiratory bronchiolitis (smoker's macrophages); emphysema
- CHRONIC HYPERSENSITIVTY PNEUMONITIS
  - Cellular infiltrates, esp. near airways
  - Loosely formed, **non-necrotizing granulomas** and/or giant cells
- CHRONIC NONSPECIFIC INTERSTITIAL PNEUMONIA (NSIP)
  - NSIP (see below) with homogenous fibrosis

OTHER HIGH YIELD POINTS
- Many diseases can become fibrosis-predominant when more advanced, so look for clues to other etiologies

---

MEDICAL LUNG DISEASE - CELLULAR INTERSTITIAL INFILTRATES

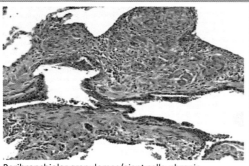

Peribronchiolar granulomas/giant cells, chronic inflammation, fibrosis

HYPERSENSITIVITY PNEUMONITIS (HP)

MORPHOLOGY
- **Airway-centric inflammation** with **peribronchiolar** granulomas/giant cells, peribronchiolar interstitial chronic inflammation, and chronic bronchiolitis
- Can see peribronchiolar metaplasia, organizing pneumonia, cholesterol clefts, fibrosis (chronic HP)

OTHER HIGH YIELD POINTS
- Due to **inhalation of small organic or chemical antigens** that stimulate an immune response
- Common antigens: Birds ("Pigeon fancier's lung"), molds ("Farmer's lung"), wood dust, certain industrial chemicals
- Often delayed diagnosis and insidious onset of dyspnea

Homogeneous thickening of alveolar septa

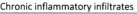

Chronic inflammatory infiltrates

NONSPECIFIC INTERSTITIAL PNEUMONIA (NSIP)

MORPHOLOGY
- A pattern of inflammation with **homogeneous, diffuse thickening** of alveolar septa by **chronic inflammatory infiltrates**
- Can see associated homogenous **fibrosis** (chronic NSIP)

OTHER HIGH YIELD POINTS
- Most commonly due to connective tissue disease (**prominent lymphoid follicles** ± geminal centers, pleuritis)
- It can also be idiopathic, medication-related, hypersensitivity pneumonitis
- Better prognosis than UIP/IPF

Path Presenter

Dense interstitial lymphoplasmacytic infiltrate

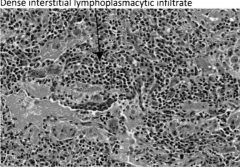

LYMPHOID INTERSTITIAL PNEUMONIA (LIP)

MORPHOLOGY
- Diffuse, dense, interstitial **lymphoplasmacytic infiltrate**
- Predominantly polymorphous **T lymphocytes**

OTHER HIGH YIELD POINTS
- Rare, idiopathic
- Must exclude other conditions, including lymphoma (esp. MALT lymphoma), autoimmune disease, HIV/AIDS, immunodeficient state (e.g., CVID)
- If numerous large lymphoid follicles surrounding airways, consider "follicular bronchiolitis"

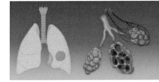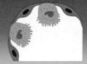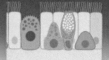
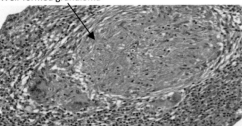
Well-formed granuloma

HOT TUB LUNG
MORPHOLOGY
- **Peribronchiolar chronic inflammation**: similar to hypersensitivity pneumonitis
- Prominent & well-formed **granulomas** (could be necrotizing)

OTHER HIGH YIELD POINTS
- Hypersensitivity pneumonia-like reaction to **mycobacterium avium complex**, which is common in water (esp. indoor hot tubs, saunas, swimming pools)

MEDICAL LUNG DISEASE - ALVEOLAR FILLING PATTERN

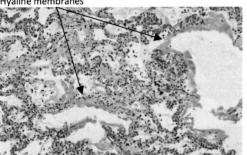
Hyaline membranes

DIFFUSE ALVEOLAR DAMAGE (DAD)
MORPHOLOGY
- **Hyaline membranes**: Due to endothelial/epithelial injury causing leakage of serum proteins
- May also show necrosis and acute inflammation (esp. with infection)

OTHER HIGH YIELD POINTS
- Histologic manifestation of **acute respiratory distress syndrome (ARDS)**: Bilateral diffuse pulmonary infiltrates, often requiring ventilation
- Can be seen in a variety of settings (**common pathologic endpoint),** including infection, sepsis, drug reactions, toxins, and shock
- If idiopathic → "Acute Interstitial Pneumonia" (AIP)

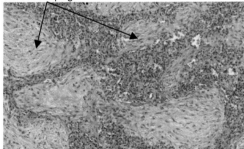
Fibroblastic plugs

ORGANIZING PNEUMONIA
MORPHOLOGY
- Accumulation of **immature myxoid material** and fibroblasts within airspaces
- May show **fibroblastic plugs**/polyps (Masson bodies) in airspaces
- Intact alveolar septa

OTHER HIGH YIELD POINTS
- Nonspecific pattern of lung injury/repair
- Can be seen after infection, injury, aspiration, connective tissue disease
- Often resolves after removing inciting agent
- If idiopathic → "Cryptogenic Organizing Pneumonia" (COP)

EOSINOPHILIC PNEUMONIA
MORPHOLOGY
- **Acute: diffuse alveolar damage** with the addition of **eosinophil-rich inflammation**; peripheral eosinophilia; eosinophils on bronchoalveolar lavage
- **Chronic:** intra-alveolar collections of eosinophils, macrophages, and edema

OTHER HIGH YIELD POINTS
- **Acute** eosinophilic pneumonia presents with fever and dyspnea of <1 month duration
  ➢ DDX: Infection (parasites), medications, cigarettes, pneumothorax, idiopathic
- **Chronic** eosinophilic pneumonia presents with insidious onset; relapsing; responds to steroids
  ➢ DDX: When idiopathic, often associated with asthma, medications, allergies

Path Presenter

Eosinophils

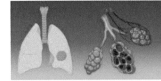 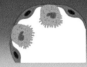 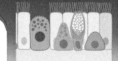

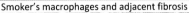

Smoker's macrophages and adjacent fibrosis

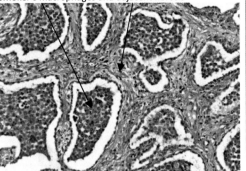

DESQUAMATIVE INTERSTITIAL PNEUMONIA (DIP) / RESPIRATORY BRONCHIOLITIS INTERSTITIAL LUNG DISEASE (RB-ILD)
MORPHOLOGY
- DIP: **Filling of alveoli by pigmented macrophages**, often associated with fibrosis and mild chronic inflammation, homogeneous involvement
- RB-ILD: **Pigmented "smoker's" macrophages** in respiratory bronchioles and adjacent alveoli (not homogeneous like DIP)

OTHER HIGH YIELD POINTS
- Need clinical symptoms/findings to label RB-ILD as **ILD**
- Spectrum of disease highly associated with **smoking**

Path Presenter

Hemosiderin-laden macrophages and hemorrhage

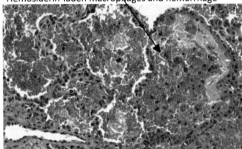

ALVEOLAR HEMORRHAGE
MORPHOLOGY
- **Hemosiderin-laden macrophages** and **fresh blood** in alveoli

OTHER HIGH YIELD POINTS
- Can be **secondary** to trauma, cardiac disease, vascular disease, medications
- **Diffuse alveolar hemorrhage** is often a result of vasculitis/capillaritis
- **Anti-GBM disease (Goodpasture syndrome)**: Autoantibodies to collagen IV in basement membrane; impacts capillaries in kidneys (crescentic glomerulonephritis) and lungs (hemorrhage)

Lipid-rich material in alveolar spaces

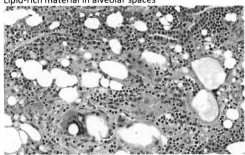

LIPOID PNEUMONIA
MORPHOLOGY
- **Lipid-rich material** and **inflammatory cells** filling alveolar spaces

OTHER HIGH YIELD POINTS
- **Endogenous/post-obstructive**: Proximal airway obstruction with an inability to clear secretions causes accumulation of **finely vacuolated macrophages** in distal airways
- **Exogenous/aspiration**: Aspiration of lipid-rich material (mineral oil) with accumulation of multinucleated giant cells containing **large lipid vacuoles**

Eosinophilic proteinaceous material in the alveoli

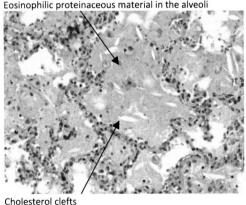

Cholesterol clefts

ALVEOLAR PROTEINOSIS
MORPHOLOGY
- Filling of alveoli by **amorphous eosinophilic, PASD(+) proteinaceous material**
- Occasional crystals and cholesterol **clefts**
- Resembles proteinaceous edema fluid (PAS-negative)

OTHER HIGH YIELD POINTS
- **"Crazy paving"** appearance on CT
- Three forms:
  - **Congenital**: Mutations of genes encoding surfactant or GM-CSF
  - **Primary**: Autoantibodies against GM-CSF causing abnormal macrophage function and accumulation of proteinaceous material
  - **Secondary**: Stem cell transplantation, solid organ transplantation
- Key histologic DDX: Pneumocystis pneumonia (**get fungal stains**, esp. if immunocompromised)

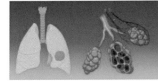

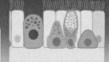

Microliths of calcium phosphate within alveoli

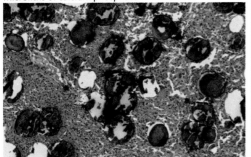

ALVEOLAR MICROLITHIASIS

MORPHOLOGY

- Lamellated **microliths of calcium phosphate** within alveoli

OTHER HIGH YIELD POINTS

- AR mutations in **SLC34A2** with dysfunctional sodium phosphate transport
- Middle-aged adults, respiratory failure, indolent with slow progression
- **"Sandstorm"** appearance on radiology
- DDX: Corpora amylacea, dystrophic calcification, ossification

PULMONARY NODULES

Degenerating food particles

ASPIRATION

MORPHOLOGY

- **Airway-centered** inflammation with **giant cells** and organizing pneumonia
- Degenerating food particles may be **polarizable** (esp. some pill particles)
- Can also see lipoid pneumonia or abscess formation

OTHER HIGH YIELD POINTS

- Due to **aspiration of food particles**; can be single or multiple
- **Risk factors**: stroke, GERD, obesity, epilepsy, alcohol, dementia

Path presenter

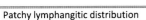
Patchy lymphangitic distribution

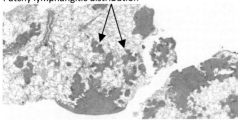

Non-necrotizing granuloma

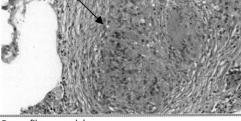

SARCOIDOSIS

MORPHOLOGY

- Tightly formed, **non-necrotizing granulomas** with giant cells
- Granulomas eventually become confluent and mass-like
- Follows **lymphangitic distribution** (not in airspaces)
- No organizing pneumonia or interstitial inflammation
- Extensive fibrosis favors infectious etiology

OTHER HIGH YIELD POINTS

- **Systemic idiopathic granulomatous disease** with frequent pulmonary involvement, diagnosis requires clinical correlation
- **Starts centrally in lung** with large airways and hilar lymphadenopathy and extends outward with **progressive fibrosis**
- Giant cells can produce some endogenous polarizable material (calcium oxalate) – do not mistake as foreign material

Path presenter

Dense fibrous nodules

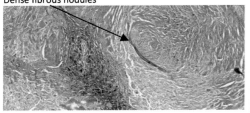

SILICOSIS

MORPHOLOGY

- Inhaled silica **engulfed by macrophages (birefringent** if polarized)
- **Form aggregates** that increasingly fibrose and hyalinize and eventually **coalesce into nodules**

OTHER HIGH YIELD POINTS

- Caused by **inhalation of silica** and related minerals
- Risk factors: Construction, manufacturing, mining

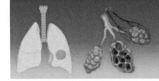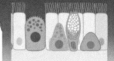

3. PULMONARY PATHOLOGY

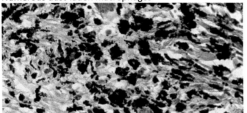
Numerous dust-laden macrophages

COAL WORKER PNEUMOCONIOSIS
MORPHOLOGY
- Numerous **dust-laden macrophages** around bronchovascular bundles
- **Haphazard fibrosis** and emphysema; can progress to large nodules with fibrosis
OTHER HIGH YIELD POINTS
- Caused by **exposure** to coal dust – **"Black Lung Disease"**
- Common to see **concurrent silica/silicosis**

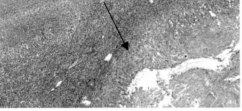
Necrotizing granulomatous inflammation

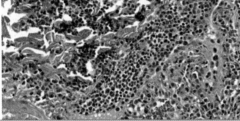
Eosinophilic granulomatosis with polyangiitis

VASCULITIS
MORPHOLOGY
- **Granulomatosis with polyangiitis (Wegener's)**
  ➢ **Necrotizing granulomatous inflammation**
  ➢ Commonly impacts lung, nasal cavity, and kidney
  ➢ **Lung:** granulomas, with geographic **central cavitating nodules**
  ➢ **Kidney:** crescentic glomerulonephritis
  ➢ **PR3-ANCA positive**
- **Eosinophilic granulomatosis with polyangiitis (Churg-Strauss)**
  ➢ **Eosinophil-rich** and necrotizing granulomatous inflammation
  ➢ Often impacts the lung; associated with asthma and eosinophilia
  ➢ **MPO-ANCA positive**
OTHER HIGH YIELD POINTS
- Dx often involves **clinical/serologic correlation**
Path Presenter

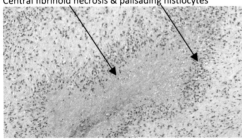
Central fibrinoid necrosis & palisading histiocytes

RHEUMATOID NODULE
MORPHOLOGY
- **Granulomatous nodules** with **central fibrinoid necrosis**
- **Palisading histiocytes** with lymphoplasmacytic inflammation
OTHER HIGH YIELD POINTS
- **Most specific** pulmonary finding for rheumatoid arthritis is above histology
- DDX: Granulomatosis with polyangiitis, infection
Path Presenter

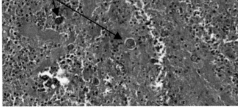
Coccidioidomycosis

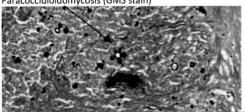
Paracoccidioidomycosis (GMS stain)

FUNGAL INFECTIONS
- Often diagnosed based on imaging and lab studies
- May be focal or diffuse (particularly if immunocompromised)
- Often cause **granulomatous response** (± necrosis)
REGARDLESS OF IMMUNE STATUS
- **Coccidioidomycosis**
  ➢ Southwestern United States in dry soil (Valley fever)
  ➢ Spherules with endospores
- **Paracoccidioidomycosis**
  ➢ South and Central America
  ➢ Fungal forms with **radial pattern**
- **Histoplasmosis**
  ➢ Mississippi/Ohio River valley in soil and caves (bat droppings)
  ➢ **Small, narrow-based buds**
  ➢ Common to have subclinical infection with burnt out hyalinized granulomas

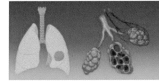
 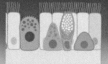
Histoplasmosis

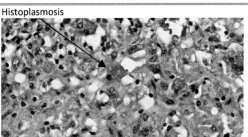

Blastomycosis

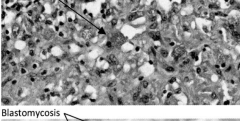

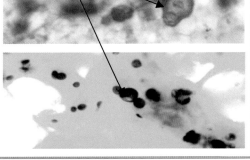

- **Blastomycosis**
  - ➢ Mississippi/Ohio River valley and Northeast in soil
  - ➢ **Broad-based buds** with round, uniform, thick double wall

IMMUNOCOMPROMISED

- **Pneumocystis pneumonia**
  - ➢ Ubiquitous; immunocompromised hosts
  - ➢ Crushed **ping pong balls** with a central dot in foamy alveolar exudate
- **Cryptococcosis**
  - ➢ Ubiquitous in soil and bird dropping
  - ➢ Round, **thick halo**; variable size; narrow budding
- **Aspergillosis**
  - ➢ Ubiquitous in soil
  - ➢ Septa hyphae with **45-degree** branching
  - ➢ Can colonize and form an aspergilloma ("fungus ball"); angioinvasive
- **Candidiasis**
  - ➢ Ubiquitous in skin (can be oral contaminant in BAL)
  - ➢ Budding yeast and pseudohyphae
- **Mucormycosis**
  - ➢ Ubiquitous; classically in poorly controlled diabetics
  - ➢ Broad ribbon-like hyphae with irregular branching

Pneumocystis jirovecii IHC

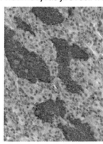

Path
Presenter

Caseating granuloma of TB

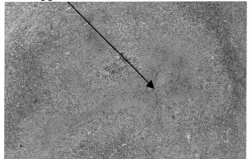

BACTERIAL INFECTIONS

Mycobacterium tuberculosis:

- Necrotizing/caseating granulomas and fibrosis (low threshold for AFB stain)
- Worldwide, many are asymptomatically infected leaving behind calcified nodules/nodes (Gohn complex), which can reactivate to cavitating infection

Nocardiosis:

- Gram-positive filamentous bacteria in immunocompromised
- Highlighted by both AFB and GMS as slender tangled strings

Path
Presenter

Actinomycosis

- Gram-positive filamentous bacteria (commensal in the oral cavity)
- Can cause abscesses with distinctive "**sulfur granules**"

Acellular hyalinized collagen

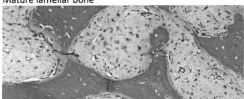

PULMONARY HYALINIZING GRANULOMA

MORPHOLOGY

- Single or multiple **slow-growing** nodules
- **Well-circumscribed**, acellular hyalinized collagen
- Scattered foci of chronic inflammation

OTHER HIGH YIELD POINTS

- The pulmonary counterpart to fibrosing mediastinitis
- Often considered an **exaggerated response to a remote infection**, most often **histoplasmosis**
- Can also be associated with **IgG4-related disease**

Mature lamellar bone

METAPLASTIC OSSIFICATION

MORPHOLOGY

- Nodule(s) of **mature lamellar bone**

OTHER HIGH YIELD POINTS

- Often incidental finding
- Often formed in response to injury, such as scar, aspiration, granulomas, apical caps, etc.

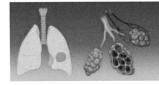

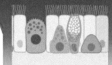
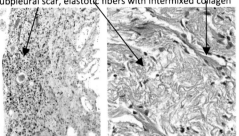

Subpleural scar, elastotic fibers with intermixed collagen

APICAL CAP
MORPHOLOGY
- **Subpleural** fibroelastotic scars
- Predominantly **elastotic fibers** with **intermixed collagen**
- Triangular-shaped with a broad pleural base
OTHER HIGH YIELD POINTS
- Seen most commonly in the apices of the upper lobes
- Unclear etiology; can radiographically mimic malignancy
- If diffuse, pleuroparenchymal fibroelastosis

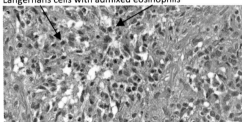

Langerhans cells with admixed eosinophils

PULMONARY LANGERHANS CELL HISTIOCYTOSIS
MORPHOLOGY
- **Eosinophils with numerous Langerhans** cells: amphophilic cytoplasm and **nuclear grooves ("coffee beans")**; IHC (+) S100, langerin (CD207), CD1a
OTHER HIGH YIELD POINTS
- Aka "eosinophilic granuloma"; strongly associated with **smoking**
- Considered a **reactive proliferation** (extrapulmonary LCH is neoplastic)
- Often presents as a cystic disease
- Electron microscopy shows Birbeck granules (tennis racket shaped)

MEDICAL LUNG DISEASE - NEAR NORMAL APPEARANCE

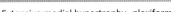

EMPHYSEMA
MORPHOLOGY
- **Airspace enlargement** due to alveolar septal destruction without significant fibrosis (common background/incidental finding)
OTHER HIGH YIELD POINTS
- Often classified by location:
  - **Centrilobular**: Destruction near small airways; associated with **smoking**, upper lobe predominant; emphysema + chronic bronchitis = COPD
  - **Panacinar**: Involves entire lobule from beginning; classically associated with **α1-antitrypsin deficiency**; lower-lobe predominant; risk of liver disease

Airspace enlargement

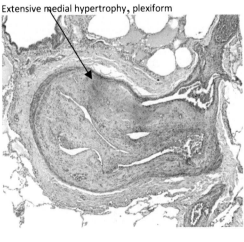

Extensive medial hypertrophy, plexiform

PULMONARY HYPERTENSION
MORPHOLOGY
- **Medial hypertrophy** of arteries and veins
- **Intimal proliferation and fibrosis**
- Plexiform lesions, fibrous webs/plugs (colander-like), emboli/thrombi
OTHER HIGH YIELD POINTS
- Usually in young females, presenting as an exercise intolerance
- **Clinical diagnosis**. Pathologic findings may not correlate with symptoms
- Increased pulmonary vascular pressure
- Common causes: heart failure, lung disease (e.g., UIP)
- Can be primary or idiopathic
- Note: recanalized thrombi (from a PE) are also plexiform
- Inactivating mutation of BMPR2 gene

Path Presenter

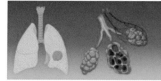 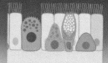
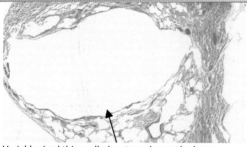
Variably sized thin-walled cysts underneath pleura

BIRT-HOGG-DUBE SYNDROME
MORPHOLOGY
- **Variably sized thin-walled cysts** underneath pleura near septa or lower lobes
OTHER HIGH YIELD POINTS
- **Multi-organ manifestations:**
  ➤ Skin: Fibrofolliculomas
  ➤ Kidney: Hybrid oncocytic neoplasms
  ➤ Lung: Cysts → Can rupture to cause pneumothorax
- **Autosomal dominant,** mutations in **folliculin gene (FLCN)**

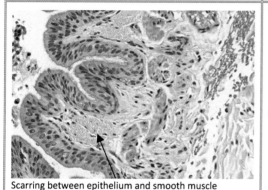
Scarring between epithelium and smooth muscle

CONSTRICTIVE (OBLITERATIVE) BRONCHIOLITIS
MORPHOLOGY
- **Fibroinflammatory scarring** of bronchioles between epithelium and smooth muscle
- Can eventually **obliterate bronchiole lumen**
- **Elastin** stain highlights elastic layer of obliterated airway (usually with a remaining paired artery)
OTHER HIGH YIELD POINTS
- **Obliterative bronchiolitis** is a term primarily used in the transplant setting
- Possible causes: Infection, fumes/toxins, medications, connective tissue disease (especially rheumatoid arthritis)

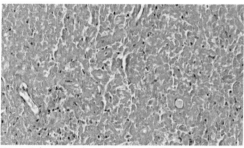
Waxy pink protein deposition (amyloid)

AMYLOIDOSIS
MORPHOLOGY
- **Waxy pink protein** deposition (**"apple green" birefringence** with Congo red)
OTHER HIGH YIELD POINTS
- Can be **localized or systemic**
- Localized pulmonary amyloidosis can be **nodular or diffuse**

Path Presenter

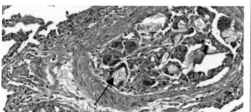
Foreign material embolism

FOREIGN MATERIAL EMBOLI
- **Intravenous drug use** associated with **microcrystalline cellulose emboli** (refractile under polarized light)
- Can also see bone marrow/fat emboli from bone fractures (especially after CPR)
Path Presenter

Intimal fibrosis of pulmonary venules
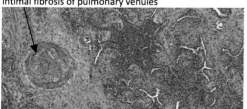

PULMONARY VENO-OCCLUSIVE DISEASE (PVOD)
MORPHOLOGY
- Pulmonary venules with **intimal fibrosis** & diffuse smooth muscle narrowing
- **Post-capillary proliferation** with interstitial and alveolar hemosiderin-laden macrophages
OTHER HIGH YIELD POINTS
- Rare cause of pulmonary hypertension
- Diagnosis confirmed by lung biopsy

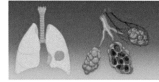
 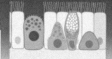
Cytomegalic cells with basophilic nuclear inclusion

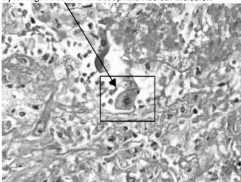

CMV PNEUMONITIS
MORPHOLOGY

- Infected cells are **large with prominent basophilic nuclear inclusion** (highlight with PAS and GMS), often with a clear halo
- Smaller basophilic cytoplasmic inclusions are also present
- Chronic inflammation, edema, pneumocyte hyperplasia, hemorrhagic necrosis
- In the lung, CMV usually infects **endothelial cells and alveolar histocytes**

OTHER HIGH YIELD POINTS

- IHC staining for CMV is confirmatory

Path Presenter

Dirofilaria organism

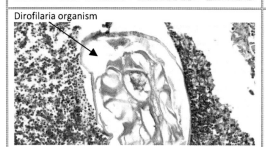

DIROFILARIA (CANINE HEARTWORM)
MORPHOLOGY

- Roundworm infection with longitudinal ridges on the cuticle

OTHER HIGH YIELD POINTS

- Blood-born parasite, can see worm moving across the **cornea in the eye**
- Serious and possibly fatal infection

Path Presenter

MEDICAL LUNG DISEASE – TRANSPLANT

Perivascular and interstitial lymphocytes

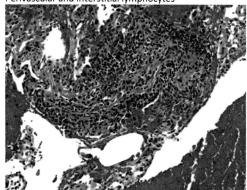

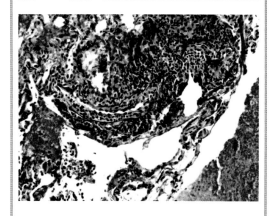

ACUTE CELLULAR REJECTION

Grading: Acute Transplant Rejection	
Alveolar Rejection	
Ax (**Ungradable**)	Inadequate sampling
A0 (**None**)	Normal pulmonary parenchyma without evidence of mononuclear cell infiltration, hemorrhage, or necrosis
A1 (**Minimal**)	Scattered, infrequent perivascular mononuclear infiltrates (particularly around venules), **< 3 cells thick**
A2 (**Mild**)	Conspicuous perivascular inflammation, **> 3 cells thick**
A3 (**Moderate**)	Conspicuous perivascular inflammation, with extension into **alveolar septa**
A4 (**Severe**)	Conspicuous perivascular inflammation, with features of **acute lung injury**
Bronchiolar Rejection	
Bx (**Ungradable**)	Inadequate sampling
B0 (**None**)	No significant airway inflammation
B1R (**Low-grade**)	**Submucosal** chronic inflammation, without significant intraepithelial inflammation or injury
B2R (**High-grade**)	Submucosal chronic inflammation with intraepithelial lymphocytes, epithelial injury, ± neutrophils, ulceration, and/or necrosis

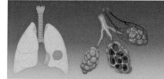
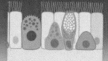
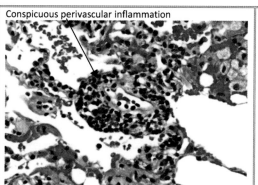
Conspicuous perivascular inflammation

MORPHOLOGY
- Based on the presence of **perivascular and interstitial T cell-rich infiltrates**
- Can also see **lymphocytic bronchiolitis** with a band-like T cell-rich chronic inflammatory infiltrate in the submucosa of bronchioles (which have no cartilage in the walls) (vs. BALT, which is well-circumscribed and B cell rich)

OTHER HIGH YIELD POINTS
- For adequate sensitivity, sampling should include **five fragments** of expanded, alveolated lung and multiple tissue levels
- Surveillance biopsies are often performed to look for rejection at regular post-transplant intervals (6, 9, 12 months)
- Perivascular/interstitial and bronchial chronic inflammation is **not specific** for rejection: Infection and PTLD can look similar, so consider other options, especially if there are many neutrophils or plasma cells

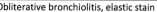
Obliterative bronchiolitis, elastic stain

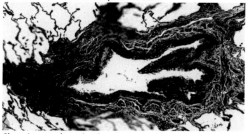
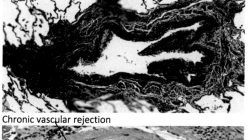

CHRONIC REJECTION
MORPHOLOGY
- **Obliterative bronchiolitis**: Progressive airway lumen obliteration by inflammation and fibrosis
- Elastic stain can be used to highlight obliterated bronchioles (synonymous with constrictive bronchiolitis in nontransplant setting)
- **Chronic vascular rejection**: Myointimal thickening and fibrosis within arteries and veins (not often seen in biopsies)

OTHER HIGH YIELD POINTS
- Hard to see on surveillance biopsies; often, a **clinical diagnosis** with reduced FEV1

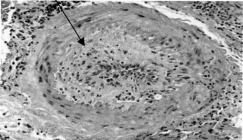
Chronic vascular rejection

GRADING: CHRONIC TRANSPLANT REJECTION	
OBLITERATIVE BRONCHIOLITIS	
C0	Absent
C1	Present
CHRONIC VASCULAR REJECTION	
D1	Absent
D0	Present

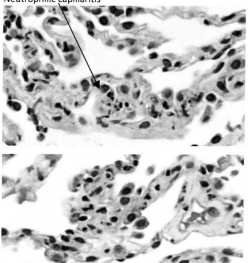
Neutrophilic capillaritis

ANTIBODY-MEDIATED REJECTION
MORPHOLOGY
- **Neutrophilic capillaritis** and neutrophilic septal margination

OTHER HIGH YIELD POINTS
- Less well-defined than in other organs
- **Requires:** Clinical dysfunction, positive circulating donor-specific antibodies (DSA), and C4d immunoreactivity
- **IHC/IF: C4d** strong, linear/donut pattern in septal capillaries

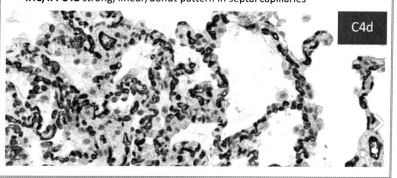
C4d

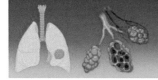 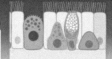

3. PULMONARY PATHOLOGY

EPITHELIAL PRECANCEROUS LESIONS AND CARCINOMAS	
Growth along airways (lepidic growth) 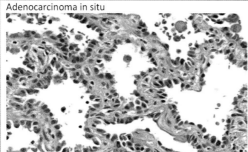	**ATYPICAL ADENOMATOUS HYPERPLASIA** MORPHOLOGY • ≤ **0.5 cm**, purely **lepidic** growth • A **localized** proliferation of mildly to moderately atypical type II pneumocytes OTHER HIGH YIELD POINTS • Often **peripheral** • Benign; cured with complete resection
Adenocarcinoma in situ 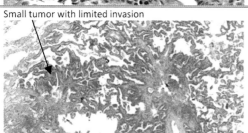	**ADENOCARCINOMA IN SITU (FORMER BRONCHOALVEOLAR CARCINOMA)** MORPHOLOGY • ≤ **3 cm**, **solitary**, localized with pure **lepidic** growth • No stromal, vascular, or pleural invasion; no spread through airspaces • **Septal widening/sclerosis** is common, mild to moderate nuclear atypia OTHER HIGH YIELD POINTS • Mostly **non-mucinous** • IHC: **(+)** CK7, TTF-1 and Napsin-A • Benign; **100% survival** if completely resected • Formerly "bronchoalveolar carcinoma" (BAC)
Small tumor with limited invasion 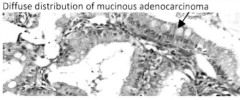	**MINIMALLY INVASIVE ADENOCARCINOMA (MIA)** MORPHOLOGY • Small tumor (≤ **3 cm**) • **Solitary**, predominantly **lepidic** growth, usually **non-mucinous** • **Invasive component ≤ 0.5 cm** in greatest dimension OTHER HIGH YIELD POINTS • By definition, the absence of lymphovascular invasion, pleural invasion, spread through air spaces, tumor necrosis • **100% survival** if completely resected
Diffuse distribution of mucinous adenocarcinoma 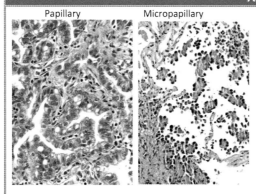 Image credits: Charles Leduc, MD	**PNEUMONIC-TYPE ADENOCARCINOMA** MORPHOLOGY • Tumors should be considered "pneumonic adenocarcinoma" if there is **diffuse distribution** as opposed to a well-defined lesion of the lung • Usually **mucinous** but can be non-mucinous • Usually, **lepidic predominant,** but there can be other patterns

ADENOCARCINOMA & VARIANTS	
Papillary Micropapillary	**ADENOCARCINOMA** MORPHOLOGY • Malignant epithelial tumor with glandular differentiation, mucin production, or pneumocyte marker expression • **Criteria for invasion**: Histologic subtype other than lepidic, desmoplastic stroma associated with tumor, vascular or pleural invasion, spread through air spaces (STAS)

Histologic patterns	
Lepidic	Tumor growth along the surface of alveolar walls (non-invasive)
Acinar	Round to oval glands with a central lumen space surrounded by tumor cells

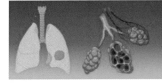

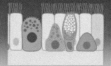

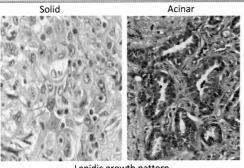

Solid | Acinar

Lepidic growth pattern

Papillary	Glands growing along central fibrovascular cores
Micropapillary	Cells growing in papillary tufts forming florets that lack fibrovascular cores (poorer prognosis)
Solid	Polygonal tumor cells growing in sheets (poorer prognosis)

OTHER HIGH YIELD POINTS
- Lung cancer is the **most common** cause of cancer-related death worldwide
- Strong association with tobacco **smoking**
- Other risk factors: Radon, air pollution, occupational exposure
- Symptoms vary, and most patients present late with advanced or metastatic disease
- CT often shows **peripherally located mass** with solid (invasive) areas of ground-glass (lepidic) areas
- **IHC: (+) TTF-1, Napsin-A, CK7**

Link   Link   Link   Link

TTF-1/Napsin	p63	p40	CK5/6	Resection Dx	Biopsy Dx
+	-	-	-	Adenocarcinoma	NSCLC favor adenocarcinoma
+	+	-	-	Adenocarcinoma	NSCLC favor adenocarcinoma
+	+	+ (focal)	-	Adenocarcinoma	NSCLC favor adenocarcinoma
+	-	-	+ (focal)	Adenocarcinoma	NSCLC favor adenocarcinoma
-	Any one of the above diffusely positive			Squamous cell carcinoma	NSCLC favor SCC
-	Any one of the above focally positive			Large cell carcinoma	NSCLC, NOS
-	-	-	-	Large cell carcinoma	NSCLC, NOS

Note: Some primary lung adenocarcinomas, including mucinous adenocarcinoma, colloid carcinoma, and enteric adenocarcinoma, can be TTF-1 negative. They can even stain with CK20 and CDX2. These cases require clinical correlation to exclude a metastasis from the GI tract.

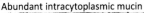
Abundant intracytoplasmic mucin
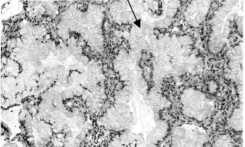

INVASIVE MUCINOUS ADENOCARCINOMA
MORPHOLOGY
- Adenocarcinoma with **abundant intracytoplasmic mucin**
OTHER HIGH YIELD POINTS
- Any growth pattern may be seen
- **KRAS mutation**
- IHC: **(+) CK7, CK20; (-) TTF-1**
- Must exclude mucinous metastasis from a non-pulmonary primary
Path Presenter

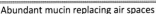
Abundant mucin replacing air spaces
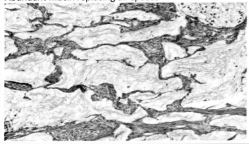

COLLOID ADENOCARCINOMA
MORPHOLOGY
- Adenocarcinoma, where **pools of mucin** replace air spaces
- Mucin **distends alveolar spaces** and destroys walls
- Tumor cells often do not entirely line the alveoli
OTHER HIGH YIELD POINTS
- IHC: **(+) CDX2, CK20; (+/-) TTF-1, CK7, Napsin-A**
Path Presenter

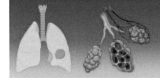 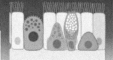
Tall columnar cells	**ENTERIC ADENOCARCINOMA**
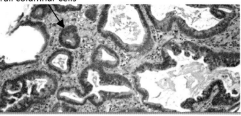	MORPHOLOGY • Adenocarcinoma **resembling colorectal-type** adenocarcinoma • Tall columnar cells with **pseudostratified** nuclei and abundant **"dirty" necrosis** OTHER HIGH YIELD POINTS • Requires careful clinical evaluation to **exclude metastasis** • Morphology and IHC identical to colorectal carcinoma
Complex glandular structures	**FETAL ADENOCARCINOMA**
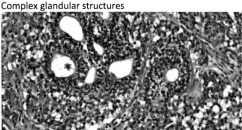	MORPHOLOGY • **Complex glandular structures** composed of glycogen-rich, non-ciliated cells (resembling the developing epithelium of the fetal lung) • Frequent **morule** formation • Variable atypia OTHER HIGH YIELD POINTS • IHC: **(+)** TTF-1; frequent **nuclear b-catenin**, neuroendocrine and germ cell marker expression

SQUAMOUS LESIONS

Squamous papillary proliferation	**SQUAMOUS PAPILLOMA**
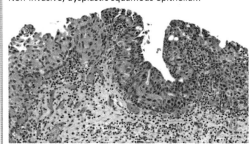	MORPHOLOGY • **Papillary fronds** covered by squamous epithelium OTHER HIGH YIELD POINTS • **HPV(+)** in the majority of laryngotracheal papillomatosis • Often presents with obstruction or hemoptysis • Rare malignant transformation Path Presenter
Non-invasive, dysplastic squamous epithelium	**SQUAMOUS CELL CARCINOMA IN SITU**
	MORPHOLOGY • Squamous dysplasia precursor lesion arising from the bronchial tree • Part of a continuum with sequential molecular abnormalities OTHER HIGH YIELD POINTS • Respiratory epithelium → **irritant/carcinogen** → hyperplasia → squamous metaplasia → squamous dysplasia → SCC in situ → invasive SCC PP Link PP Link
Well-differentiated SCC with keratinization	**SQUAMOUS CELL CARCINOMA**
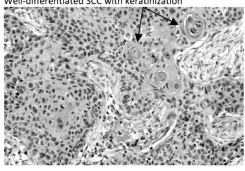	MORPHOLOGY • **Keratinization**, **intercellular bridges**, or expression of squamous differentiation by IHC • Can be non-keratinizing OTHER HIGH YIELD POINTS • Strongly associated with **smoking**, often **centrally located** • IHC: **(+) p40, p63, CK5/6**; **(-)** TTF-1, Napsin-A

ADENOCARCINOMA	SQUAMOUS CELL CARCINOMA
TTF-1	p40 (most specific)
Napsin A	CK5/6
CK7 (less specific)	p63 (less specific)

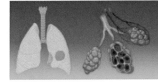 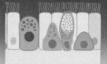

Peripheral palisading, lobular architecture

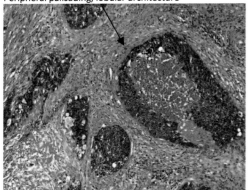

BASALOID SQUAMOUS CELL CARCINOMA
MORPHOLOGY
- Small cells with a **high N:C ratio**, distinct borders
- **Lobular** architecture with **peripheral palisading**; hyaline or mucoid stroma
- Lacks overt squamous histomorphology, numerous **mitoses**

OTHER HIGH YIELD POINTS
- Must comprise **> 50% of tumor**
- IHC: **(+/-) p40, p63, CK5/6**; **(-)** TTF-1, Napsin-A; Ki67 often 50-80%
- **Worse prognosis** than conventional SCC

Path Presenter

NEUROENDOCRINE TUMORS

Polygonal cells with "salt and pepper" chromatin

TYPICAL CARCINOID
MORPHOLOGY
- Organoid or trabecular growth, **uniform polygonal cells**, finely granular **"salt and pepper"** chromatin, inconspicuous nucleoli, and eosinophilic cytoplasm
- **< 2 mitoses per 2 mm²**, lacking necrosis, > 0.5 cm tumor size
- If <0.5 cm, designated as **"tumorlet"**

OTHER HIGH YIELD POINTS
- **Low-grade**; often arises near the **central airway** and can grow into the airway

Path Presenter

Necrosis   Mitotic activity

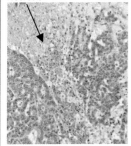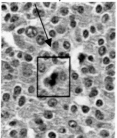

ATYPICAL CARCINOID
MORPHOLOGY
- A tumor with "carcinoid morphology"
- **2-10 mitoses per 2 mm²** and/or **necrosis (often punctate)**

OTHER HIGH YIELD POINTS
- **Intermediate-grade** malignancy; worse prognosis than typical carcinoid

Path Presenter

Proliferation of neuroendocrine cells along the airway

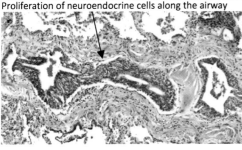

DIFFUSE IDIOPATHIC PULMONARY NEUROENDOCRINE CELL HYPERPLASIA
MORPHOLOGY
- Generalized proliferation of pulmonary **neuroendocrine cells along airways**

OTHER HIGH YIELD POINTS
- Often **older patients**
- May **invade locally**
- **Chronic progressive disease**
- Patients often present with cough and wheezing

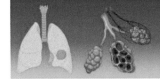

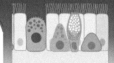
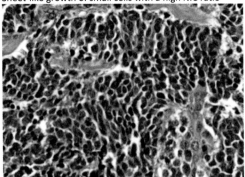
Sheet-like growth of small cells with a high N:C ratio

SMALL CELL CARCINOMA
MORPHOLOGY
- **Small cells** (smaller than 3 resting lymphocytes), scant cytoplasm, molding
- **Densely cellular sheet-like growth**, finely granular chromatin (**no** nucleoli)
- High mitotic rate: **>10 mitoses per 2 mm²**, frequent **necrosis**, Ki67 often approaching 100%

OTHER HIGH YIELD POINTS
- Often **centrally located** in major airways/hilar region
- Present with **rapid growth, metastases**
- Strongest association with heavy **smoking, very poor prognosis**

Path Presenter

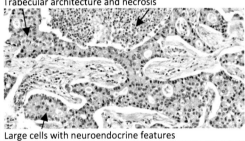
Trabecular architecture and necrosis

Large cells with neuroendocrine features

LARGE CELL NEUROENDOCRINE CARCINOMA
MORPHOLOGY
- **Neuroendocrine** morphology (architecture: organoid, nesting, palisading, rosettes, trabeculae)
- Cytologic features: **large cells** with abundant cytoplasm, vesicular chromatin, and **prominent nucleoli**
- **High mitotic rate, necrosis**   Path Presenter

OTHER HIGH YIELD POINTS
- **Smoking**-related, often **peripheral, aggressive**

	Typical carcinoid	Atypical carcinoid	Large cell NE carcinoma	Small cell carcinoma
Smoking association	No	Maybe	Yes	Yes
Mitoses/2mm²	0-1	2-10	>10 (median 70)	>10 (median 80)
Necrosis	No	Focal, if any	Yes	Yes, extensive
NE morphology	Yes	Yes	Yes	Yes
Ki-67	Up to 5%	Up to 20%	40-80%	Almost 100%
TTF-1 expression	Usually not	Usually not	~50%	~85%
Non-small cell component	No	No	Sometimes	Sometimes

- **IHC markers for neuroendocrine differentiation**: Synaptophysin, chromogranin, INSM1, CD56 (sensitive but less specific), NSE; Cytokeratin IHC often show perinuclear "dot-like" staining.
- Note: lung neuroendocrine neoplasms are **graded based on mitoses and necrosis** (counted in a hotspot). Ki67 may be helpful for confirmation but cannot be utilized for grading currently.

OTHER CARCINOMAS

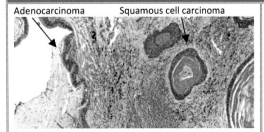
Adenocarcinoma   Squamous cell carcinoma

ADENOSQUAMOUS CARCINOMA
MORPHOLOGY
- Carcinoma with both **squamous component and adenocarcinoma component**
- Each must constitute **at least 10%**

OTHER HIGH YIELD POINTS
- Diagnosis can only be made on resection specimens (not biopsy)

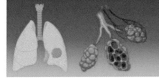 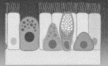
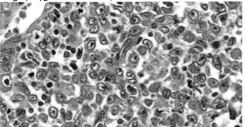

Large polygonal cells with prominent nucleoli

LARGE CELL CARCINOMA
MORPHOLOGY
- **Undifferentiated, non-small cell carcinoma** that lacks cytologic, architectural, and IHC features of small cell carcinoma, adenocarcinoma, or SCC
- Sheets or nests of **large polygonal cells** with vesicular nuclei and **prominent nucleoli**
OTHER HIGH YIELD POINTS
- **Diagnosis of exclusion**, prevalence is decreasing
- IHC: **(+) cytokeratin, (-)** TTF-1, p40, synaptophysin, chromogranin

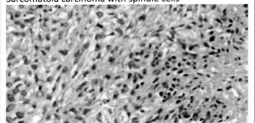

Sarcomatoid carcinoma with spindle cells

SARCOMATOID CARCINOMA
MORPHOLOGY
- **Spindle cell carcinoma**: Almost entirely composed of pure spindle cells
- **Giant cell carcinoma**: Numerous giant cells
- **Pleomorphic carcinoma**: Contains >10% giant cell or spindle cell carcinoma
- **Carcinosarcoma**: A mixture of NSCLC and sarcoma (poor prognosis)
OTHER HIGH YIELD POINTS   Path Presenter
- Diagnosis only on resection specimens; IHC variable

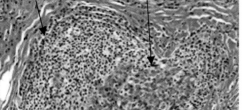

Lymphoid infiltrates   Carcinoma

LYMPHOEPITHELIOMA-LIKE CARCINOMA
MORPHOLOGY
- Carcinoma with **marked lymphoid infiltrate**
- **Large cells** with syncytial growth, large vesicular nuclei, and prominent nucleoli
OTHER HIGH YIELD POINTS   Path Presenter
- **EBV infection** of neoplastic cells; **EBER ISH(+)**
- IHC: **(+)** cytokeratin AE1/AE3, CK5/6, p40, p63

MULTIPLE TUMORS
- When **more than one tumor nodule is identified** in resection samples, always attempt to distinguish synchronous primary tumors from a tumor with intrapulmonary metastasis
- **Consider it a second primary (and stage each separately) if:**
  - Tumors have different histologic types (e.g., one squamous and one adenocarcinoma)
  - Tumors are dramatically different morphologically after a comprehensive review
  - Tumors are two squamous carcinomas, with each having an in situ component
- **Consider an intrapulmonary metastasis if:** Identical genetic abnormalities are detected
- **Relative arguments that favor a second primary:**
  - Different biomarker pattern
  - Absence of nodal or systemic metastases
- **Relative arguments that favor intrapulmonary metastasis:**
  - Matching appearance after a comprehensive review
  - Same biomarker pattern
  - Significant nodal or systemic metastases

PLEURAL INVASION
- If the tumor is approaching the visceral pleura, get an Elastin stain (EVG) to see if it crosses the elastic layer for staging purposes

Stage	Depth of invasion
PL0	Tumor does not completely traverse the elastic layer
PL1	Tumor extends through the elastic layer but not to the visceral pleural surface
PL2	Tumor extends to the visceral pleural surface
PL3	Tumor invades parietal pleura

SPREAD THROUGH AIR SPACES (STAS)
- **Definition:** Micropapillary clusters, solid nests, or single cells of tumor extending beyond the edge of the tumor into the air spaces of the surrounding lung parenchyma
- No strict distance cut-off
- If present, **it cannot** be considered AIS or minimally invasive adenocarcinoma
- Associated with an **increased incidence of recurrence** in tumors that have undergone limited resection
- Should not be incorporated into measurement of tumor size

MOLECULAR PATHOGENESIS
- ~70% of lung cancers are inoperable; diagnosis and testing performed on biopsy or FNA
- Must test adenocarcinoma for: **EGFR, ALK, ROS1** in all cases (molecular/FISH/IHC); **PD-L1** (IHC)
- Considering testing for BRAF, KRAS, HER2, RET
- Can consider some of these tests in non-adenocarcinoma if mixed histology or small biopsy

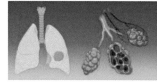 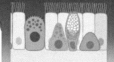

CLASSIFICATION OF LUNG CARCINOMAS WITH LIMITED TISSUE

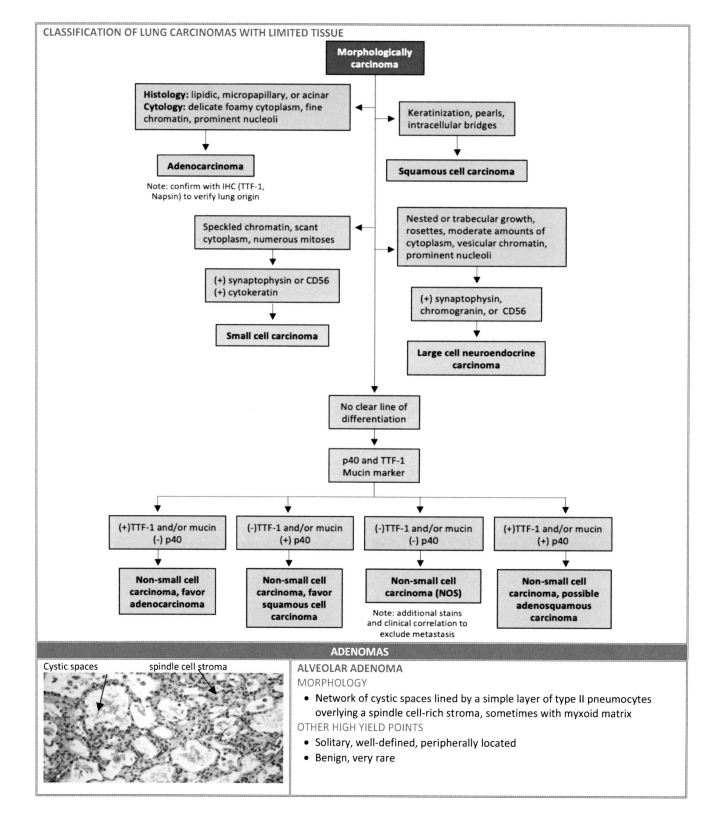

Morphologically carcinoma

Histology: lipidic, micropapillary, or acinar
Cytology: delicate foamy cytoplasm, fine chromatin, prominent nucleoli

→ **Adenocarcinoma**

Note: confirm with IHC (TTF-1, Napsin) to verify lung origin

Keratinization, pearls, intracellular bridges

→ **Squamous cell carcinoma**

Speckled chromatin, scant cytoplasm, numerous mitoses

→ (+) synaptophysin or CD56 (+) cytokeratin

→ **Small cell carcinoma**

Nested or trabecular growth, rosettes, moderate amounts of cytoplasm, vesicular chromatin, prominent nucleoli

→ (+) synaptophysin, chromogranin, or CD56

→ **Large cell neuroendocrine carcinoma**

No clear line of differentiation

→ p40 and TTF-1 Mucin marker

(+)TTF-1 and/or mucin (-) p40	(-)TTF-1 and/or mucin (+) p40	(-)TTF-1 and/or mucin (-) p40	(+)TTF-1 and/or mucin (+) p40
Non-small cell carcinoma, favor adenocarcinoma	**Non-small cell carcinoma, favor squamous cell carcinoma**	**Non-small cell carcinoma (NOS)** Note: additional stains and clinical correlation to exclude metastasis	**Non-small cell carcinoma, possible adenosquamous carcinoma**

ADENOMAS

Cystic spaces   spindle cell stroma

ALVEOLAR ADENOMA
MORPHOLOGY
- Network of cystic spaces lined by a simple layer of type II pneumocytes overlying a spindle cell-rich stroma, sometimes with myxoid matrix

OTHER HIGH YIELD POINTS
- Solitary, well-defined, peripherally located
- Benign, very rare

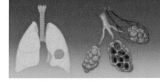
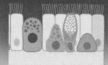

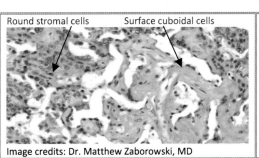
Round stromal cells   Surface cuboidal cells

Image credits: Dr. Matthew Zaborowski, MD

SCLEROSING PNEUMOCYTOMA
MORPHOLOGY
- Pneumocytic origin with **dual cell populations**:
  - ➢ Small surface cuboidal cells: (+) cytokeratin, TTF-1, Napsin-A
  - ➢ Large stromal cells: (+) TTF-1, (-) cytokeratin
- Four growth patterns: solid, papillary, sclerotic, hemorrhagic
OTHER HIGH YIELD POINTS
- Benign, often asymptomatic, more commonly in women

OTHER ADENOMAS
MORPHOLOGY
- Glandular papilloma:
  - ➢ Benign, papillary, glandular tumor lined by ciliated or non-ciliated columnar cells with varying numbers of cuboidal and goblet cells
- Papillary adenoma:
  - ➢ Benign, circumscribed, papillary neoplasm that consists of cytologically bland, cuboidal to columnar cells covering fibrovascular cores
- Mucinous gland adenoma:
  - ➢ Benign, exophytic, well-circumscribed tumor of tracheobronchial seromucinous glands/ducts; microacini, glands, and tubules of bland cells

SALIVARY GLAND TUMORS
MORPHOLOGY
- **Mucoepidermoid carcinoma**: Triphasic tumor with mucin-secreting cells, squamous cells, and intermediate cells (MAML rearrangement)
- **Adenoid cystic carcinoma**: Basaloid carcinoma with epithelial and myoepithelial cells arranged in variable configurations (MYB rearrangement)
- **Epithelial-myoepithelial carcinoma**: Ducts of epithelial cells surrounded by myoepithelial cells, clear to spindled morphology
- **Pleomorphic adenoma**: Epithelial and myoepithelial cells intermingled with myxoid to chondroid stroma (PLAG1 rearrangement)
OTHER HIGH YIELD POINTS
- Arise from salivary-like glands in bronchi, often in the **central airway**

MESENCHYMAL TUMORS

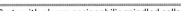
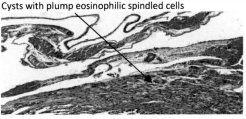
Pulmonary hamartoma with fat and smooth muscle

PULMONARY HAMARTOMA
MORPHOLOGY
- At least two mesenchymal elements (e.g., **cartilage, fat**, smooth muscle, etc.) combined with **entrapped epithelium**
OTHER HIGH YIELD POINTS
- **Relatively common**
- Asymptomatic, benign, solitary, well-circumscribed
- Usually peripheral with **"popcorn" calcifications**
- Frequent **HMGA2 fusion**

Cysts with plump eosinophilic spindled cells

LYMPHANGIOLEIOMYOMATOSIS (LAM)
MORPHOLOGY
- Thin-walled cysts with **plump spindled cells** with pale eosinophilic/clear cytoplasm
OTHER HIGH YIELD POINTS
- Perivascular epithelioid cell tumor (**PEComa**)
- **Diffuse, bilateral, multicystic proliferation**, low-grade
- Exclusively young women and associated with **tuberous sclerosis**
- IHC: (+) **HMB45**, MelanA, MITF, SMA, desmin

Path Presenter

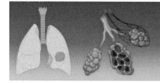
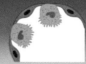
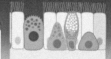

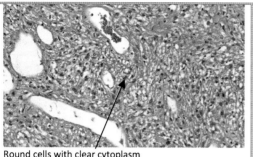

Round cells with clear cytoplasm
Image credits: Farres Obeidin, MD, Northwestern University - Feinberg School of Medicine

CLEAR CELL ("SUGAR") TUMOR
MORPHOLOGY
- Well-circumscribed lesion composed of round to oval cells with **abundant clear or eosinophilic cytoplasm** (PAS+ cytoplasmic glycogen)

OTHER HIGH YIELD POINTS
- Rare, benign, solitary, peripherally localized **PEComa**
- IHC: (+) **HMB45**, MelanA, MiTF, MART-1, SMA, desmin   **Image: MART-1**

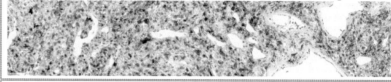

A patternless pattern of bland spindle cells

SOLITARY FIBROUS TUMOR (SFT)
MORPHOLOGY
- **A patternless pattern** of bland spindled cells with variable cellularity
- Collagenized stroma and **"staghorn" vessels** (dilated, thin-walled, branching)
- Can be hyalinized or myxoid

OTHER HIGH YIELD POINTS
- IHC: (+) **STAT6**, CD34, CD99   Path Presenter
- Molecular: **NAB2-STAT6 gene fusion**
- Can also be seen as a tumor of the pleura

INTIMAL SARCOMA
MORPHOLOGY
- Variably **pleomorphic spindled cells** with **necrosis and mitoses**

OTHER HIGH YIELD POINTS
- Malignant, arises in large blood vessels, characteristic **intraluminal growth** with obstruction of blood flow and tumor seeding
- IHC: (+) MDM2. Molecular: **Amplification of MDM2/CDK4**

Path Presenter

Variably pleomorphic cells with frequent mitoses

Bland spindle cells with fascicular / storiform pattern

INFLAMMATORY MYOFIBROBLASTIC TUMOR
MORPHOLOGY
- **Bland spindled to stellate cells** in myxoid to hyalinized stroma
- Can have **loose, fascicular, or storiform growth**
- Prominent lymphoplasmacytic infiltrate

OTHER HIGH YIELD POINTS
- Relatively **indolent**, usually solitary, frequently asymptomatic
- IHC: Variable staining with actin/desmin; **ALK(+)** with ALK gene rearrangements in ~50%

Path Presenter

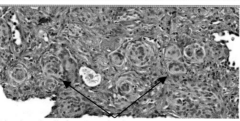

Bland oval cells forming whorls

MENINGOTHELIAL-LIKE NODULE
MORPHOLOGY
- Monotonous, **bland, ovoid to spindle cells** within septa
- Indistinct cell borders, oval nuclei, **nuclear pseudoinclusions**
- **Whorled** architecture

OTHER HIGH YIELD POINTS
- Benign, common, incidental, often multiple, and small (1-4 mm)
- IHC: (+) **SSTR2A**, PR, EMA, CD56; (-) CK, S100, TTF1

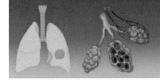 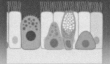

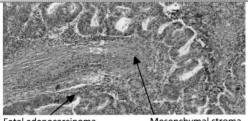

Fetal adenocarcinoma   Mesenchymal stroma

PULMONARY BLASTOMA

MORPHOLOGY
- **Biphasic tumor** with low-grade fetal adenocarcinoma and primitive mesenchymal stroma

OTHER HIGH YIELD POINTS
- Uncommon, usually in **adult patients**
- Poor prognosis

Small round primitive cells, sarcomatous differentiation

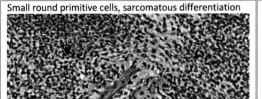

PLEUROPULMONARY BLASTOMA

MORPHOLOGY
- **Small round primitive cells** with variable **sarcomatous** differentiation
- Can be solid or cystic

OTHER HIGH YIELD POINTS
- Sarcoma of the lung in **infancy/childhood**
- **DICER1 mutations**   (Image courtesy: Adriana Zucchiatti, MD)

Sheets of undifferentiated epithelioid cells

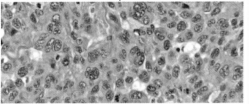

SMARCA4-DEFICIENT THORACIC SARCOMA

MORPHOLOGY
- **Diffuse sheets** of mildly discohesive, **undifferentiated epithelioid cells** with prominent nucleoli

OTHER HIGH YIELD POINTS
- Malignant, centered in the thorax, very **aggressive**
- IHC: (+) **CD34**, SALL4, (+/-) CK
- Molecular: **SMARCA4 mutations**

Strands and cords of round to spindle cells

PULMONARY MYXOID SARCOMA WITH EWSR1-CREB1 TRANSLOCATION

MORPHOLOGY
- Lobules of **delicate, lace-like strands and cords** of round to spindled cells within **myxoid stroma**

OTHER HIGH YIELD POINTS
- Malignant; usually arises in airways
- IHC: Generally negative except vimentin
- **EWSR1 rearrangements** with FISH

Uniform spindled cells with scant cytoplasm

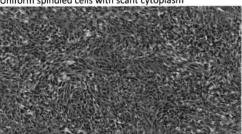

SYNOVIAL SARCOMA

MORPHOLOGY
- Malignant **spindle cell neoplasm** with uniform nuclei, scant cytoplasm, and frequent **staghorn vessels**
- **Monophasic** (spindled only) or **biphasic** (spindled & epithelioid components)

OTHER HIGH YIELD POINTS
- t(X;18), **SS18-SSX gene fusions**   Path Presenter
- IHC: (+) **CD99, TLE-1**; patchy EMA and CK
- **Poor prognosis**, usually young adults

MISCELLANEOUS PULMONARY TUMORS

MALT lymphoma of the lung

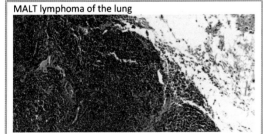

- **Metastasis**
  - Always a consideration in the lung, especially if multiple or bilateral
- **MALT Lymphoma**
  - Thought to arise secondary to inflammatory conditions or autoimmune process

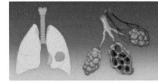

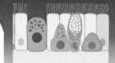

Lymphomatoid granulomatosis

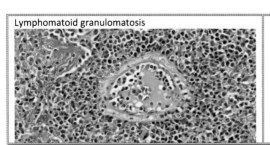

- **Lymphomatoid Granulomatosis**
  - ➢ Pulmonary nodules composed of angiocentric and angiodestructive polymorphous lymphoid infiltrates, including reactive T cells and EBV(+) B cells
- **Germ Cell Tumors**
  - ➢ Mature teratoma most common   Path Presenter
- **Intrapulmonary Thymoma**
- **Melanoma**

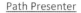

NON-NEOPLASTIC LESIONS OF THE PLEURA & PERITEONEUM

REACTIVE MESOTHELIAL HYPERPLASIA	MESOTHELIOMA
Absence of stromal invasion - beware of entrapment and tangential sectioning	Stromal invasion is usually apparent - highlight with pancytokeratin staining
Cellularity may be prominent	Dense cellularity
Simple papillae; single cell layers	Complex papillae; tubules, and cellular stratification
Loose sheets of cells without stroma	Cells surrounded by stroma
Necrosis rare	Necrosis occasionally present
Inflammation common	Minimal inflammation
Uniform growth	Expansile nodules, disorganized growth

Simple papillae with single cell layer

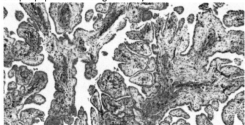

Courtesy: Laura G. Pastrián, MD

REACTIVE MESOTHELIAL HYPERPLASIA
MORPHOLOGY
- **A reactive proliferation** of mesothelial cells with **several architectural patterns** (solid, nested, papillary, cord-like, etc.)
- Common **worrisome findings**: high cellularity, mitoses, cytologic atypia, papillary groups, and entrapment of mesothelial cells (mimicking invasion)
OTHER HIGH YIELD POINTS
- Reactive mesothelial cells responding to inflammation/irritation
- Can **histologically mimic mesothelioma/carcinoma**

Hypocellular fibrous tissue deposition

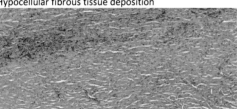

FIBROUS PLEURISY
MORPHOLOGY
- Deposition of **bland, hypocellular fibrous tissue** in the pleura
OTHER HIGH YIELD POINTS
- Often involves the **visceral pleura** and may produce apical fibrous "capping"
- Severe cases can obliterate the pleural space
- May be associated with connective tissue disorders and chronic inflammation
- Can **mimic desmoplastic mesothelioma**

Hypocelluar dense collagen

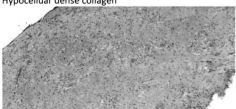

PLEURAL PLAQUE
MORPHOLOGY
- **Hypocellular, dense bundles of hyalinized collagen**, often with a "basket weave" arrangement
- Often dystrophic **calcifications**, variable chronic inflammation
OTHER HIGH YIELD POINTS
- Usually on **parietal pleura**, particularly on the diaphragm; **asbestos** exposure

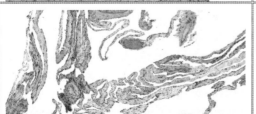

PERITONEAL INCLUSION CYST
MORPHOLOGY
- Single or multiple, **small, thin-walled, translucent, unilocular cysts**
- Attached or free in the peritoneal cavity
- Lined by a **single layer** of flattened, benign-appearing mesothelial cells
OTHER HIGH YIELD POINTS
- Often discovered **incidentally**, more common in **women**

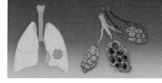

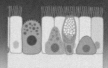

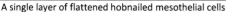

A single layer of flattened hobnailed mesothelial cells

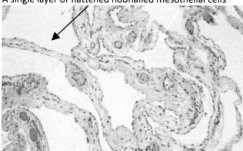

BENIGN MULTICYSTIC PERITONEAL MESOTHELIOMA
MORPHOLOGY
- Grossly: often **large, multiple, thin-walled, translucent, unilocular** cysts that may be attached or free floating
- Often fibrous tissue in septa with sparse inflammation
- Cysts are lined by a **single layer** of flattened to cuboidal mesothelial cells with a hobnailed appearance

OTHER HIGH YIELD POINTS
- Young to middle-aged **women** in the peritoneum/pelvis
- **Associations:** Previous abdominal surgery, pelvic inflammatory disease, and endometriosis; strong tendency to recur

Chronic inflammation and fibrosis

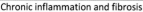

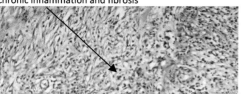

SCLEROSING MESENTERITIS
MORPHOLOGY
- Varying degrees of **fat necrosis, chronic inflammation, and fibrosis,** usually involving the **mesentery**

OTHER HIGH YIELD POINTS
- Rare, idiopathic, forms a **distinct mass** involving the small bowel mesentery

Bowel encapsulated by fibrous tissue

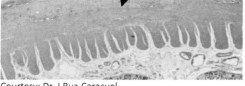

Courtesy: Dr. I Ruz-Caracuel

SCLEROSING PERITONITIS
MORPHOLOGY
- **Encasement of the bowel** by fibrous tissue

OTHER HIGH YIELD POINTS
- Rare, causes **bowel obstruction**
- Can be idiopathic or seen with intraperitoneal dialysis, VP shunts, and fibrothecomas of the ovary

Gland-like microcystic spaces with flattened cells

ADENOMATOID TUMOR
MORPHOLOGY
- **Irregularly shaped gland-like microcystic spaces** composed of flattened or cuboidal cells with associated fibrous stroma
- Bland cytologic features and **thread-like bridging strands**

OTHER HIGH YIELD POINTS
- Solitary, localized, most commonly in the **female genital/genitourinary tract** but can also be pleural

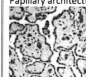 Path Presenter

Papillary architecture with a single layer of cells

WELL-DIFFERENTIATED PAPILLARY MESOTHELIOMA
MORPHOLOGY
- Gross: **Velvety** appearance
- Prominent **papillary architecture with myxoid cores** covered by a single layer of flattened to cuboidal bland epithelioid cells

OTHER HIGH YIELD POINTS
- Rare, indolent, most cases cured by excision but may recur

Image credits: Gladell Paner, MD

MALIGNANT MESOTHELIAL TUMORS
- **Demonstration of tissue invasion** is often key for the diagnosis but is not required when a substantial amount of solid tumor is present
- Common histologic patterns: **solid, tubulopapillary, trabecular**
- Special studies: **Use IHC to confirm mesothelial** and not a metastatic carcinoma (**always use a panel**)
- **IHC: BAP1 or MTAP loss, FISH: CDKN2A deletion;** multigene expression profiling panels.
- These studies support the diagnosis of mesothelioma with good (but not great) specificity
- Look for cytokeratin-positive malignant cells in regions in which they would not normally be present: adipose tissue, skeletal muscle deep to the parietal pleura, or lung tissue
- Benign processes tend to be well-circumscribed. Malignant processes tend to be poorly circumscribed and invasive

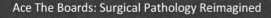

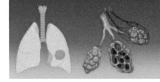 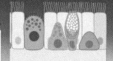

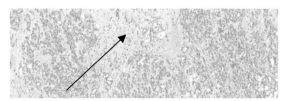

Tissue Invasion

IMMUNOHISTOCHEMISTRY PANEL

Metastatic adenocarcinoma	Squamous cell carcinoma	Mesothelial cells
BerEP4	p40	Calretinin
B72.3	p63	D2-40
MOC31	MOC31	WT-1
Claudin-4	Claudin-4	CK5/6

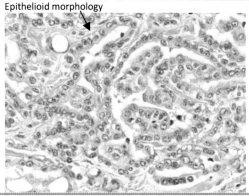

Epithelioid morphology

EPITHELIOID MESOTHELIOMA
MORPHOLOGY
- **Malignant** proliferation of mesothelial cells with **epithelioid morphology**
- Often bland cytologically with eosinophilic cytoplasm and vesicular chromatin

OTHER HIGH YIELD POINTS
- Usually **diffuse** (circumferential, rind-like) with a **poor prognosis**
- Rarely, localized with a better prognosis
- Most common in **elderly males**; **asbestos exposure**; insidious onset

Path Presenter

[QR code]

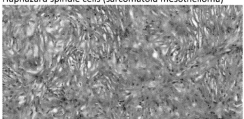

Haphazard spindle cells (sarcomatoid mesothelioma)

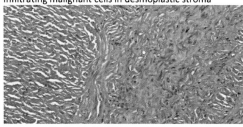

Infiltrating malignant cells in desmoplastic stroma

MESOTHELIOMA VARIANTS
MORPHOLOGY
- **Sarcomatoid mesothelioma**
  - ➤ **Spindle cells arranged in fascicles** or haphazardly
  - ➤ Can see **heterologous elements** (e.g., rhabdomyosarcoma)
- **Desmoplastic mesothelioma**
  - ➤ **Dense collagenized tissue** with malignant mesothelial cells
  - ➤ Must be **>50% of the tumor**
  - ➤ Patternless or storiform pattern
  - ➤ **Invasion into fat** is most helpful to differentiate from organizing pleuritis
- **Biphasic mesothelioma**
  - ➤ Contains **both epithelioid and sarcomatoid patterns**, each >10%

OTHER HIGH YIELD POINTS
- Stroma invasion is often difficult to recognize
- **IHC: (+) pancytokeratin** (at least focally), helpful to demonstrate invasion
- **Loss of BAP1 is very uncommon in these types**
- **Worse prognosis** than epithelioid mesothelioma (desmoplastic <6 months)

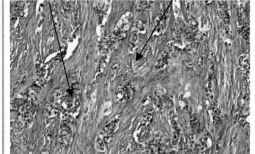

Basaloid nests of tumor cells in desmoplastic stroma

DESMOPLASTIC SMALL ROUND CELL TUMOR
MORPHOLOGY
- **Basaloid nests** of small, uniform cells surrounded by **desmoplastic stroma**
- Hyperchromatic chromatin, scant cytoplasm, **frequent mitoses** & apoptosis

OTHER HIGH YIELD POINTS
- Malignant tumor of uncertain histogenesis; often in the peritoneal cavity of young men; poor prognosis
- IHC: (+) **Cytokeratins**, **desmin** (perinuclear dot-like pattern), EMA
- Molecular: **EWSR1-WT1 translocation**

Path Presenter

[QR code]

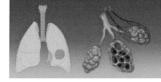 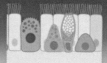

Hypocellular collagenized tissue 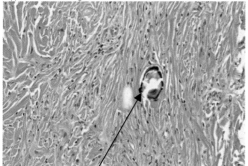 Psammomatous calcification	**CALCIFYING FIBROUS TUMOR** MORPHOLOGY • Paucicellular collagenized fibrous tissue with associated psammomatous or dystrophic calcifications • **Circumscribed** but not encapsulated OTHER HIGH YIELD POINTS • Rare, **benign**, occurs in visceral pleura/peritoneum and **does not invade** underlying tissue • More common in **younger women** • IHC: (+) CD34; (-) STAT6, ALK, β-catenin Path Presenter
Infiltrating uniform, small spindle cells 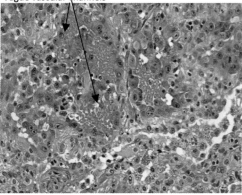	**DESMOID-TYPE FIBROMATOSIS** MORPHOLOGY • **Infiltrative growth** into surrounding structures (skeletal muscle) • **Broad, sweeping fascicles** of uniform spindled cells with pinpoint nucleoli • Moderate amounts of **collagen** surrounding cells, slightly myxoid background OTHER HIGH YIELD POINTS • Benign, but **infiltrative** with a **high recurrence rate** (>50%) • IHC: **(+) nuclear b-catenin**; (+/-) actin • **Molecular:** mutations of FAP and APC/b-catenin (CTNNB1) pathway Path Presenter
Vague vascular channels 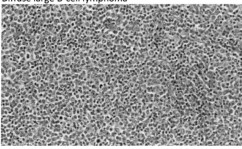	**ANGIOSARCOMA** MORPHOLOGY • **Variable degrees of vascular differentiation** • Some areas show well-formed anastomosing vessels, while other areas show solid sheets of high-grade cells • Can be **epithelioid or spindled** cells, often with extensive **hemorrhage** • Significant cytologic atypia, necrosis, and mitotic figures OTHER HIGH YIELD POINTS • Malignant, very **aggressive**, usually **elderly** patients • IHC: (+) CD31, ERG, FLI1, often CD34 Path Presenter

Diffuse large B-cell lymphoma	**LYMPHOPROLIFERATIVE DISORDERS**
	• **Diffuse large B cell lymphoma associated with chronic inflammation**
	  ➤ **Resembles other forms of DLBCL** with large vesicular nuclei & prominent nucleoli
	  ➤ Occurs in patients with **long-standing pyothorax** or other chronic inflammatory processes; usually in **body cavities**; **aggressive**
	  ➤ **EBV-associated**, (+) B cell markers
	
	Path Presenter

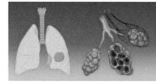
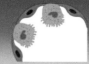
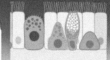

Immunoblastic appearance of PEL

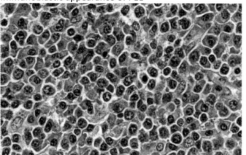

- **Primary Effusion Lymphoma (PEL)**
  - ➤ **Large, atypical B cells** with an **immunoblastic appearance** (basophilic cytoplasm, round nucleus with prominent nucleolus, variable pleomorphism)
  - ➤ Rare, presents as **effusion without solid tumor mass**
  - ➤ Usually, in **immunocompromised** patients; a **poor prognosis**
  - ➤ **Positive for HHV8**, often **coinfection with EBV**
  - ➤ IHC: (+) CD45, CD30, CD138, EMA, HHV8
    - (-) CD19, CD20, PAX5, CD79a (**negative for pan B cell markers**)

Endocervicosis (endocervical-like epithelium)

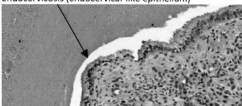

MULLERIAN LESIONS OF THE PERITONEUM
- **Mullerianosis**
  - ➤ **Endosalpingiosis**: Glands lined by benign **tubal-type (ciliated)** epithelium involving the peritoneum or pelvic/para-aortic lymph nodes; likely secondary as associated with salpingitis
  - ➤ **Endometriosis**: Benign endometrial glands and stroma; often accompanying hemosiderin-laden macrophages
  - ➤ **Endocervicosis**: Benign endocervical-type epithelium

Decidual cells (deciduosis)

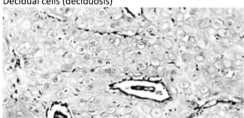

- **Deciduosis**
  - ➤ **Ectopic decidual cells**: Epithelioid with abundant pale pink granular cytoplasm and bland nuclei
  - ➤ Arranged individually, in nodules, or in plaques
  - ➤ Seen during **pregnancy**; may have associated hemorrhage/inflammation

Peritoneal serous borderline tumor

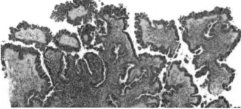

- **Primary peritoneal serous borderline tumor**
  - ➤ **Identical to noninvasive peritoneal implants** of ovarian serous borderline tumors
  - ➤ **Diagnosis of exclusion**: Only when the ovaries are uninvolved or with only minimal surface involvement
  - ➤ Likely arises from endosalpingiosis, generally **good prognosis**
  - ➤ Can get primary peritoneal low-grade serous carcinoma (sample well)

Peritoneal high-grade serous carcinoma

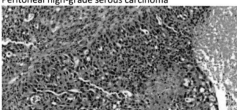

- **Primary peritoneal high-grade carcinoma**
  - ➤ **Identical** to the primary tubo-ovarian high-grade serous carcinoma
  - ➤ **Diagnosis of exclusion**: Both tubes and both ovaries grossly and microscopically uninvolved (when examined entirely)
  - ➤ Diagnosis can only be made at primary surgery prior to any chemotherapy

Path Presenter

TUMORS OF THE MEDIASTINUM

GENERAL
- **Mediastinum**: Anatomic region located between the lungs, sternum, spine, thoracic inlet, and diaphragm
- About **half of tumors are asymptomatic** and identified incidentally on imaging
- If symptomatic: Cough, pain, dyspnea, **superior vena cava syndrome** (face swelling & distended neck veins due to blockage of SVC)
- Tumors in adults: Carcinoma or lymphoma most common; tumors in children: Leukemia/lymphoma most common

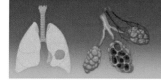

3. PULMONARY PATHOLOGY

 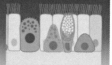

DIFFERENTIAL DIAGNOSIS BY LOCATION			
ANTERIOR	**SUPERIOR**	**MIDDLE**	**POSTERIOR**
Thymic tumors	Thymic tumors	Pericardial cyst	Neurogenic tumors
Germ cell tumors	Thyroid tumors	Bronchial cyst	Schwannoma
Thyroid tumors	Lymphoma	Lymphoma	Neurofibroma
Parathyroid tumors	Parathyroid tumors		Ganglioneuroma
Lymphoma			MPNST
Paraganglioma			Neuroblastoma
Hemangioma			Gastrointestinal cyst
Lipoma			Bronchogenic cyst

The classic **5 "T's"** of anterior mediastinal masses:

Thymus
Thyroid
Teratoma
Terrible lymphoma
Thoracic aorta (aneurysm)

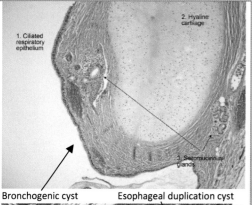

DEVELOPMENTAL CYSTS
- Congenital anomalies that arise during embryogenesis
- **Bronchogenic cyst** (Image courtesy: Chandra Krishnan, MD)
  - Well-formed, unilocular cystic structures **resembling bronchus**
  - Contain: **Ciliated epithelium**, **cartilage**, submucosal glands, smooth muscle, and/or degenerative changes
  - Abnormal tracheobronchial tree branching
  - Cured by excision, risk of infection if not excised
  - Hard to distinguish from esophageal duplication cysts if no cartilage ("foregut cyst")
- **Gastrointestinal duplication cyst**
  - Attached to the GI tract, with epithelium that resembles some part of the GI tract and a well-developed double layer of smooth muscle
  - No cartilage (distinguishes from bronchogenic cyst)
  - **Esophageal duplication cyst:** Columnar, squamous, or mixed epithelium
  - **Enteric duplication cyst:** Variable epithelium, usually gastric/duodenal
  - Can contain heterotopic lung or thyroid

Bronchogenic cyst   Esophageal duplication cyst

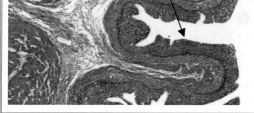

Link   Link

Path Presenter

THYMOMA				
Type	**Composition**	**Proportion epithelium**	**Proportion lymphocytes**	**Prognosis**
Type A	Bland spindled to ovoid cells, few or no admixed lymphocytes	Predominant Spindled/oval	Few/none	Excellent
Type AB	Both lymphocyte poor (Type A) and lymphocyte-rich (Type B) components, with a significant proportion of immature T cells	Significant	Significant	Very good
Type B1	Predominantly lymphocytes with dispersed epithelial cells (no clusters)	Low No clusters, polygonal	Predominant	Very good
Type B2	Predominantly lymphocytes, with small clusters of epithelial cells	Low Small clusters	Significant	Fair
Type B3	Predominantly atypical polygonal epithelial cells in sheets	Predominant Epithelioid	Few	Fair, often high stage
Micronodular with lymphoid stroma	Multiple tumors with bland spindled cells surrounded by lymphoid stroma	Significant Spindled	Significant B and T cells No epithelial cells	Excellent
Metaplastic	Biphasic tumor with solid polygonal epithelial cells in a background of bland spindled cells	Predominant Epithelioid/spindled	Few/none	Very good

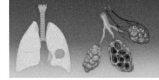 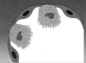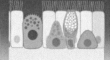

GENERAL
- Thymic epithelial neoplasms display a **variety of histologic patterns**
  - ➢ Heterogeneous and can show multiple patterns of growth; quantify subtype patterns by percentage (%)
  - ➢ Care should be taken if attempting to subtype on a small biopsy specimen (likely best diagnosis is "thymoma" and describe the patterns present)
- Overall **rare**, but **most common mediastinal tumor in adults**
- **Multiple subclassifications**, but <u>stage</u> is most important prognostically
- Frequent association with **paraneoplastic syndrome (myasthenia gravis** most common)
- Immunohistochemistry:
  - ➢ Most do not require IHC for subtyping; helpful to differentiate from non-thymus tumors
  - ➢ Thymic epithelial cells: (+) AE1/AE3, P63, PAX8, P40
  - ➢ T cells in the thymus: (+) CD5, CD3, TdT (immature thymic T cells)

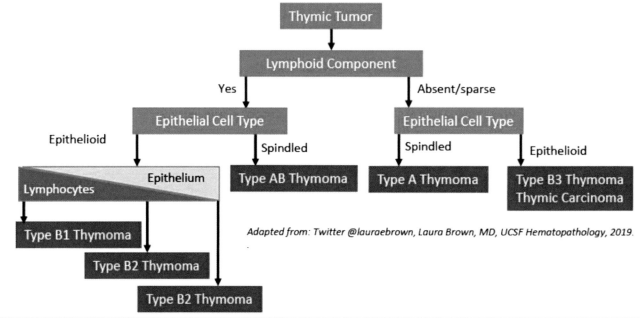

Adapted from: Twitter @lauraebrown, Laura Brown, MD, UCSF Hematopathology, 2019.

Bland, oval cells with powdery chromatin	TYPE A THYMOMA

TYPE A THYMOMA
MORPHOLOGY
- **Spindled to oval cells** with few or no admixed immature lymphocytes
- Bland nuclei with **powdery chromatin**
- Can have a **microcystic** appearance

OTHER HIGH YIELD POINTS
- Usually **low stage**, often lobulated and **circumscribed**/encapsulated
- **Excellent prognosis**

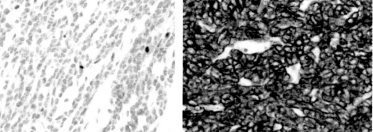

Image credits: Sanjay Mukhopadhyay, MD

TdT: No/sparse immature lymphoid cells, CK AE1/AE3 diffusely positive

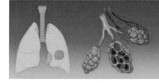
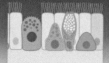
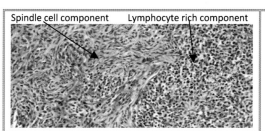

Spindle cell component   Lymphocyte rich component

TYPE AB THYMOMA
MORPHOLOGY
- **Two components**: lymphocyte-poor spindle cell component and lymphocyte rich component

OTHER HIGH YIELD POINTS
- Varying proportions, but >10% of tumor with moderate infiltrate of immature TdT (+) T cells
- Usually low stage, lobulated, very good prognosis

Resemblance of normal thymus

TYPE B1 THYMOMA
MORPHOLOGY
- **Closely resembles normal thymus**: Dispersed epithelial cells without clusters in a **dense background of immature T cells** mimicking thymic cortex
- Also has areas of medullary differentiation (nodular pale areas, ± Hassall's corpuscles, mostly TdT (+) T cells with numerous B cells)

OTHER HIGH YIELD POINTS
- Usually nodular; **very good prognosis**   Path Presenter

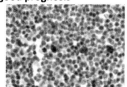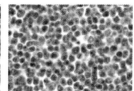

CKAE1/AE3, PAX8, P40   Image credits: Kevin Kuan, MD

Polygonal epithelial cells

TYPE B2 THYMOMA
MORPHOLOGY
- **Polygonal neoplastic epithelial cells** set in a background of numerous **immature T cells**
- Epithelial cells denser than B1, usually clustered with round vesicular nuclei

OTHER HIGH YIELD POINTS
- Often encapsulated, fair to good prognosis

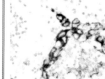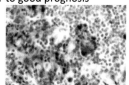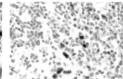

CKAE1/AE3, PAX8, P40   Image credits: Kevin Kuan, MD

Polygonal, pink epithelial cells

TYPE B3 THYMOMA
MORPHOLOGY
- Mild or moderately **atypical polygonal pink epithelial cells** with lobules of sheet-like or solid growth with fibrous septa; few intermingled T cells

OTHER HIGH YIELD POINTS
- **Poorly circumscribed** with extension into mediastinal fat/organs
- Most patients have **local symptoms** (chest pain or SVC syndrome)
- Fair prognosis, frequent recurrences

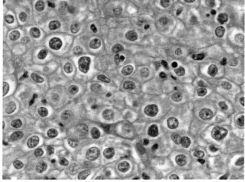

Courtesy: Lucas Massoth, MD

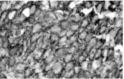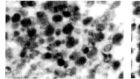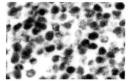

CKAE1/AE3, PAX8, P40   Image credits: Kevin Kuan, MD

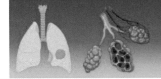 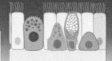

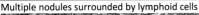

Multiple nodules surrounded by lymphoid cells

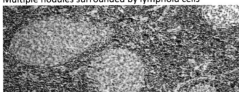

MICRONODULAR THYMOMA WITH LYMPHOID STROMA
MORPHOLOGY
- Multiple epithelial nodules surrounded by prominent lymphoid stroma containing mature B and T cells and devoid of epithelial cells
- May contain germinal centers and/or plasma cells

OTHER HIGH YIELD POINTS
- Excellent prognosis

Image credits: Jake Bledsoe, MD

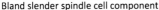

Bland slender spindle cell component

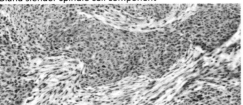

METAPLASTIC THYMOMA
MORPHOLOGY
- **Biphasic**: composed of alternating areas of solid epithelial cells and bland slender spindle cells
- Absent or very few lymphocytes

OTHER HIGH YIELD POINTS
- Very rare, no paraneoplastic syndrome
- **YAP1-MAML2 gene fusions**

Image credits: @Andy_pathology

MISCELLANEOUS THYMOMAS
- **Microscopic thymoma** – Multifocal thymic epithelial proliferations, < 1mm, composed of bland spindled to polygonal cells in well-circumscribed nodules embedded in the medulla or cortex (very rare)
- **Sclerosing thymoma** – Abundant collagen-rich stroma in an otherwise conventional thymoma
- **Lipofibroadenoma** – Benign thymic tumor that resembles fibroadenoma of the breast (very rare)

Resembles conventional carcinomas

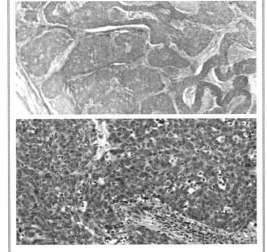

THYMIC CARCINOMA
MORPHOLOGY
- **Malignant** thymic epithelial tumor that lacks thymic organization
- **Resembles conventional carcinomas** in other organs
- Often unequivocal cytologic atypia
- Unencapsulated, no fibrous septa, variable T cell infiltrate

OTHER HIGH YIELD POINTS
- IHC: (+) AE1/AE3, p63, PAX8, CD5, CD117, Glut1, MUC1

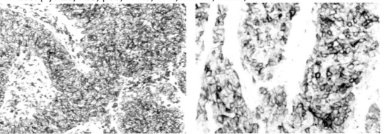

CD5 and CD117. Image credits: Lucas Massoth, MD (@LucasMassoth)

TYPES OF THYMIC CARCINOMA	
Squamous Cell Carcinoma	**Most common**; lacks normal thymic structure; frankly invasive into nearby structures; often eosinophilic cytoplasm and abundant stroma
Basaloid Carcinoma	**High N:C ratio** with cystic/papillary architecture and **peripheral palisading**; numerous mitoses and necrosis; very **aggressive**
Mucoepidermoid Carcinoma	Histologically similar to MEC in other organs; **MAML2 translocation**
Lymphoepithelioma-like Carcinoma	**Poorly differentiated SCC** with rich lymphoplasmacytic infiltrate; often **EBV positive**
Clear Cell Carcinoma	Composed of cells with **vacuolated clear cytoplasm**
Sarcomatoid Carcinoma	Completely or partly spindle cells; if heterologous elements → carcinosarcoma
NUT Carcinoma	Monomorphic round cells with **characteristic abrupt keratinization**, often stain with squamous markers; **NUT gene arrangement**; extremely **aggressive**
Adenocarcinoma	Heterogenous group showing **glandular and/or mucin production**
Undifferentiated Carcinoma	Large cell thymic carcinoma with inflammatory reaction resembling Castleman disease; indolent behavior

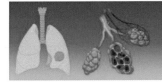
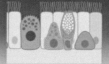
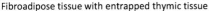
Fibroadipose tissue with entrapped thymic tissue

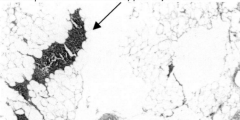

Mature fat and hyperchromatic spindled cells

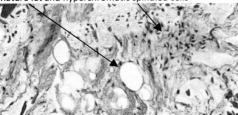

Infiltrating fibrosis (sclerosing mediastinitis)

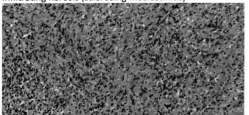

SOFT TISSUE TUMORS/LESIONS

- **Thymolipoma**
  - ➤ Encapsulated tumor with mature adipose tissue
  - ➤ Interspersed normal thymic tissue
  - ➤ Rare, benign, cured with excision
- **Liposarcoma**
  - ➤ Most common sarcoma of the mediastinum; poor prognosis
  - ➤ Ring or giant marker chromosomes derived from chromosome 12q13
  - ➤ MDM2 and CDK4 amplification
  - ➤ **Well-differentiated liposarcoma:** variable lipoblasts and hyperchromatic atypical cells in a background of adipocytes and fibrous tissue; morphologic variability
  - ➤ **Dedifferentiated liposarcoma:** Well-differentiated liposarcoma component with abrupt transition to an undifferentiated pleomorphic sarcoma
- **Sclerosing (Fibrosing) Mediastinitis**
  - ➤ **Non-neoplastic** fibrosis of mediastinum compressing and infiltrating normal structures
  - ➤ May be caused by prior infection/response to Histoplasma or TB; IgG4-related disease; autoimmune diseases; or prior radiation
  - ➤ Bland spindled cells with lymphoplasmacytic infiltrate ± calcifications
- **Other soft tissue/mesenchymal tumors of the mediastinum:**
  - ➤ Synovial sarcoma
  - ➤ Solitary fibrous tumor
  - ➤ SMARCA4-deficient thoracic sarcoma
  - ➤ Angiosarcoma

Link   Link

Small round blue cell tumor with pseudorosettes (NB)

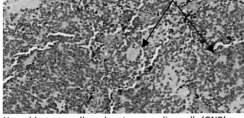

Neuroblastoma cells and mature ganglion cells (GNB)

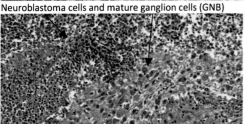

Mature ganglion cells and spindled cells (GN)

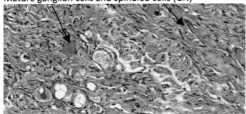

NEUROGENIC TUMORS

- **Schwannoma**
  - ➤ Biphasic tumor with hypercellular compact areas (Antoni A) and hypocellular cystic areas (Antoni B)
  - ➤ Verocay bodies: Rows of nuclear palisading
  - ➤ Hyalinized blood vessels, chronic inflammatory infiltrates
- **Malignant peripheral nerve sheath tumor (MPNST)**
  - ➤ Spindled cells arranged in sweeping fascicles
  - ➤ Densely cellular spindle cells in sweeping fascicles
  - ➤ Admixed areas with less cellularity, giving a marble-like effect
  - ➤ Geographic necrosis and/or brisk mitotic activity (>10/10 HPF)
- **Neuroblastoma (NB)**
  - ➤ Undifferentiated small round blue cell tumor, ± Homer-Wright pseudorosettes, neurofibrillary matrix
  - ➤ IHC: (+) Synaptophysin, chromogranin, CD56, neurofilament
- **Ganglioneuroblastoma (GNB)**
  - ➤ Intermediate differentiation
  - ➤ Composed of both neuroblastic cells (small round blue cells) and ganglion cells (large, mature appearing) in a Schwannian background
- **Ganglioneuroma (GN)**
  - ➤ Benign, most mature differentiation
  - ➤ Admixed spindled cells and large mature ganglion cells in a fibrillary stroma

Link   Link   Link   Link   Link

Path Presenter

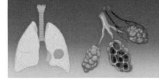
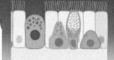
Teratoma with mixture of well-differentiated tissue types

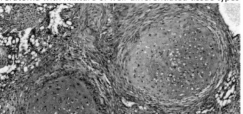

GERM CELL TUMORS
- Associated with Klinefelter syndrome (XXY)
- Morphologically identical to counterparts in the gonads
  - ➤ Teratoma – most common mediastinal GCT
  - ➤ Seminoma – large polygonal cells with background lymphocytes
  - ➤ Yolk Sac Tumor – Schiller-Duval bodies and elevated serum AFP
  - ➤ Embryonal Carcinoma – large primitive appearing cells
  - ➤ Choriocarcinoma – abundant hemorrhage

Reed-Sternberg (RS) cells in Classical Hodgkin Lymphoma

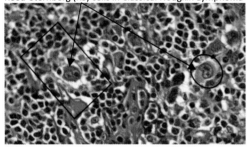

Diffuse growth of large lymphoid cells (DLBCL)

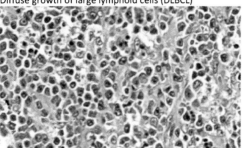

Oval tumor cells, background lymphocytes (FDCL)

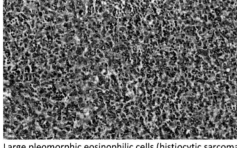

Large pleomorphic eosinophilic cells (histiocytic sarcoma)

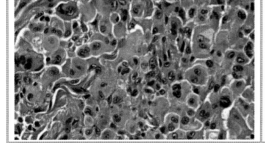

HEMATOLYMPHOID TUMORS
- **Classic Hodgkin Lymphoma**
  - ➤ Most common type of primary mediastinal lymphoma
  - ➤ RS cell IHC: (+) CD30, CD15, MUM1, characteristic weak PAX5
    (-) CD20, CD45
- **Primary Mediastinal Large B Cell Lymphoma**
  - ➤ Aggressive large B cell lymphoma arising in the mediastinum
  - ➤ Diffuse growth of large cells with abundant, often clear cytoplasm
  - ➤ Requires clinical exclusion of widespread extrathoracic disease as morphology and IHC identical to DLBCL
- **T Lymphoblastic Leukemia/Lymphoma**
  - ➤ Medium-sized cells with scant cytoplasm and fine chromatin; numerous mitoses
  - ➤ IHC/Flow: (+) TdT, CD34, CD1a, CD99, CD3
- **Germ Cell Tumor with Associated Hematologic Malignancy**
  - ➤ Coexisting clonally related mediastinal germ cell tumor and a hematologic malignancy, which can be systemic or localized
  - ➤ Can be any type of heme malignancy, often acute leukemia
  - ➤ Very poor prognosis

Link Link Link Link Path Presenter

HISTIOCYTIC AND DENDRITIC CELL TUMORS
- Follicular Dendritic Cell Lymphoma
- Histiocytic Sarcoma
- Langerhans Cell Histiocytosis

THYMIC NEUROENDOCRINE TUMORS
- Rare; classified using the same criteria as in the lung

THYROID AND PARATHYROID TUMORS
- **Thyroid tumors often arise as an extension** from the neck (as opposed to ectopic thyroid tissue)
- Identical histology, IHC, and behavior to the tumor in the neck
- Parathyroid tumors are often formed from **ectopic parathyroid tissue**, usually near the thymus (shared origin – 3rd branchial pouch)

METASTASIS
- Always a consideration
- Lung is most common (also consider breast, esophageal, stomach, etc.)

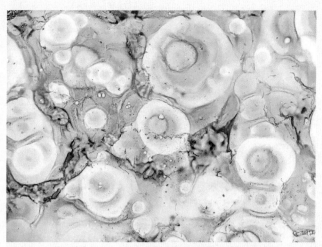

Thick colloid from a Pap-stained FNA of benign
thyroid. Image courtesy: Ziad El Zaatari, MD

CHAPTER 4: ENDOCRINE PATHOLOGY

Maricel Reyes, MD
Vishwajeeth Pasham, MD
Jared T. Ahrendsen, MD, PhD

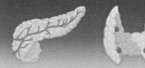
PITUITARY

Sheets of monomorphic cells

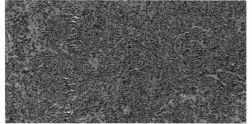

Monomorphic epithelioid neuroendocrine cells

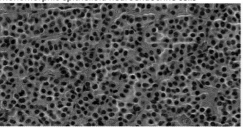

Disrupted reticulin network

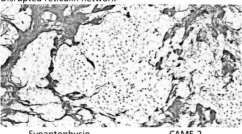

Synaptophysin   CAM5.2

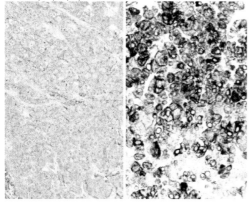

PITUITARY ADENOMA
MORPHOLOGY
- Monomorphic neuroendocrine cells with round nuclei
- Cystic structures can be present, particularly in gonadotroph adenomas
- Gonadotroph adenomas can have clear-cell changes and oncocytic changes
- Variety of histologic growth patterns: diffuse, papillary, trabecular
- Can have eosinophilic or basophilic cytoplasm
- May show perivascular orientation, "endocrine atypia" and occasional mitoses
- Touch prep shows cellular, discohesive, homogenous neuroendocrine proliferation

OTHER HIGH YIELD POINTS
- **Most common tumor of Sella** turcica; usually seen in **adults**
- Neoplasm of anterior pituitary hormone-producing cells (adenohypophysis)
- IHC: **(+) synaptophysin**, chromogranin; (-) S100
- **Reticulin** stain shows disruption of normal network
- Classification by hormone secretion - typically accomplished by **IHC panel**
- **Functional adenomas secrete hormones** - often present early with symptoms/tumor syndrome
- Among functioning adenomas, **prolactin secreting adenomas are most common (up to 50% of all adenomas)**; sex - variable presentation with females having galactorrhea/amenorrhea and males presenting with sexual dysfunction and mass effect
- ACTH secreting adenomas → **Cushing's disease**
- GH secreting adenomas → **gigantism and/or acromegaly**
- Thyrotroph adenomas are very rare but can present with hyperthyroidism
- Silent adenomas do not secrete hormones, but still stain with hormone IHC
- Gonadotroph secreting adenomas are most often clinically silent
- **Non-functional adenomas typically present with mass effect** – compression of optic chiasm leads to bitemporal hemianopsia, diplopia, and headache
- **Most are sporadic**; few associated with tumor syndromes
  - MEN1 syndrome, DICER1 syndrome
- Most common genetic defect in sporadic tumors is **GNAS gene mutations**, found in 40% of somatotroph adenomas
- **Benign**, but can invade adjacent structures
- Tumors can grow into cavernous sinuses, anteriorly into sphenoid sinuses, or invade into bone of sellar floor
- Treatment: Trans-sphenoidal resection with option for pharmacotherapy or radiation

Path Presenter

Mitotic activity and nuclear pleomorphism

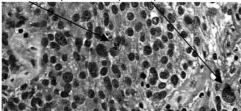

PITUITARY CARCINOMA
MORPHOLOGY
- **Resembles pituitary adenoma by histology and IHC**
- Generally with more mitoses and higher proliferation index; however, these can be relatively low as well
- There are **no morphologic criteria for pituitary carcinoma**; diagnosis is based on metastasis or non-contiguous intracranial spread

OTHER HIGH YIELD POINTS
- Very rare; relatively poor prognosis

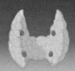 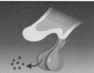
THYROID

Large nodule without distinct capsule

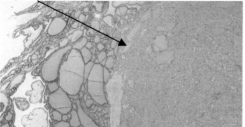

Variably dilated follicles filled with colloid

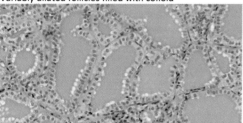

MULTINODULAR GOITER

MORPHOLOGY

- Gross: **enlarged and nodular exterior surface** with gelatinous cut surfaces, occasional calcifications
- **Large nodules with variably dilated follicles** filled with colloid and lined with low cuboidal epithelium
- **Papillary fronds** with basal nuclei are also present
- May have a pseudocapsule, oxyphilia, nuclear atypia, degenerative changes

OTHER HIGH YIELD POINTS

- **Most common disease of the thyroid gland**; presents as multiple nodules
- **Adults** with a wide age range, more common in **females**
- Majority are **asymptomatic** and with **normal thyroid levels**
- **Iodine deficiency** is most common cause worldwide; **autoimmune** etiology (**Hashimoto's thyroiditis**) most common in USA
- **Increased risk (~3.5%) of thyroid cancer**, predominantly follicular variant of papillary thyroid carcinoma

Path Presenter

Lymphoplasmacytic aggregates with germinal centers

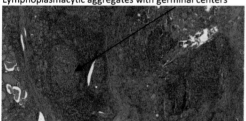

Hurthle cell metaplasia

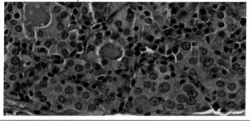

CHRONIC LYMPHOCYTIC (HASHIMOTO'S) THYROIDITIS

MORPHOLOGY

- **Gross: diffusely enlarged, lobulated thyroid gland** with white cut surfaces
- **Lymphoplasmacytic aggregates** with **germinal centers**, Hurtle cell metaplasia, and areas of **fibrosis**

OTHER HIGH YIELD POINTS

- Commonly middle-aged **females**
- Presents as a diffusely enlarged thyroid and variable hyper/hypothyroidism
- May **coexist with other autoimmune diseases**
- **Autoantibodies** to TSH receptor, thyroglobulin, and thyroid peroxidase
- Lab test: Serum antithyroglobulin and antithyroperoxidase (TPO) antibodies
- Increased incidence of lymphoma

Path Presenter

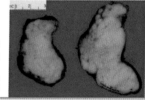

Diffusely enlarged thyroid with white cut surface

Image courtesy of Cory Nash, MS, PA(ASCP)

Papillary infoldings

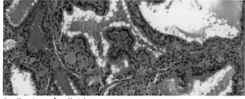

Scalloping of colloid

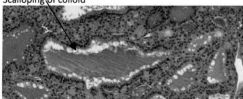

GRAVES DISEASE

MORPHOLOGY

- Gross: Diffusely enlarged, beefy red thyroid
- Hyperplastic follicular epithelium with eosinophilic cytoplasm, papillary infoldings, scalloping of colloid, and a patchy lymphocytic infiltrate

OTHER HIGH YIELD POINTS

- Commonly middle-aged **females**
- **Hyperthyroidism** due to circulating anti-TSH receptor antibodies
- Risk factor: High iodine intake
- Labs: Elevated T3 and free T4, decreased TSH
- Associated with polymorphisms in HLA-DR3 and CTLA-4 gene

Path Presenter

4. ENDOCRINE PATHOLOGY

Nuclear groove | Nuclear clearing

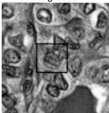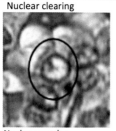

Nuclear pseudoinclusion | Nuclear overlap

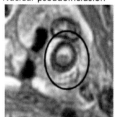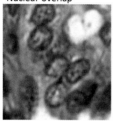

Conventional (classic) PTC with papillae

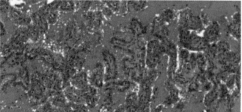

Papillary microcarcinoma (≤1 cm)

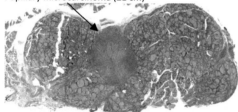

Tall cell variant

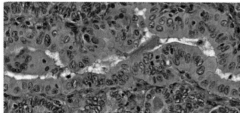

Gross image of Papillary Thyroid Carcinoma

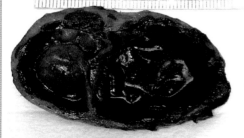

PAPILLARY THYROID CARCINOMA
MORPHOLOGY
- Gross: **ill-defined mass with infiltrative border**; may have gritty areas corresponding to calcifications
- **Papillary or follicular** architectures are most common
- **Nuclear Features:**
  - Nuclear **enlargement** and elongation
  - Nuclear **overlap**
  - **Irregular nuclear contours**
  - Nuclear **pseudoinclusions**
  - Longitudinal **nuclear grooves**
  - **Chromatin clearing**
- **Conventional (classic) PTC**: Papillary architecture with occasional follicular features; frequent **psammoma bodies**; occasional squamous metaplasia; cystic degeneration; densely eosinophilic colloid
- Histologic Variants:
  - **Papillary microcarcinoma**: ≤1 cm; often missed grossly or incidentally identified; malignant but excellent prognosis
  - **Encapsulated**: Completely surrounded by a fibrous capsule (intact or focally infiltrated); excellent prognosis
  - **Follicular**: Exclusively (or almost exclusively) follicular architecture; can be infiltrative or encapsulated with invasion
  - **Tall cell**: Cells are 2-3x tall as they are wide; abundant eosinophilic cytoplasm; must account for ≥ 30% of tumor; more aggressive
  - **Columnar cell**: Rare; columnar cells with prominent pseudo stratification; lacks conventional nuclear features; resembles endometrioid/intestinal adenocarcinoma; IHC (+) CDX-2
  - **Diffuse sclerosing**: Rare; diffuse involvement with sclerosis and solid nests of tumor cells; background lymphocytic inflammation and psammoma bodies
  - **Cribriform-morular**: Mixture of cribriform, follicular, papillary, trabecular, and solid growth with round squamoid structures (morules); frequent vascular invasion; almost always females; association with FAP (nuclear β-catenin); IHC (+) LEF-1
  - Other variants: Hobnail, solid/trabecular, oncocytic, spindle cell, clear cell, Warthin-like, and PTC with fibromatosis/fasciitis-like stroma
- IHC: (+) TTF-1, thyroglobulin, PAX8, CK7, CK19

OTHER HIGH YIELD POINTS
- **Most common type of thyroid cancer** in adults and children
- Usually presents as **painless thyroid nodule** or mass in neck or cervical node, usually cold on scan
- **Female** predilection; often present with **painless thyroid mass**
- Risk factors: **Radiation exposure**, high dietary iodine intake, Carney complex, familial adenomatous polyposis (FAP), presence of benign thyroid disease
- Molecular: **BRAF V600E (most common)**, NRAS, HRAS, KRAS, EIF1AX, TERT, RET gene fusions, copy number alterations
- Prognosis: Overall **excellent prognosis** with a life expectancy similar to general population

Link Link

Path Presenter

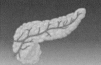 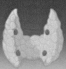
Solid, completely encapsulated nodule

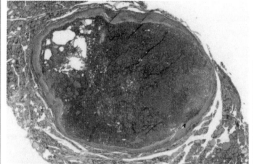

Uniform cuboidal cells lacking PTC nuclear features

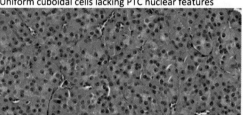

FOLLICULAR ADENOMA
MORPHOLOGY
- Gross: solid encapsulated mass
- **Completely surrounded** by **intact fibrous capsule** (must submit entire capsule to rule out capsular and vascular invasion)
- Cuboidal cells with round, basally located nuclei, **smooth nuclear contours, uniform chromatin** (lacks PTC-type nuclear features, see below)
- Variable architecture but usually one predominant pattern: Microfollicular, macrofollicular, trabecular, insular, spindled, organoid, papillary, etc.
- Variants:
  - Hyperfunctioning – Hyperthyroidism; papillary projections
  - Lipoadenoma – Mature adipose tissue sprinkled throughout
  - Signet-ring cell – Cells with cytoplasmic vacuoles
  - Other variants: Clear cell, spindle cell, black

OTHER HIGH YIELD POINTS
- **Benign**; usually presents as a **solitary painless nodule**
- IHC: (+) TTF-1, thyroglobulin, PAX8
- Molecular: **RAS mutations** most common

Path Presenter

Capsular invasion with mushroom appearance

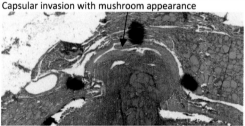

Vascular invasion

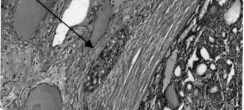

Lacks PTC nuclear features

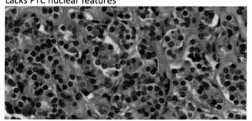

Cytology: Follicular neoplasm

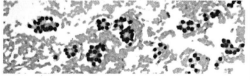

FOLLICULAR CARCINOMA
MORPHOLOGY
- **Lacks nuclear features of PTC**
- Must demonstrate either **capsular or vascular invasion**; cytologic features are otherwise identical to follicular adenoma
- Often surrounded by a thick capsule:
  - For capsular invasion, must **penetrate the entire capsule**, often with a mushroom appearance
- For vascular invasion, tumor cells must be **adherent to vascular wall** either with **covering endothelium** or **associated with a fibrin thrombus**

OTHER HIGH YIELD POINTS
- Presents as an **asymptomatic/painless mass**
- **Risk factors**: Ionizing radiation, insufficient iodine intake
- **Gross**: Tan to brown solid cut surface, can have cystic changes and hemorrhage, permeation of the capsule can be seen grossly
- **Subclassified into 3 groups:**
  - **Minimally invasive** – Capsular invasion only; excellent prognosis
  - **Encapsulated angioinvasive** – Risk of hematogenous metastasis (often bone or lung)
  - **Widely invasive** – Extensive involvement of thyroid and soft tissues, often with prominent vascular invasion
- 4% familial (associations: PTEN hamartoma tumor (Cowden) syndrome, Carney complex)
- IHC: (+) TTF-1, PAX8, thyroglobulin, CK7
- Molecular: **RAS mutations, PAX8-PPAR gamma fusion**
- **Poor prognostic factors**: tumor size greater than 4 cm, distant metastases, age greater than 45 years, large size, extensive vascular invasion, extrathyroidal extension

Path Presenter

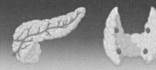
Is that good enough for capsular invasion?
- Most require complete transgression of the capsule; however, some criteria are more lenient
- When in doubt, get multiple deeper tissue levels
- Sometimes, as the tumor grows, it can induce a desmoplastic stromal reaction, inducing a secondary fibrous band:
  - ➢ Look at the gland contour: If the invasive tongue of the tumor extends outside of the usual contour (even if there is a thin capsule), many would consider this invasive

Is that good enough for vascular invasion?
- PTC usually spreads via lymphatics (no RBCs, highlight with D2-40 IHC) to lymph nodes
- Follicular carcinoma spreads via veins (luminal RBCs, use CD31 IHC) hematogenously to lungs/bones
- Vascular invasion must be outside of the tumor: Either in the capsule or beyond
- According to the WHO, tumor cells should be adherent to the vessel wall either with covering endothelium or in a thrombus with fibrin
  - ➢ Newer data suggests that tumor cells within vascular lumina unassociated with a thrombus and tumor cells underlying intact endothelium could represent "pseudoinvasion" given the fenestrated endothelial network of endocrine organs
- Stricter CAP unequivocal definition: invasion of tumor cells through a vessel wall accompanied by fibrin thrombus; correlates more closely with aggressive disease
- *** This example is controversial: WHO criteria say this is sufficient for vascular invasion, but stricter CAP criteria would say negative for vascular invasion

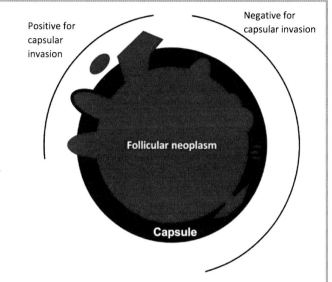

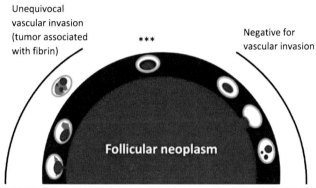

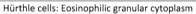
Hürthle cells: Eosinophilic granular cytoplasm

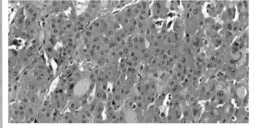

Capsular invasion in Hürthle cell carcinoma

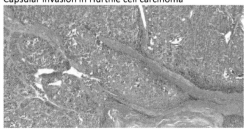

HÜRTHLE CELL (ONCOCYTIC) TUMORS
MORPHOLOGY
- Neoplasms composed of **oncocytic cells with abundant eosinophilic granular cytoplasm**, central nuclei, and prominent nucleoli
- Oncocytic cells **must comprise >75% of the tumor**; otherwise, you can say "Hurtle cell features"
- Variable architecture: Follicular, trabecular, solid
- **Hurtle cell adenoma:**
  - ➢ Essentially a follicular adenoma composed of Hurtle cells; encapsulated and benign
- **Hurtle cell carcinoma:**
  - ➢ Contains capsular and/or vascular invasion (essentially a follicular carcinoma composed of Hurtle cells)

OTHER HIGH YIELD POINTS
- Worse prognosis and has a greater tendency to extend to soft tissue and have lymph node metastasis than follicular carcinoma
- IHC: (+) TTF-1, thyroglobulin, PAX8, cytokeratin
- Molecular: TP53 and PTEN alterations

Path Presenter

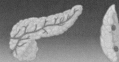 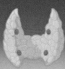 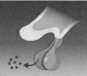
TUMORS OF UNCERTAIN MALIGNANT POTENTIAL

- Some encapsulated neoplasms with follicular architecture can have **questionable capsular/vascular invasion** or **nuclear changes that are mild**, where it is unclear if they are sufficient to justify a diagnosis of papillary thyroid carcinoma
- In such uncertain cases, one can use the diagnosis "**uncertain malignant potential**" (UMP)
  - ➤ E.g., tumor cells invade into, but not completely across, the capsule
  - ➤ E.g., tumor cells are in a blood vessel, but they are not covered by endothelium or thrombus

- **Follicular Tumor of Uncertain Malignant Potential:**
  - ➤ Encapsulated to well-circumscribed follicular-patterned tumor lacking PTC nuclear features with equivocal capsular or vascular invasion (essentially between follicular adenoma and follicular carcinoma)
- **Well-differentiated Tumor of Uncertain Malignant Potential:**
  - ➤ Encapsulated to well-circumscribed follicular-patterned tumor with well-developed or partially developed PTC-type nuclear changes and with questionable capsular or vascular invasion
  - ➤ If invasion is completely excluded → NIFTP (see below)

		Capsular/Vascular Invasion		
		Present	Questionable	Absent
Nuclear features of PTC	Present	Invasive Encapsulated Follicular Variant of PTC	Well-differentiated Tumor of Uncertain Malignant Potential	Non-Invasive Follicular Thyroid Neoplasm with Papillary-like Nuclear Features (NIFTP)
	Questionable	Well-Differentiated Carcinoma, NOS		
	Absent	Follicular Carcinoma	Follicular Tumor of Uncertain Malignant Potential	Follicular Adenoma

Nuclear alteration	Findings
Size & Shape (+1 point)	Nuclear enlargement, overlap/crowding, elongation
Nuclear membrane irregularities (+1 point)	Irregular contours, grooves, pseudo-inclusions
Chromatin characteristics (+1 point)	Clearing with margination, glassy nuclei

PTC nuclear features (enlargement, clearing)

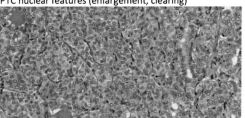

Insular growth

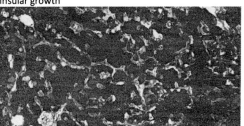

NON-INVASIVE FOLLICULAR THYROID NEOPLASM WITH PAPILLARY-LIKE NUCLEAR FEATURES (NIFTP)

MORPHOLOGY
- Diagnostic requirements:
  - ➤ **Encapsulated** or clear demarcation
  - ➤ Follicular pattern of growth with no true papillae, no psammoma bodies, and <30% solid/trabecular/insular growth pattern
  - ➤ Nuclear features of PTC (score of 2 or 3, see table)
  - ➤ No capsular or lymphovascular invasion (submit entire capsule)
  - ➤ No tumor necrosis
  - ➤ No significant mitotic activity (<3 mitoses/10 high power fields)
- **Nuclear features of PTC are often only partially developed in NIFTP; if they are very well-developed, consider BRAF testing** (present in PTC, absent in NIFTP)

Path Presenter

OTHER HIGH YIELD POINTS
- Very low risk of progressive disease
- Treatment with lobectomy alone
- Molecular: **RAS** mutations (like follicular adenoma/carcinoma); **lacks BRAF V600E** mutation (useful to differentiate from PTC)

POORLY DIFFERENTIATED THYROID CARCINOMA

MORPHOLOGY
- **Turin criteria:**
  - ➤ Carcinoma of follicular cell origin
  - ➤ **Solid, trabecular, or insular growth**
  - ➤ Absence of nuclear features of conventional PTC
  - ➤ **At least <u>one</u> of the following**:
    - o Convoluted nuclei (dedifferentiated PTC nuclear features)
    - o ≥3 mitoses / 10 high power fields
    - o Tumor necrosis

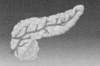 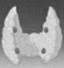
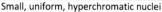
Small, uniform, hyperchromatic nuclei

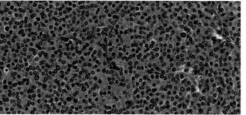

Convoluted nuclei, mitoses
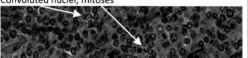

- Tumor cells are small, uniform, and hyperchromatic
- Mitoses common; extensive tumor necrosis can give peritheliomatous pattern

OTHER HIGH YIELD POINTS
- Morphology, genetics, and behavior between differentiated carcinoma (i.e., papillary, and follicular) and anaplastic carcinoma
- Some arise via dedifferentiation of PTC or follicular carcinoma, while others appear to arise de novo
- Often widely invasive into soft tissues and vessels
- Intermediate prognosis

Path Presenter

Malignant spindle cells

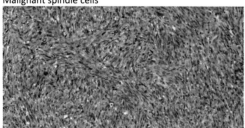

Mitosis   Nuclear pleomorphism
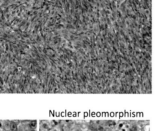
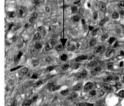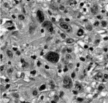

ANAPLASTIC THYROID CARCINOMA
MORPHOLOGY
- Variable histology with **3 primary patterns:**
  - **Sarcomatoid** – spindle cells resembling pleomorphic sarcoma
  - **Giant cell** – highly pleomorphic cells, some with multinucleation
  - **Epithelial** – squamous nests
- Common findings: **Mitoses, necrosis, invasive growth**
- Often with inflammatory cells

OTHER HIGH YIELD POINTS
- Many seem to arise from dedifferentiation of a pre-existing thyroid tumor (history of long-standing nodule)
- Classically, older women with rapidly growing, firm, fixed neck mass → pain, dysphagia, hoarseness
- IHC: PAX8 usually retained; frequent loss of TTF-1, cytokeratin
- Molecular: Frequent TP53 mutations; also, BRAF, PTEN, RAS alterations
- Highly aggressive, very poor prognosis, survival usually < 1 year

Path Presenter

SQUAMOUS CELL CARCINOMA
MORPHOLOGY
- Malignant epithelial tumor with entirely squamous differentiation
- Often extensive infiltration of soft tissue/vessels

OTHER HIGH YIELD POINTS
- Clinical features and prognosis are similar to anaplastic carcinoma
- Notably, both PTC and anaplastic carcinoma can have areas of squamous differentiation, so the tumor should be sampled well to exclude squamous differentiation of another tumor

---

THYROID CARCINOMA IMMUNOHISTOCHEMISTRY

	CK	Thyroglobulin	TTF-1	PAX8	Ki67	P53	Synaptophysin
Normal thyroid follicular cells	+	+	+	+	<3%	Wildtype	-
Well-differentiated thyroid carcinoma	+	+	+	+	<10%	Wildtype	-
Poorly differentiated thyroid carcinoma	+	-/+	+	+	10-30%	Mutant	-
Anaplastic thyroid carcinoma	+/-	-	-/+	-/+	>30%	Mutant	-
Medullary carcinoma	+	-	+	+/-		Wildtype	+

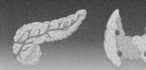

Neuroendocrine tumor with stromal amyloid

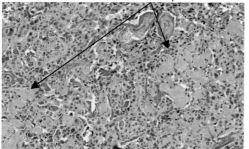

Round nuclei with salt 'n pepper chromatin

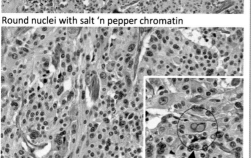

Nuclear pseudoinclusions

MEDULLARY THYROID CARCINOMA
MORPHOLOGY
- Malignant tumor of the thyroid with **parafollicular C-cell** differentiation
- **Wide morphologic spectrum**: Common patterns include solid, lobular, trabecular, and/or insular
- Tumor cells can appear round, plasmacytoid, or spindled
- Nuclei are **round with speckled "salt 'n pepper" chromatin**, occasional pseudoinclusions
- Cytoplasm is eosinophilic to amphophilic and granular
- **Frequent stromal amyloid**
OTHER HIGH YIELD POINTS
- Painless neck mass; lymph node involvement common at presentation; **elevated serum calcitonin**
- Mostly sporadic but associated with MEN2A/B (germline RET mutation)
  - In familial tumors, more likely to be multifocal with C-cell hyperplasia
- IHC: **(+) calcitonin (most specific)**, synaptophysin, chromogranin, CD56, TTF-1; (+/-) PAX8; (-) thyroglobulin
- Molecular: **Frequent RET mutations**; occasional RAS mutations
- Intermediate prognosis

Path Presenter

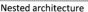

Calcitonin
Image credits:
@Patholwalker

Nested architecture

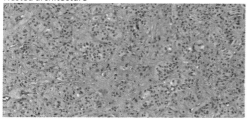

Polygonal cells with granular eosinophilic cytoplasm

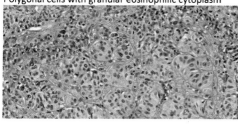

HYALINIZING TRABECULAR TUMOR
MORPHOLOGY
- Solid, well-circumscribed nodule
- **Wide trabeculae** and nests separated into **bundles** by stroma
- Large, **polygonal/elongated cells**; eosinophilic **finely granular cytoplasm**; occasional **perinuclear yellow bodies**
- Round nuclei with vesicular chromatin, **frequent nuclear grooves, inclusions, and membrane irregularities** (can be mistaken for PTC on FNA)
- Cells may be enveloped by **hyalinized PAS-d (+) basement membrane material**
- Absence of capsular, vascular, and parenchymal invasion
OTHER HIGH YIELD POINTS
- Rare, follicular derived neoplasm
- IHC: (+) TTF-1, thyroglobulin; (-) calcitonin; **unique membranes staining with MIB1 (Ki67 clone)**
- Excellent prognosis

Path Presenter

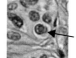 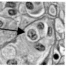

Nuclear groove, inclusion

Mucoepidermoid carcinoma

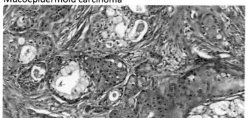

OTHER THYROID TUMORS
- **Mucoepidermoid carcinoma**
  - **Very rare**; favored to represent metaplastic differentiation of follicular derived carcinoma
  - Two cell types: Squamoid cells and mucin-producing goblet cells
  - Occasional MAML2 gene rearrangements
- **Sclerosing mucoepidermoid carcinoma with eosinophilia (SMECE)**
  - Rare; strong female predilection
  - Consistently associated with **sclerosing Hashimoto's thyroiditis**
  - Small nests/strands of **epidermoid cells infiltrating sclerotic stroma** with interspersed mucin-secreting cells

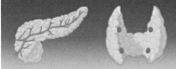
SMECE

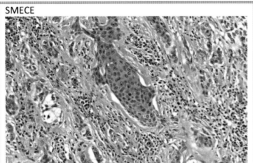

Image credits: Tristan D Rutland MBBS FRCPA (@TristanRutland7)

- ➤ Rich inflammatory infiltrate with **prominent eosinophils**
- **Mucinous carcinoma**
  - ➤ Malignant; extremely rare
  - ➤ Abundant **pools of mucin** with **floating trabeculae/tumor clusters**
  - ➤ **Must exclude metastatic mucinous carcinoma**
- **Ectopic thymoma**
  - ➤ Typical mediastinal thymoma histology
  - ➤ Arises from ectopic thyroid tissue
- **Spindle epithelial tumor with thymus-like differentiation (SETTLE)**
  - ➤ Malignant; intermediate behavior
  - ➤ Highly cellular; lobulated architecture; spindled epithelial cells that merge into glandular structures
- **Intrathyroid thymic carcinoma**
  - ➤ Formerly known as "carcinoma showing thymus-like differentiation" (CASTLE)
  - ➤ Identical to thymic carcinoma of mediastinum

OTHER THYROID TUMORS

- Paraganglioma
- Peripheral nerve sheath tumors
- Hemangioma/Angiosarcoma
- Smooth muscle tumors
- Solitary fibrous tumor
- Langerhans cell histiocytosis

- Rosai-Dorfman disease
- Follicular dendritic cell sarcoma
- Diffuse large B cell lymphoma
- MALT lymphoma
- Teratoma
- Metastasis

PARATHYROID

Chief cells, oxyphil cells, and fat

NORMAL PARATHYROID
MORPHOLOGY
- Three main components:
  - ➤ **Chief cells:** main cell type; round central nucleus, clear to amphophilic cytoplasm
  - ➤ **Oxyphil cells:** large cells with abundant pink cytoplasm
  - ➤ **Fat** and fibrous tissue: divides cells into lobules
OTHER HIGH YIELD POINTS
- Regulates calcium levels with parathyroid hormone (PTH)

Path Presenter

Hypercellular parathyroid without fat

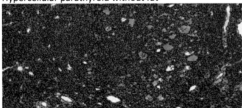

Proliferation of chief cells

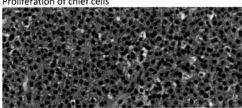

PRIMARY PARATHYROID HYPERPLASIA
MORPHOLOGY
- Increased parathyroid cellularity - **usually chief cells** but less commonly oncocytes and clear cells, **no rim of residual normal parathyroid**
- Can have atypia and occasional mitoses; fat is absent
OTHER HIGH YIELD POINTS
- Usually **all four glands** involved, but can have asymmetric involvement
- Typically, middle aged females with increased serum PTH and calcium, decreased serum phosphate
- Familial cases associated with **MEN1/2A syndromes**
- **Clinical context is key** in differentiating adenoma vs hyperplasia - look at imaging to see if one markedly enlarged gland or negative localization studies

Path Presenter

Well-circumscribed mass

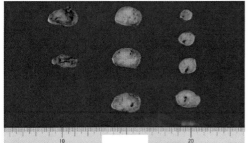

Image credit: Takashi Fujisawa M.D., Ph.D
@Patholwalker

Expanded monomorphic population, no fat present

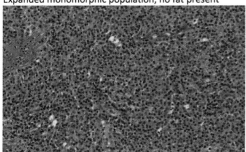

PARATHYROID ADENOMA
MORPHOLOGY
- **Well-circumscribed**, often encapsulated
- Composed of expanded population of **chief cells (most common)**, oncocytes, or a mixture (uncommon)
- Cells have round, central nuclei with dense chromatin
- Can have follicular architecture; rare mitoses and/or pleomorphism
- Unlike normal parathyroid, **no fat present**

OTHER HIGH YIELD POINTS
- **Benign** encapsulated parathyroid neoplasm; relatively **common**
- Usually involvement is limited to one gland
- Often present with **primary hyperparathyroidism** leading to **hypercalcemia** (metabolic bone disease, kidney stones, fatigue, etc.)
- Minority of cases associated with **MEN1/2A**
- IHC: (+) PTH, GATA3, synaptophysin, chromogranin; **Ki67 <4%**
  (-) TTF-1, thyroglobulin, calcitonin; (+/-) PAX8
- **Many variants** - oncocytic, water-clear cell, lipoadenomas (fat and other parenchymal elements)
- May not be able to distinguish on FNA from follicular thyroid lesions
- Remember to **weigh the specimen**!

Path Presenter

Vessel Invasion

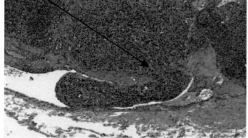

Variable pleomorphism, mitoses

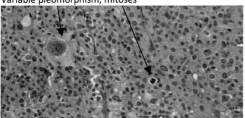

Fibrous band

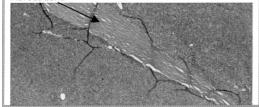

PARATHYROID CARCINOMA
MORPHOLOGY
- Requires evidence of **one of the following**:
  - ➢ **Invasive growth** involving adjacent structures
  - ➢ **Invasion of vessels** in capsule or beyond (attached to wall)
  - ➢ **Metastases**
- Perineural invasion is a helpful feature; variable pleomorphism/mitoses
- Usually subdivided by broad **fibrous bands**

OTHER HIGH YIELD POINTS
- Rare, malignant neoplasm derived from parathyroid cells
- Usually presents with **hyperparathyroidism** and hypercalcemia
- IHC: (+) PTH, GATA3, synaptophysin, chromogranin; **Ki67 <6-8%**
- Association with **hyperparathyroidism-jaw tumor syndrome** (HPT-JT) - inherited condition with hyperparathyroidism and hypercalcemia
- **"Atypical Parathyroid Adenoma"**
  - ➢ Adenomas that exhibit <u>some</u> features of parathyroid carcinoma but **lack unequivocal invasive growth**
  - ➢ **Frequent findings**: fibrous bands, adherence to adjacent structures, tumor within capsule, solid/trabecular growth, nuclear atypia, increased mitoses
  - ➢ Usually, benign clinical course with close follow up

Path Presenter

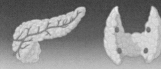

ADRENAL

Nests of lipidized (clear) tumor cells

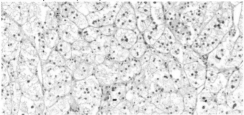

Cords of lipid-poor (pink) tumor cells

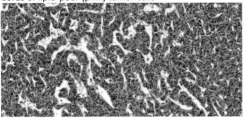

Path Presenter

ADRENOCORTICAL ADENOMA
MORPHOLOGY
- Gross: circumscribed **golden yellow mass**
- Tumor cells can be lipid-rich (clear) or lipid-poor (pink), arranged in nests & cords separated by abundant vasculature
- Occasional lipofuscin pigment
- Nuclei are generally small and round but extreme "endocrine atypia" can be encountered
- Low to absent mitotic activity
- "Spironolactone bodies" (spherical eosinophilic structures) in aldosterone secreting adenomas treated with spironolactone

OTHER HIGH YIELD POINTS
- Benign, very common, often incidental and unilateral
- On a spectrum and may be difficult to differentiate from hyperplastic nodules (more often multifocal and bilateral)
- IHC: (+) SF1, inhibin, Melan-A, calretinin, synaptophysin
  (-) chromogranin, cytokeratin, S100
- Associated with MEN1, FAP, Carney Complex, Beckwith-Wiedemann
- Can be non-functional (85%) or functional (15%)
  - ➢ **Aldosterone** producing → **Conn syndrome:** hypertension and hypokalemia
  - ➢ **Cortisol** producing (ACTH-independent) → **Cushing syndrome:** central obesity, moon facies, hirsutism, poor healing, striae
  - ➢ **Sex-hormone** producing (rare, more common in carcinoma) → virilization or feminization depending on patient's sex

Varied architecture with fibrous bands

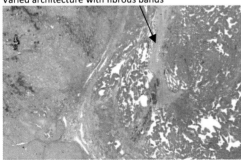

Large nests of oncocytic tumor cells

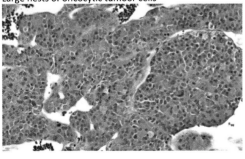

ADRENAL CARCINOMA
MORPHOLOGY
- Gross: lobulated, large tumors that are yellow, orange, tan, or brown with cystic change, hemorrhage, and/or necrosis
- Solid, broad trabeculae or large nested growth (larger nests than adenoma)
- Thick fibrous capsule with occasional fibrous bands
- Frequent tumor necrosis, vascular or capsular invasion, and increased mitotic activity
- Variants: oncocytic, myxoid, sarcomatoid

OTHER HIGH YIELD POINTS
- Malignant, more common in older adults
- Can present as an incidental unilateral mass or with an endocrinopathy
- Mostly sporadic but can be associated Li Fraumeni

Path Presenter

Lobulated tumor with tan-brown cut surface

Necrosis, mitoses

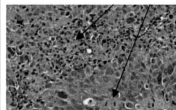

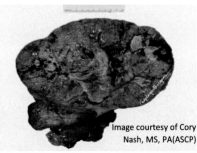

Image courtesy of Cory Nash, MS, PA(ASCP)

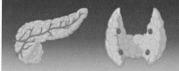

DISTINGUISHING BETWEEN ADRENOCORTICAL ADENOMA AND CARCINOMA
WEISS CRITERIA
- Most widely used system but doesn't work well with borderline cases or variants
- Presence of **≥3 criteria correlate with malignant behavior**
- Cannot be used for oncocytic adrenal neoplasms or pediatric adrenal tumors (see below)
- Features only seen in metastasizing tumors:
  - ≥6 mitoses per 50 high power fields
  - Atypical mitoses
  - Invasion of venous structures

"MODIFIED" WEISS CRITERIA
- Designed to be more reproducible
- Total score of **3 or greater** correlated with malignant behavior

RETICULIN ALGORITHM
- Check intactness of reticulin network; **if intact throughout → adenoma**; if disrupted, then:
- **Malignancy is identified by at least one of the following:**
  - Tumor necrosis
  - High mitotic rate (>5/50 HPF)
  - Venous invasion

Although distinction between adenoma and carcinoma is usually straight forward, in some borderline cases, it may be more appropriate to categorize as **"Uncertain Malignant Potential"**

Although not fitting into the above schemes, Ki67 can be helpful, too. The proliferation index in adenomas is usually <5% whereas carcinomas tend to have a proliferation index >5%.

WEISS CRITERIA (≥ 3 = MALIGNANT)
High nuclear grade (based on Fuhrman criteria)
Mitotic rate >5 per 50 high power fields
Atypical mitotic figures
<25% clear cells
Diffuse architecture
Tumor necrosis
Venous invasion
Sinusoidal invasion
Capsular invasion

"MODIFIED WEISS CRITERIA	POINTS
Mitotic rate >5 per 50 HPF	2
<25% clear cells	2
Atypical mitotic figures	1
Tumor necrosis	1
Capsular invasion	1

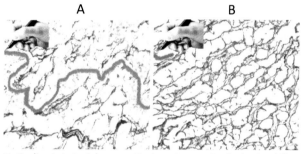

Reticulin stain in Adrenocortical carcinoma, Squiggle sign (A) vs normal staining pattern (B):, image courtesy: Matthew Zaborowski, MD (@Mattzaborowski1)

Lu-Weiss-Bisceglia Criteria	
Major criteria	>5 mitoses per 50 HPF
	Atypical mitotic figures
	Venous invasion
Minor criteria	Size >10 cm and/or weight >200 grams
	Tumor necrosis
	Sinusoidal invasion
	Capsular invasion

ONCOCYTIC ADRENOCORTICAL NEOPLASMS
MORPHOLOGY
- Cells with abundant granular eosinophilic cytoplasm
- >90% of tumor to be considered oncocytic
- Often with areas of nuclear pleomorphism, intranuclear pseudoinclusions, and prominent nucleoli
OTHER HIGH YIELD POINTS
- Mostly non-functional
- Cannot use Weiss criteria, use **Lu-Weiss-Bisceglia Criteria** instead
  - **1 major criteria → Malignant carcinoma**
  - **1-4 minor criteria → Uncertain malignant potential**
  - **No major and minor criteria → Benign adenoma**

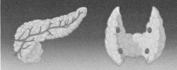
Hematopoietic tissue and adipose tissue

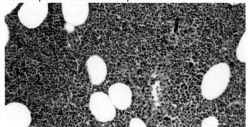

MYELOLIPOMA
MORPHOLOGY
- Composed of **mature fat** and **bone marrow elements**
OTHER HIGH YIELD POINTS
- Benign; second most common adrenal neoplasm
- Often older adult presenting with incidental asymptomatic mass
- Can often diagnose on imaging due to fat content

Path Presenter

Oval mass with gray cut surface and areas of hemorrhage

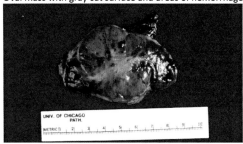

Image credits: Cory Nash, MS, PA(ASCP), Dept. of Pathology, University of Chicago; Used with permission.

Sharply circumscribed mass

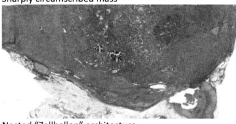

Nested "Zellballen" architecture

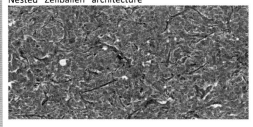

PHEOCHROMOCYTOMA
MORPHOLOGY
- Gross: unicentric round/oval mass, sharply circumscribed with gray-white cut surfaces and areas of hemorrhage
- Classically, **nested ("Zellballen") architecture**; can also show trabecular or diffuse growth
- Polygonal cells with amphophilic to purple cytoplasm
- **Richly vascular**, often with hemorrhage and/or hemosiderin
- Frequent **intranuclear pseudoinclusions** and **intracytoplasmic hyalin globules** (PASD+)
- Nuclear pleomorphism can be prominent but mitotic figures are rare
OTHER HIGH YIELD POINTS
- Tumor of chromaffin cells that arises from **adrenal medulla**
- All are **malignant** but only **~10% metastasize**
  - No current standardized test to assess tumor risk
- Can occur at any age but usually adults
- ~50% are asymptomatic and discovered incidentally
- Can make **catecholamines**
  - Hypertension, headache, tachycardia, sweating
  - Sustained or paroxysmal symptoms
  - Can detect in urine or serum metanephrine testing
- IHC: **(+) diffuse chromogranin** and synaptophysin, **sustentacular S100** and SOX10; (-) cytokeratins, SF1, inhibin, Melan-A, calretinin
- **At least 30% are familial due to germline mutations** (genetic testing is recommended for all patients)
  - Common mutations: SDH, RET, NF1
  - Higher risk of metastasis with SDHB mutations
- Complete resection is only cure; can have metastasis many years later

Path Presenter

PARAGANGLIOMA
- Arise from **extra-adrenal paraganglia**, but **morphologically and functionally like pheochromocytoma** (also frequently hereditary!)
- **Head and neck paragangliomas:**
  - Arise from parasympathetic nerves
  - Most common sites: carotid body and jugulotympanicum
- Generally non-functional and good prognosis (<5% risk of metastasis)
- **Sympathetic paragangliomas:**
  - Arise from vertebral and paravertebral sympathetic chains and sympathetic nerves (mainly in the abdomen)
  - Frequently functional
  - Risk similar to pheochromocytoma; SDHB mutation associated with increased risk of metastasis
- **Composite paraganglioma:**
  - Rare
  - Combined with ganglioneuroma, ganglioneuroblastoma, neuroblastoma or peripheral nerve sheath tumor
  - Most common locations: adrenal, urinary bladder and retroperitoneum

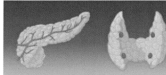
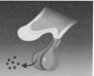
NEUROBLASTOMA	GANGLIONEUROBLASTOMA	GANGLIONEUROOMA
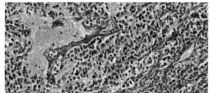	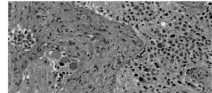	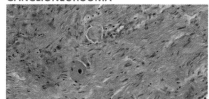

MORPHOLOGY
- Small round blue cells +/- rosettes
- Neurofibrillary matrix without Schwannian stroma
- Most primitive/aggressive
- Malignant

Path Presenter

MORPHOLOGY
- Small round cells (neuroblastoma) intermixed with Schwannian stroma, including ganglion cells
- Intermediate differentiation
- Malignant

Path Presenter

MORPHOLOGY
- Ganglion cells set in abundant fibrillary Schwannian stroma
- No neuroblastoma or neuropil
- Most mature
- Benign

Path Presenter

OTHER HIGH YIELD POINTS
- Derived from neural crest cells. The tumor sites reflect path of migration of neural crest cells. Most common site being adrenal gland, followed by abdominal ganglia, thoracic ganglia, and pelvic ganglia
- Neuroblastoma is **3rd most common pediatric tumor** (after leukemia and brain tumors)
- Most common neoplasm in first year of life; ~**90% occur within the first 5 years of life**
- Neuroblastoma IHC: (+) synaptophysin, chromogranin, PGP9.5, CD56, NB84, PHOX2B
- Ganglioneuroma IHC: Schwann cells (+) S100; Ganglion cells (+) synaptophysin, neurofilament
- **Favorable versus unfavorable histology** is determined by age, degree of neuroblast differentiation, nodular pattern, degree of Schwannian stromal development, and mitotic-karyorrhexis index (MKI)
- Molecular genetics:
  - ➤ **MYCN is a major oncogenic driver; amplification → higher risk**
  - ➤ Whole chromosome copy number gains without structural abnormalities **(hyperploidy) have an excellent prognosis**

COMPOSITE PHEOCHOMOCYTOMA/PARAGANGLIOMA	OTHER HIGH YIELD POINTS
MORPHOLOGY • A pheochromocytoma or paraganglioma combined with a developmentally related neurogenic tumor such as ganglioneuroma, ganglioneuroblastoma, neuroblastoma, or peripheral nerve sheath tumor	• Each component looks and stains like it would by itself • Can occur in the setting of NF1 • If surgically resected, good prognosis

FAMILIAL ENDOCRINE TUMOR SYNDROMES
Multiple Endocrine Neoplasia (MEN) 1 & 2

	MEN1	MEN2A	MEN2B
Gene	Menin, autosomal dominant	RET, autosomal dominant	RET, autosomal dominant
Most common conditions	Parathyroid hyperplasia Pituitary adenoma Pancreatic/duodenal neuroendocrine tumor *Think "3 P's"*	Parathyroid hyperplasia Pheochromocytoma Medullary thyroid carcinoma *Think "2 P's, 1 M"*	Pheochromocytoma Medullary thyroid carcinoma Mucosal neuromas Marfanoid features *Think "1 P, 3 M's"*
Other conditions	Adrenal cortex, thymus, lungs, stomach tumors	Hirschsprung disease	Ganglioneuromas

Often multiple tumors in each organ (e.g., diffuse pancreatic microadenomatosis with several larger dominant nodules)

Familial Paraganglioma-Pheochromocytoma Syndromes
- Caused by mutations in genes encoding subunits of **succinate dehydrogenase (SDH)**
- Autosomal dominant; can see mutations in SDHA, **SDHB (most common)**, SDHC, SDHD, or SDHAF2

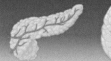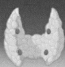

- Immunoreactivity for SDHB is lost in SDH-deficient tumors caused by mutations in any of the subunits → can be used to screen for SDH mutations in paragangliomas, pheochromocytomas, and unusual GISTs and RCCs
- **Most common tumor: paraganglioma/pheochromocytoma**, can be multifocal
- Tumors associated with SDHB mutations are often more aggressive and present at a younger age
- Other specific tumors:
  - ➢ **SDH-deficient Gastrointestinal Tumor (GIST)** – usually occurs in kids or young adults; epithelioid morphology and can be multifocal or plexiform; metastasize to lymph nodes; not responsive to RTK inhibitor therapy (no CKIT mutations!); overall more indolent
  - ➢ **SDH-deficient Renal Cell Carcinoma (RCC)** – eosinophilic cytoplasm with "flocculent" cytoplasm/inclusions; neuroendocrine-like nuclei (round, evenly dispersed chromatin, solid to nested architecture); young age and good prognosis
  - ➢ **Carney Triad** – generally non-hereditary SDHC promoter hypermethylation; paraganglioma + SDH-deficient GIST + pulmonary chondroma
  - ➢ **Carney-Stratakis Syndrome** – paraganglioma + SDH-deficient GIST

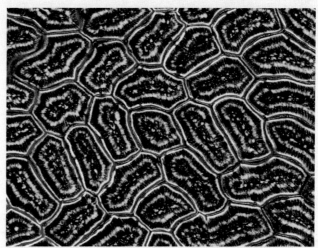

Fluorescence microscopy, intestinal villi. Image
courtesy: Amy Engevik, MD

CHAPTER 5: GASTROINTESTINAL
PATHOLOGY

Upasana Joneja, MD
Manju Ambelil, MD
Satyapal Chahar, MD
Binny Khandakar, MD
Aastha Chauhan, MD

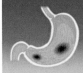
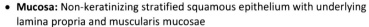
ESOPHAGUS

NORMAL HISTOLOGY
STRUCTURE

- **Mucosa:** Non-keratinizing stratified squamous epithelium with underlying lamina propria and muscularis mucosae
- **Submucosa:** Loose connective tissue containing blood vessels, lymphatics, mucous glands, nerve fibers, and ganglion cells; submucosal glands are connected to the lumen by squamous epithelium-lined ducts
- **Muscularis propria:** Inner circular and outer longitudinal layer of smooth muscles, and myenteric plexus
- **Adventitia:** Loose connective tissue
- **Squamocolumnar junction/Z-line** is the mucosal junction of squamous and columnar epithelium whereas **gastroesophageal junction (GEJ)** between the tubular esophagus and proximal stomach is marked by rugal folds

BENIGN INCIDENTAL FINDINGS

- **Gastric inlet patch:** Heterotopic gastric mucosa in the upper 1/3rd of the esophagus
- **Pancreatic metaplasia/heterotopia:** Benign pancreatic acini and ducts
- **Glycogenic acanthosis:** Epithelial hyperplasia with abundant glycogen accumulation in the superficial squamous cells; endoscopic appearance of solitary/scattered white plaques; extensive involvement of the esophagus may be a manifestation of **Cowden syndrome**

Path Presenter   Path Presenter

Heterotopic gastric mucosa (Inlet patch)

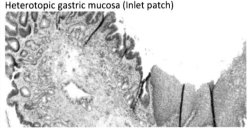

Glycogenic acanthosis

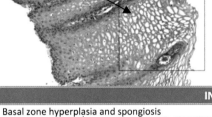

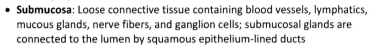
INFLAMMATORY/NON-NEOPLASTIC CONDITIONS

Basal zone hyperplasia and spongiosis

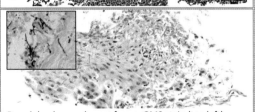

GASTROESOPHAGEAL REFLUX DISEASE (GERD)
MORPHOLOGY

- Endoscopy: Variable findings from normal to erythema/hyperemia to erosion/ulceration depending upon the severity
- Characteristic but non-specific pattern of injury includes intercellular edema/**spongiosis**, **basal cell hyperplasia,** elongation of the vascular papilla, mucosal capillary ectasia, **scattered intraepithelial inflammatory cells** (including eosinophils, lymphocytes, and neutrophils)
- Usually more prominent in the distal aspect near the GEJ

CANDIDA ESOPHAGITIS
MORPHOLOGY

- Endoscopy: **White plaques**, usually easily scraped off to reveal erythematous or ulcerated underlying mucosa
- **Fungal pseudohyphae and budding yeast** forms with squamous debris or active esophagitis or necrosis/ulceration
- Stains with GMS and PAS special stains

Path Presenter

Pseudohyphae and yeast forms, GMS stain (top left)

Herpes Simplex esophagitis (viral cytopathic effect)

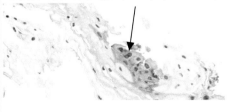

HERPES SIMPLEX VIRUS ESOPHAGITIS
MORPHOLOGY

- Endoscopy: **Shallow ulcers** and vesicles
- Ulcer with necrotic exudate and viral cytopathic effects in the epithelial cells featuring ground glass nuclei due to **margination of chromatin, multinucleation,** and **nuclear molding (3Ms)**

 Path Presenter

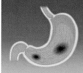

CMV esophagitis (viral inclusions)

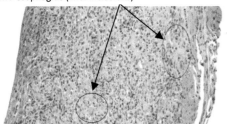

CYTOMEGALOVIRUS ESOPHAGITIS
MORPHOLOGY
- Endoscopy: Erythema, erosions, or **ulceration**
- Ulcer with active esophagitis and viral cytopathic effects in the mesenchymal cells featuring enlarged cells with nucleomegaly and inclusions
- Characteristic **owl's-eye intranuclear inclusions** and **granular intracytoplasmic inclusions**   Path Presenter

Polarizable foreign material (microcrystalline cellulose)

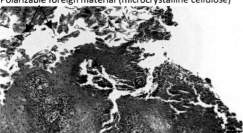

PILL/MEDICATION-INDUCED ESOPHAGITIS
MORPHOLOGY
- Endoscopy: Ulceration
- Ulceration, inflammatory exudate (neutrophils), and polarizable foreign material/ pill-filler material (refractile, transparent **microcrystalline cellulose** and/or purple-pink **crospovidone**)

Path Presenter

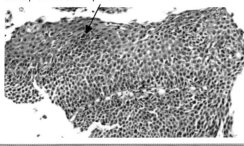

Esophageal 'trachealization"
Intraepithelial eosinophils

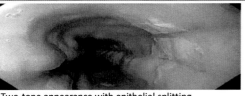

EOSINOPHILIC ESOPHAGITIS
MORPHOLOGY
- Endoscopy: **Concentric rings** or linear furrows (trachealization/felinization), and white plaques or exudates
- Increased intraepithelial **eosinophils (≥15 per HPF)**, eosinophilic microabscesses, superficial concentration of eosinophils with degranulation, and surface desquamation
- Other minor histologic features include basal cell hyperplasia, intercellular edema/spongiosis, elongated papillae, and lamina propria fibrosis

OTHER HIGH YIELD POINTS
- Immune/antigen-driven type 2 helper (Th2) T-cell mediated chronic disorder of children and adults
- **Clinicopathologic diagnosis** based on clinical features (dysphagia, food impaction, and feeding intolerance), endoscopic appearance, ≥15 intraepithelial eosinophils per HPF, and exclusion of other causes of eosinophilia
- Associated with "Atopic Triad" (**Allergies, Asthma, Eczema**)
- Often diffuse involvement of the esophagus/worse proximally

Path Presenter

Two-tone appearance with epithelial splitting

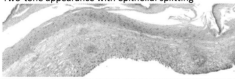

ESOPHAGITIS DISSECANS SUPERFICIALIS (SLOUGHING ESOPHAGITIS)
MORPHOLOGY
- Endoscopy: White plaques of peeling and **sloughing epithelium**
- Characteristic two-tone appearance, **superficial hypereosinophilic/necrotic epithelium with parakeratosis** and underlying viable uninflamed/minimally inflamed deeper layers, reactive basal zone hyperplasia
- Edema and vacuolization of this interface will eventually lead to **splitting** of the squamous epithelium   Path Presenter

OTHER HIGH YIELD POINTS
- Variable associations including multiple medications, autoimmune bullous dermatoses, thermal and chemical injury, heavy smoking, alcohol, and patients with multiple comorbidities

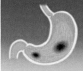

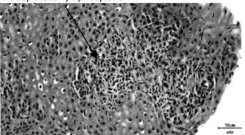

Intraepithelial lymphocytosis

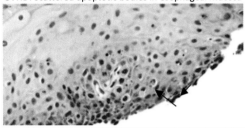

GVHD: Scattered apoptotic bodies in esophageal mucosa

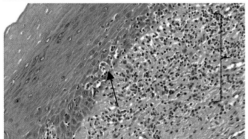

Civatte body (arrow)   Band-like infiltrate

LYMPHOCYTIC ESOPHAGITIS

MORPHOLOGY

- Endoscopy: May mimic eosinophilic esophagitis including rings, furrows, and while plaques
- **Increased intraepithelial lymphocytes** concentrated around dermal papillae
- Associated **intercellular edema/spongiosis** and **dyskeratotic epithelial cells**

OTHER HIGH YIELD POINTS

- This pattern of injury is seen in **GERD, Crohn disease, Celiac disease, achalasia, and other types of dysmotilities, lichen planus, common variable immunodeficiency, and graft-versus-host disease (GVHD)**
- **Lichen planus:**
  - ➤ Intraepithelial lymphocytosis
  - ➤ Band-like (lichenoid) lymphocytic infiltrate at interface between epithelium and lamina propria
  - ➤ Dyskeratotic keratinocytes (Civatte bodies)
  - ➤ Associated with cutaneous lichen planus, medications, viral infections, and rheumatologic disorders
  - ➤ Risk of dysplasia and progression to squamous cell carcinoma has been described
- **GVHD:**
  - ➤ Intraepithelial lymphocytosis with dyskeratotic keratinocytes and scattered apoptotic bodies
  - ➤ Typically presents with rash, diarrhea, and/or elevated liver enzymes

Path Presenter

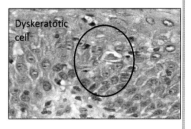

Dyskeratotic cell

BARRETT'S ESOPHAGUS, PRECURSOR LESIONS, AND CARCINOMAS

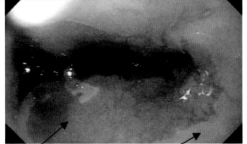

Salmon-colored mucosa   Esophageal squamous mucosa

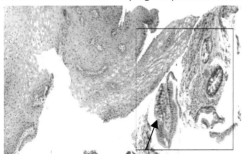

Goblet cells in gastroesophageal mucosa

BARRETT'S ESOPHAGUS (BE)

- **Extension of salmon-colored mucosa into the tubular esophagus extending ≥1 cm proximal to the GEJ on endoscopy, with biopsy confirmation of intestinal metaplasia (defined by presence of goblet cells)**
- Risk factors: Chronic GERD, male gender, Caucasians, central obesity, smoking, and age >50 years
- Pathogenesis: Chronic GERD induced tissue damage→ **Upregulation of columnar transcription factors (SOX9)** induces columnar differentiation→ Upregulation of intestinal differentiation factors (CDX2) → Intestinal metaplasia→ Molecular alterations→ Low-grade dysplasia→ Additional mutations like *TP53* and DNA aneuploidy→ High-grade dysplasia and carcinoma   Path Presenter
- **Alcian-blue/PAS stain**: highlights goblet cells (blue color)
- True goblet cells: rounded/ovoid shape, clear to slightly blue-tinged cytoplasmic mucin, eccentrically located nucleus, and typically randomly distributed

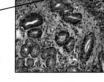

- **Multilayered epithelium**: Immature squamoid cells in the basal layer and superficial acid mucin containing non-goblet columnar cells; considered a marker of GERD and potential precursor to Barrett's esophagus

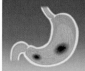

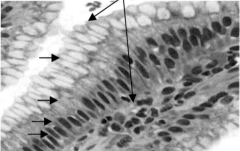

Preserved cell polarity featuring 4 lines

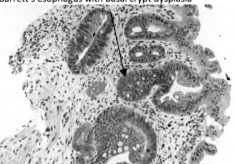

Barrett's esophagus with basal crypt dysplasia

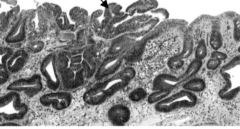

Barrett's esophagus with low-grade dysplasia

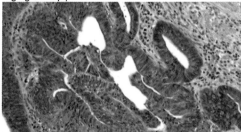

High-grade dysplasia

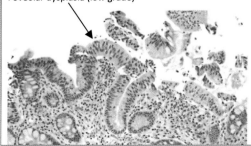

Foveolar dysplasia (low grade)

DYSPLASIA IN BARRETT'S ESOPHAGUS
MORPHOLOGY

Negative for dysplasia:
- Surface maturation and preserved cell polarity showing the four lines (best seen in well-aligned tissue)
  - Apical neutral mucin cap
  - Base of the mucin cap
  - Eosinophilic cytoplasm below the mucin
  - Row of nuclei
- Endoscopic surveillance interval of every 3-5 years

Indefinite for dysplasia:
- Used when it is uncertain whether the changes (nuclear enlargement and hyperchromasia) seen are reactive/reparative versus neoplastic
- Significant inflammation is obscuring the findings
- Technical artifacts and thermal effect on tissues limit the interpretation
- Treat for GERD and repeat biopsy in 3-6 months

Low-grade dysplasia: Adenoma-like or intestinal type
- Cytological abnormality with little or no architectural complexity
- Nuclear enlargement, hyperchromasia, and stratification with retained nuclear polarity
- The findings extend to surface epithelium and often show abrupt transition from non-dysplastic to dysplastic area
- Managed by endoscopic mucosal ablation

High-grade dysplasia:
- Greater degree of cytological atypia often along with architectural abnormality; no surface maturation
- Marked nuclear enlargement, pleomorphism, irregular nuclear contours, loss of polarity, and hyperchromasia
- Crowded crypts with variable size and shape, cribriforming, and back-to-back arrangement

Foveolar (non-intestinal) dysplasia:
- Few, if any, goblet cells
- Typically composed of a single layer of foveolar type columnar cells with prominent cytoplasmic mucin
- Hyperchromatic slightly enlarged nuclei without stratification
- High-grade foveolar dysplasia shows markedly increased nuclear size and open chromatin, prominent nucleoli, and increased mitoses

Basal crypt dysplasia:
- Marked cytological atypia at the base of the crypt that matures at the surface

OTHER HIGH YIELD POINTS
- **Aberrant p53 immunohistochemical stain** expression is considered significant for dysplasia
  - Overexpression: Strong and diffuse positivity in every nucleus
  - Null phenotype: Absent staining

Path Presenter   Path Presenter

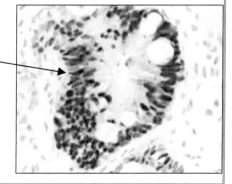

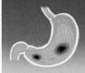

Tubular pattern

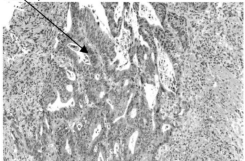

Mucinous pattern

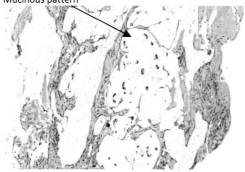

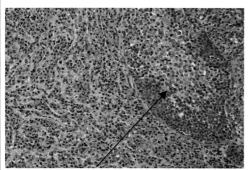

Signet-ring cell pattern

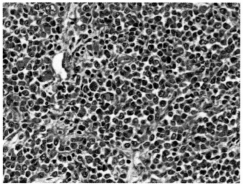

Undifferentiated carcinoma with rhabdoid morphology

ADENOCARCINOMA

MORPHOLOGY

- Gross: Polypoid, fungating, ulcerated or diffuse infiltrative lesions
- Microscopy: Shows gastric, intestinal and mixed lineage with tubular, papillary, mucinous or signet-ring cell growth pattern
- **Tubular pattern**: Most common, characterized by irregular single or anastomosing glandular structures
- **Papillary pattern**: Form papillae, rare cases show micropapillary pattern
- **Mucinous pattern**: Tumor cells float in abundant extracellular mucin
- **Signet-ring cell pattern**: Worse prognosis

OTHER HIGH YIELD POINTS

- Presence of invasive features such as tumor budding (defined as the presence of detached, isolated groups of 1–5 cells) and irregular angulated glands into lamina propria and muscularis mucosae are defined as pT1a or intramucosal carcinomas
- Glandular luminal necrosis, prominent nucleoli, and glands growing parallel to the surface are other features of early intramucosal carcinoma
- Hints that deep invasion is present on mucosal biopsies: Prominent desmoplasia and/or pagetoid extension of carcinoma cells in the squamous epithelium
- Endoscopic resection with or without radiofrequency ablation is the standard of treatment for pT1 esophageal adenocarcinomas that do not show adverse pathological features
- **Adverse pathological features include submucosal invasion (pT1b) to a depth > 500 μm, poor differentiation, lymphovascular invasion, and positive margins**
- **Muscularis mucosae is commonly duplicated** and thickened in the setting of Barrett's esophagus and invasion of this layer should not be misinterpreted as invasion of muscularis propria
- Advanced carcinomas require esophagectomy, possibly after chemoradiation
- **HER2 testing** is done routinely and if amplified is approved for treatment with Trastuzumab
- The immunotherapy agent pembrolizumab has shown promising early results for the treatment of advanced and metastatic esophagogastric junction adenocarcinomas
- It can be difficult to distinguish a poorly differentiated adenocarcinoma from a poorly differentiated squamous cell carcinoma (SCC), particularly in biopsy specimens
- Undifferentiated carcinoma should be considered if the immunohistochemical pattern is equivocal or if there are no definite morphologic features

IHC panel for Adenocarcinoma versus SCC	
Adenocarcinoma	**Squamous cell carcinoma**
CK7+	CK7- (usually)
CK5/6, p63, and p40-	CK5/6, p63, and p40+
PAS and mucin+	PAS and mucin-

Path Presenter

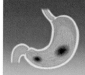

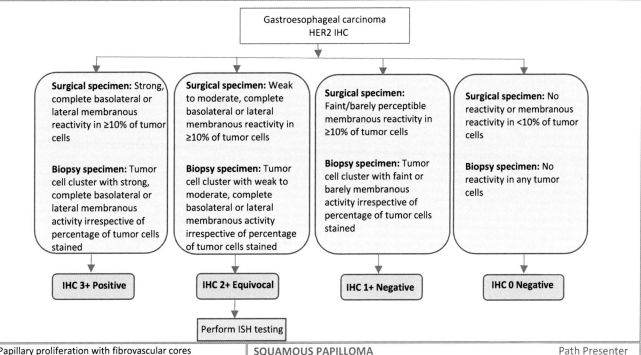

Gastroesophageal carcinoma
HER2 IHC

Surgical specimen: Strong, complete basolateral or lateral membranous reactivity in ≥10% of tumor cells

Biopsy specimen: Tumor cell cluster with strong, complete basolateral or lateral membranous activity irrespective of percentage of tumor cells stained

Surgical specimen: Weak to moderate, complete basolateral or lateral membranous reactivity in ≥10% of tumor cells

Biopsy specimen: Tumor cell cluster with weak to moderate, complete basolateral or lateral membranous activity irrespective of percentage of tumor cells stained

Surgical specimen: Faint/barely perceptible membranous reactivity in ≥10% of tumor cells

Biopsy specimen: Tumor cell cluster with faint or barely membranous activity irrespective of percentage of tumor cells stained

Surgical specimen: No reactivity or membranous reactivity in <10% of tumor cells

Biopsy specimen: No reactivity in any tumor cells

IHC 3+ Positive

IHC 2+ Equivocal

IHC 1+ Negative

IHC 0 Negative

Perform ISH testing

Papillary proliferation with fibrovascular cores

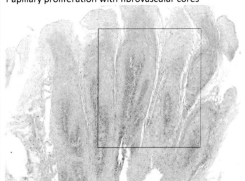

SQUAMOUS PAPILLOMA Path Presenter

MORPHOLOGY

- Gross: Usually small **polypoid lesions** with a warty surface
- **Benign papillary proliferation of the squamous epithelium with fibrovascular core of lamina propria**
- Vacuolated cells with morphological features of **koilocytes** can be seen without atypical nuclear features
- Usually exophytic, but can be flat/endophytic

OTHER HIGH YIELD POINTS

- Result from mucosal irritation, caused by GERD, trauma, or HPV infection, stimulating a hyper-regenerative response
- Typically, in distal esophagus in the US population, but in Asian population more frequently seen in the mid esophagus

---

Low grade dysplasia

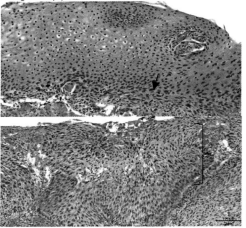

High grade dysplasia

SQUAMOUS DYSPLASIA Path Presenter

MORPHOLOGY

- Gross: Flat lesions are better **highlighted by Lugol iodine solution**
- Diagnosis requires both cytologic and architectural atypia
  - ➤ Cytologic atypia: Nuclear enlargement, pleomorphism, hyperchromasia, loss of polarity, and nuclear overlap
  - ➤ Architectural Atypia: Abnormal epithelial maturation
- **Low-grade and High-grade dysplasia (two-tier)** are the WHO recommended grading system
- **Low-grade dysplasia:** Involvement of the **lower half of the epithelium** only with mild atypia
- **High-grade dysplasia:** Involvement of **more than half of the epithelium or severe cytologic atypia** is present regardless of the extent of the epithelial involvement

OTHER HIGH YIELD POINTS

- Risk factors are similar to those of esophageal squamous cell carcinoma

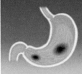

Ulcerated lesion

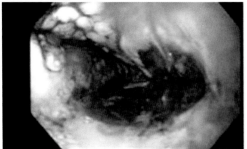

Squamous cell carcinoma with keratinization

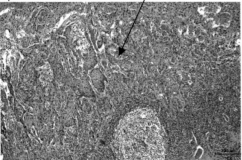

Basaloid squamous cell carcinoma

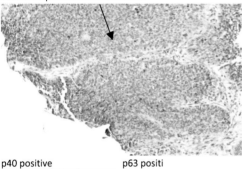

p40 positive   p63 positi

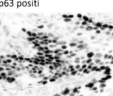

SQUAMOUS CELL CARCINOMA (SCC)   Path Presenter

MORPHOLOGY

- Gross: Exophytic or ulcerated mass lesion
- Malignant epithelial neoplasm showing squamous differentiation characterized by keratinocyte-type cells with intercellular bridges and/or keratinization
- Grading is based on the degree of cytological atypia, mitotic activity, and presence of keratinization

SUBTYPES:

- **Verrucous SCC:** Exceedingly well-differentiated squamous cells with minimal cytological atypia, minimal mitotic activity, surface papillary projections, and invasive front characterized by **broad bulbous pushing projections**
  - ➢ Often arises in the setting of chronic irritation, esophagitis, or previous injury
- **Spindle cell SCC:** Polypoid growth pattern with biphasic pattern of neoplastic squamous epithelium and spindle cells
  - ➢ Squamous elements are usually well to moderately differentiated or may be carcinoma in situ alone
  - ➢ The spindle cell component is a high-grade malignancy, which may show osseous, cartilaginous, or skeletal muscle differentiation
- **Basaloid SCC:** Solid or nested growth pattern of basaloid cells, sometimes with central comedo necrosis and occasionally with pseudoglandular/cribriform formations
  - ➢ Unlike basaloid SCC in the oropharynx, **esophageal one has no association with HPV infection**

OTHER HIGH YIELD POINTS

- Risk factors: Tobacco, alcohol, drinking hot beverages, dietary and genetic factors, medical conditions like Plummer-Vinson syndrome, achalasia, and radiotherapy, caustic ingestion, and HPV infection
- In most cases, HPV appears to be an innocent bystander; viral integration and transcription is uncommon, and the current consensus is that HPV infection is unlikely to be a substantial risk factor
- Accumulating genetic abnormalities drive progression from normal→ low-grade dysplasia→high-grade dysplasia→invasive carcinoma
- *TP53* mutation is a key early driver mutation
- **Tylosis**, an autosomal dominant keratosis disorder caused by a missense mutation in *RHBDF2*, is associated with familial early onset esophageal SCC
- **Epidermoid metaplasia/Esophageal leukoplakia:** Characterized by prominent granular layer with keratohyalin granules, like in epidermis of skin, along with surface orthokeratosis - possible association with squamous dysplasia / carcinoma

STOMACH

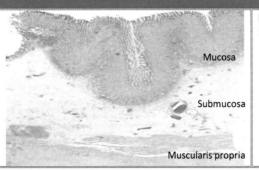

Mucosa

Submucosa

Muscularis propria

NORMAL

HISTOLOGY

- **Mucosa:** Comprised of lining epithelium, lamina propria, and muscularis mucosa
- Gastric pits and deep glands are the two compartments of mucosa
  - ➢ Gastric pits or surface invaginations: Lined by neutral mucin containing foveolar cells throughout the stomach
  - ➢ Deep glands: Vary with anatomic regions
  - ➢ Cardiac and antrum/pylorus: Comprised of mucus secreting glands
  - ➢ Fundus and body (Oxyntic mucosa): Comprised of pink parietal cells that

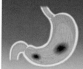
Gastric oxyntic/body mucosa

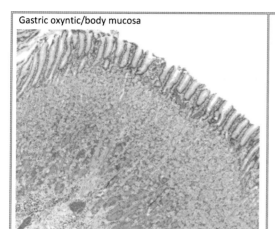

Pink=parietal cells, blue-chief cells

produce acid and intrinsic factor (for B12 absorption) and purple chief cell that produce pepsinogen

- Endocrine cells are present throughout mucosa, but gastrin-secreting **G-cells** are normally found only in the antrum
- **Submucosa:** Loose connective tissue containing blood vessels, lymphatics, nerve fibers, and ganglion cells   Arrows mark the G-cells
- **Muscularis propria:** Inner oblique, middle circular and outer longitudinal layer of smooth muscles, and myenteric plexus
- **Subserosa and serosa:** thin layer of collagen and lining mesothelium

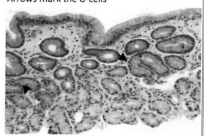

INFLAMMATORY/NON-NEOPLASTIC CONDITIONS

Congested mucosal capillaries with hemorrhage

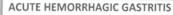
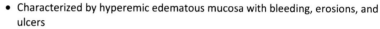

Path Presenter

ACUTE HEMORRHAGIC GASTRITIS

- Characterized by hyperemic edematous mucosa with bleeding, erosions, and ulcers
- Microscopy: **Dilatation and congestion of mucosal capillaries, edema, lamina propria hemorrhage**, and superficial erosions with fibrin and neutrophils
- Usual etiologic factors include severe stress, trauma, shock, binge drinking, caustic agents, large doses of NSAIDs, steroids, and doxycycline

OTHER HIGH YIELD POINTS

- **Fibrinoid necrosis of superficial capillaries can be seen in the setting of doxycycline gastritis**
- Adjacent epithelium may show reactive changes with mucin depletion

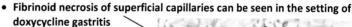
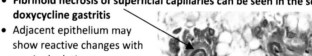

Superficial mononuclear inflammatory infiltrate

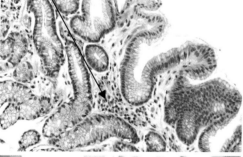

H.pylori immunohistochemical stain

HELICOBACTER PYLORI GASTRITIS (H. Pylori gastritis)
MORPHOLOGY

- Most common treatable form of chronic gastritis caused by gram negative curved rods
- Endoscopy: Varies from erythema, erosions, hypertrophy or atrophic changes
- **Superficial mononuclear (lymphoplasmacytic) inflammatory infiltrate** with prominent lymphoid follicles and musical neutrophils
- Slender curved bacilli are typically seen in the mucin coat of lining epithelial cells and intracellular invasion has been seen in patients who have received proton pump inhibitor therapy (PPI); coccoid forms can also be seen after PPI treatment
- After successful eradication therapy, acute inflammation disappears rapidly, however chronic inactive inflammation persists longer

OTHER HIGH YIELD POINTS

- Commonly colonize the antrum first but can eventually progress to pangastritis→ mucosal atrophy→ intestinal metaplasia→ dysplasia→ carcinoma
- Major **risk factor for development of extranodal marginal zone lymphoma** of mucosa-associated lymphoid tissue

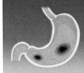

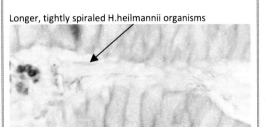

Longer, tightly spiraled H.heilmannii organisms

- *Helicobacter heilmannii* gastritis: Infection acquired from farm animals and household pets, therefore more common in children, histologic findings are similar to H.pylori gastritis but usually less severe
  - ➤ **Longer, more tightly spiraled bacilli** seen in the lumen
Path Presenter

 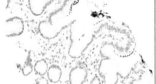

Early phase: Dense lamina propria inflammation and patchy loss of oxyntic cells (see box)

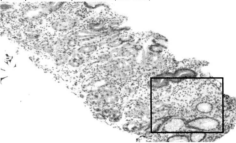

Florid phase: Atrophic oxyntic mucosa with intestinal metaplasia and chronic inflammation

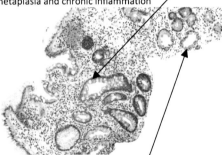

Residual parietal cells

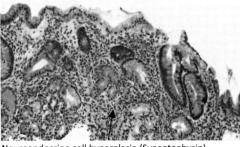

Neuroendocrine cell hyperplasia (Synaptophysin)

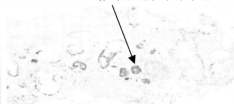

AUTOIMMUNE GASTRITIS
MORPHOLOGY
- Gastric **oxyntic mucosa-restricted** chronic atrophic gastritis
- Associated with circulating **anti-parietal cell** and **anti-intrinsic factor antibodies**
- Antrum may be normal or features reactive gastropathy changes and G- cell hyperplasia
- Endoscopy: Atrophic body mucosa with the absence of rugal folds; hyperplastic polyps can be seen in advanced disease
- Early, florid and end stage are the three pathologic phases identified in the course of disease
- **Early phase**:
  - ➤ Diffuse or multifocal, dense lamina propria lymphoplasmacytic infiltration often mixed with eosinophils and mast cells
  - ➤ Patchy lymphocytic infiltration with destruction of individual oxyntic gland may be seen
  - ➤ Patchy pseudo-pyloric metaplasia and hypertrophic changes of the residual parietal cells
  - ➤ Intestinal metaplasia is rare
- **Florid phase**:
  - ➤ Marked atrophy of oxyntic glands
  - ➤ Lamina propria with diffuse lymphoplasmacytic infiltration
  - ➤ Extensive pseudopyloric metaplasia
  - ➤ Prominent intestinal metaplasia
- **End stage**:
  - ➤ Marked reduction in oxyntic glands, foveolar hyperplasia and hyperplastic polyp formation
  - ➤ Increasing degrees of pseudopyloric, pancreatic, and intestinal metaplasia
  - ➤ Parietal cells are hard to detect, and inflammation is reduced
  - ➤ Linear or nodular enterochromaffin-like (ECL) cell hyperplasia secondary to achlorhydria→ physiologic hypergastrinemia
- Can **progress to intramucosal and invasive neuroendocrine tumors**
OTHER HIGH YIELD POINTS
- Lack of intrinsic factor→ B12 deficiency→ Pernicious anemia
- Gastrin stain can help confirm that sample came from gastric body (negative) and not antrum (positive)
- Synaptophysin and chromogranin stain highlight ECL hyperplasia
Path Presenter

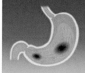

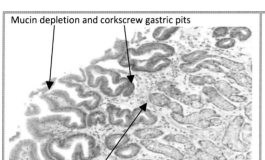

Mucin depletion and corkscrew gastric pits

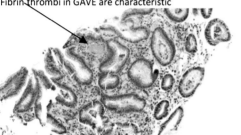

Smooth muscle bands in the lamina propria
Fibrin thrombi in GAVE are characteristic

REACTIVE (CHEMICAL) GASTROPATHY
MORPHOLOGY
- Endoscopy: Mucosal erythema and edema
- **Foveolar hyperplasia (tortuous/corkscrew gastric pits)**
- **Mucin depletion**, edema, and ectatic capillaries
- **Extension of smooth muscle bands in the lamina propria** and minimal inflammation

OTHER HIGH YIELD POINTS
- Often caused by chemical irritation by bile reflux, chronic use of medications like NSAIDs and iron, alcohol or chemoradiation therapy
- **Gastric antral vascular ectasia (GAVE)**: Endoscopic appearance of **watermelon stomach** due to hyperemic mucosal streaks converging on antrum; Overall resembles reactive gastropathy with antral vascular ectasia and **intravascular fibrin thrombi**
- **Portal hypertensive gastropathy**: Occurs in cirrhotic or non-cirrhotic portal hypertension, endoscopically **mosaic or snake-skin pattern** of edematous mucosa, histology like reactive gastropathy with dilated capillaries and veins in mucosa and submucosa   Path Presenter

Increased eosinophils in gastric mucosa

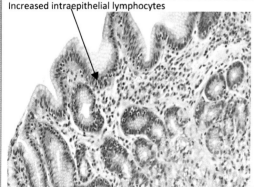

Strongyloides in gastric mucosal biopsy

EOSINOPHILIC GASTRITIS/GASTROENTERITIS
MORPHOLOGY
- Increased eosinophilic infiltration of the gastrointestinal tract (stomach, small intestine, or colon)
- Although there is no established cut-off to diagnose the entity, **>30 eosinophils/HPF in five HPFs** is likely too many
- **Presence of intraepithelial eosinophils with eosinophilic crypt abscesses and eosinophils in the muscularis mucosae and submucosa are abnormal**
- Other associated findings include edema, erosion, reactive epithelial changes, and mast cell infiltration

OTHER HIGH YIELD POINTS
- Etiology is unknown for primary eosinophilic gastrointestinal disorder and is a diagnosis of exclusion
- Secondary gastric tissue eosinophilia is seen in food allergies, H. pylori, parasitic (*Strongyloides* and *Anisakis* spp.) infections, medications, inflammatory bowel disease, and connective tissue diseases/vasculitis

Path Presenter

Increased intraepithelial lymphocytes

LYMPHOCYTIC GASTRITIS   Path Presenter

- Chronic gastritis characterized by increased numbers of mature **intraepithelial (surface and foveolar) lymphocytes**
- Endoscopy: Varies from normal to mucosal nodularity with erosions (varioliform gastritis)
- **Increased intraepithelial lymphocytes (> 25 per 100 epithelial cells),** along with mixed lymphoplasmacytic infiltration of lamina propria
- Lack of lymphoepithelial lesions

OTHER HIGH YIELD POINTS
- Associated with celiac disease, H. pylori infection, HIV, medications (Ticlopidine, Immune-check point inhibitors, NSAIDs), Crohn disease, Ménétrier disease, and lymphocytic and collagenous colitis

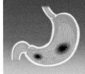

Thickened subepithelial collagen layer

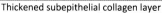

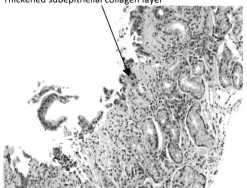

COLLAGENOUS GASTRITIS
MORPHOLOGY
- **Diffuse or patchy thickened subepithelial collagen band (trichrome+)**, having a thickness of **> 10 μm, often with entrapped inflammatory cells and capillaries** in the collagen band; other findings include increased intraepithelial lymphocytosis and lamina propria lymphoplasmacytic infiltration with intermixed eosinophils

OTHER HIGH YIELD POINTS
- Pediatric patients and young adults usually present with anemia, upper GI symptoms, and disease related to gastric mucosa
- Adults may present with associated collagenous/lymphocytic colitis, celiac disease, and lymphocytic gastritis

Path Presenter

Gastric mucosal granuloma

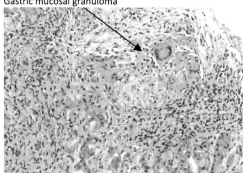

GRANULOMATOUS GASTRITIS
MORPHOLOGY
- Histologic pattern of disease entity characterized by multiple gastric mucosal granulomas
- Number, location, and type of granuloma are variable depending upon the etiology

OTHER HIGH YIELD POINTS
- Usual etiologies include **infections (tuberculosis, fungal, parasitic), systemic conditions (sarcoidosis, Crohn's disease, common variable immunodeficiency, rarely Langerhans cell histiocytosis), foreign bodies, and lymphoma**

Path Presenter

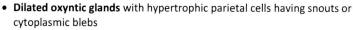

PROTON PUMP INHIBITOR THERAPY EFFECT
MORPHOLOGY
- **Dilated oxyntic glands** with hypertrophic parietal cells having snouts or cytoplasmic blebs

OTHER HIGH YIELD POINTS
- Associated with any type of proton pump inhibitor use
- Increases gastrin levels through feedback, causing parietal cell hypertrophy
- Long term therapy may lead to fundic gland polyps

Path Presenter

Thickened folds characterized by marked foveolar hyperplasia

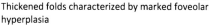

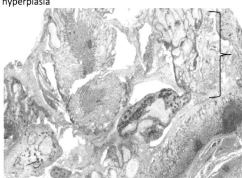

MÉNÉTRIER DISEASE
MORPHOLOGY
- Hyperplastic gastropathy characterized by thickened body/fundus folds, low acid production, and **protein-losing enteropathy**
- **Marked foveolar hyperplasia** with tortuous gastric pits and cystically dilated atrophic glands
- Lamina propria with edema and variable inflammation

OTHER HIGH YIELD POINTS
- Pathogenetic mechanisms include increased signaling of epidermal growth factor (EGFR) and viral infections

Path Presenter

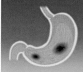

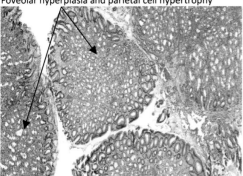
Foveolar hyperplasia and parietal cell hypertrophy

ZOLLINGER-ELLISON SYNDROME   Path Presenter

MORPHOLOGY
- Gastric mucosal hypertrophy and increased acid secretion caused by serum hypergastrinemia due to pancreatic or duodenal neuroendocrine tumor (Gastrinoma)
- Enlarged gastric body/fundus mucosal folds and duodenal ulcers
- Foveolar hyperplasia with dilated oxyntic glands and parietal cell hypertrophy; can progress to secondary ECL-cell hyperplasia, dysplasia, and gastric neuroendocrine tumors

OTHER HIGH YIELD POINTS
- Can develop in the setting of **multiple endocrine neoplasia (MEN)-type 1 syndrome**

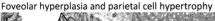
BENIGN/PRECURSOR NEOPLASMS AND MALIGNANCIES

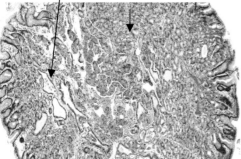
Cystically dilated oxyntic glands

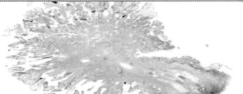
Fundic gland polyp with low grade dysplasia

FUNDIC GLAND POLYPS

MORPHOLOGY
- Benign hyperplastic expansion of deep oxyntic mucosa with **cystically dilated oxyntic glands** and parietal cell hyperplasia
- Foveolar hyperplasia can be seen
- **Most common type of gastric polyp, usually sporadic, and often associated with PPI use**
- Presence of numerous polyps in a young patient should raise the possibility of a polyposis syndrome

OTHER HIGH YIELD POINTS
- Associated polyposis syndromes include **familial adenomatous polyposis (FAP), Zollinger-Ellison syndrome, and gastric adenocarcinoma and proximal polyposis of the stomach (GAPPS)**
- Sporadic polyps are devoid of *APC* mutations but can have mutations in *CTNNB1* (encoding β-catenin)
- Polyps in the setting of FAP and GAPPS harbor *APC* mutations and have increased incidence of dysplasia
- Even in FAP-associated fundic gland polyps, adenocarcinoma and high-grade dysplasia are rare
- Dysplasia in sporadic polyps is rare (<1%)   Path Presenter

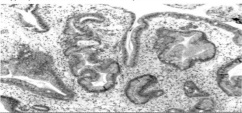
Hyperplastic surface foveolar epithelium

GASTRIC HYPERPLASTIC POLYPS   Path Presenter

MORPHOLOGY
- Benign epithelial lesions featuring elongated, tortuous, **hyperplastic foveolar epithelium** and **cystically dilated glands** (not lined by two-cell types)
- Stromal edema, inflammation, and surface erosions are often seen
- Small, haphazardly distributed smooth muscle bundles extending to the surface may be present

OTHER HIGH YIELD POINTS
- Second most common gastric polyp and arises as a hyperproliferative response to tissue injury
- Polypoid foveolar hyperplasia is regarded as a precursor to gastric hyperplastic polyps
- There is a strong association with **chronic gastritis, including H. pylori gastritis and post-gastrectomy gastritis**

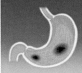

Pyloric adenoma: high power magnification

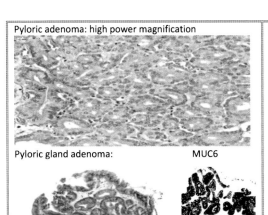

Pyloric gland adenoma: MUC6

MUC5AC

PYLORIC GLAND ADENOMA (PGA)
MORPHOLOGY
- Polypoid proliferation of closely packed pyloric-type glands, lined by cuboidal to low-columnar epithelial cells
- Cells feature clear or lightly eosinophilic ground-glass cytoplasm with basally located nuclei and lack well-formed apical mucin cap
- PGAs can develop high-grade dysplasia and adenocarcinomas
- IHC: Diffuse MUC6 and variable MUC5AC expression

OTHER HIGH YIELD POINTS
- Sporadic cases are associated with **autoimmune atrophic gastritis**
- Can also arise in polyposis syndromes like **FAP, GAPPS, McCune–Albright syndrome, juvenile polyposis,** and **Lynch syndrome**
- Both sporadic and FAP–associated PGAs feature activating *GNAS* and/or *KRAS* mutations and **inactivating *APC* mutations**

Path Presenter

IHC images courtesy of Dr. Maryam Pezhouh; used with permission

---

Low-grade dysplasia in the background of intestinal metaplasia

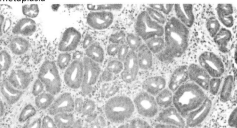

High-grade dysplasia

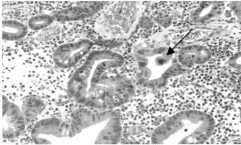

Indefinite for dysplasia

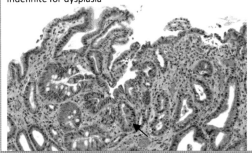

GASTRIC DYSPLASIA
MORPHOLOGY
- Neoplastic change of gastric epithelium without stromal invasion
- Subtypes recognized include intestinal-type, foveolar/gastric-type, gastric pit/crypt dysplasia, and serrated dysplasia
- Endoscopically appear as flat, depressed, or polypoid lesion
- Graded as low-grade or high-grade, based on degree of nuclear atypia, mitotic activity, cytoplasmic differentiation, and architectural distortion

Low-grade	High-grade
Relatively preserved architecture	Complex architecture with back-to-back glands and marked distortion
Nuclei maintain polarity (basally located) Intestinal - type: hyperchromatic, elongated (cigar-shaped) nuclei Foveolar - type: round to oval nuclei	Loss of nuclear polarity (atypical nuclei extends to the luminal surface) Enlarged nuclei with a high nuclear to cytoplasmic ratio, sometimes prominent nucleoli

OTHER HIGH YIELD POINTS
- Risk factors: **H. pylori (most common),** smoking, radiation exposure, and occupation in rubber manufacturing
- Indefinite for dysplasia: Not a biologic entity; used when there are questions as to if a lesion is neoplastic or reactive
  - ➢ Often applied for biopsies with marked inflammation
- Intramucosal carcinoma: Neoplasm that invades lamina propria or muscularis mucosae and is characterized by glandular crowding, excessive branching, and budding
  - ➢ Helpful findings to look for include single-cell infiltration, trabecular growth, intraglandular necrotic debris, and irregular gland fusions

Path Presenter

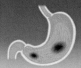

5. GASTROINTESTINAL PATHOLOGY

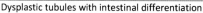
Dysplastic tubules with intestinal differentiation

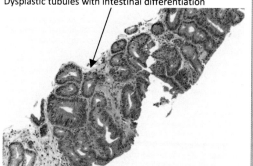

INTESTINAL-TYPE GASTRIC ADENOMA

- Localized polypoid lesion with **dysplastic intestinal-type epithelium**
- Polypoid dysplastic tubules lined by columnar epithelium showing intestinal differentiation (like colorectal adenomas) with varying degrees of Paneth and goblet cells
- Risk factors include **any cause of gastric intestinalization (e.g., H. pylori and autoimmune gastritis)** and genetic syndromes
- Third most common type of gastric polyp
- Intestinal type gastric adenoma is more prone to progress to gastric cancer than foveolar-type gastric adenoma   Path Presenter

Dysplastic foveolar epithelum with mucin-cap

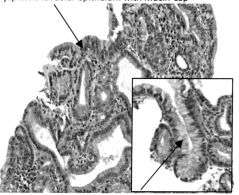

Mucin-cap (differentiating feature)

FOVEOLAR-TYPE ADENOMA   Path Presenter

MORPHOLOGY

- Polypoid lesion with dysplastic foveolar epithelium, mostly occurs in the oxyntic compartment (body/fundus)
- Dysplastic foveolar-type epithelium shows stratified nuclei and a **distinctive PAS-positive apical neutral mucin cap**
- Background gastric mucosa is usually without inflammation, atrophy, or metaplasia

OTHER HIGH YIELD POINTS

- **Usually syndrome associated like FAP and GAPPS**; may coexist with fundic gland polyps and pyloric gland adenomas, and their **rate of cancer progression is consistently low**
- Foveolar-type adenoma with hybrid phenotype (both intestinal and gastric differentiation) carries a higher risk of cancer progression

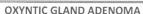
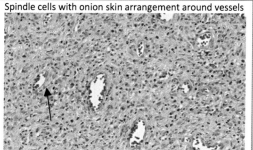
Polyp composed of chief cells only in the gastric body
Image courtesy of Dr. Adam L. Booth @ALBoothMD

OXYNTIC GLAND ADENOMA   Path Presenter

MORPHOLOGY

- Benign gastric neoplasm composed of columnar cells with pale basophilic cytoplasm and mild nuclear atypia, **mimicking oxyntic glands (mainly chief cells)**
- Occurs predominantly in the upper 1/3rd of the stomach and there is a high risk of progression to adenocarcinoma (gastric adenocarcinoma of fundic-gland type)
- IHC: **(+)** Pepsinogen I and MUC6 (chief cell) and H+/K+ ATPase (parietal cell); **(-)** MUC5AC

OTHER HIGH YIELD POINTS

- Missense or nonsense mutations in the **WNT/β-catenin signaling pathway** are seen

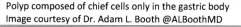
Spindle cells with onion skin arrangement around vessels

INFLAMMATORY FIBROID POLYP
MORPHOLOGY

- Benign lesion occurs throughout the gastrointestinal tract, **most commonly in the stomach**
- Characterized by **submucosal** proliferation of vascular fibrous tissue
- Bland spindle cells with characteristic **onion skin arrangement around small vessels**
- **Eosinophil rich** inflammatory infiltrate
- Edematous background
- IHC: **(+) expression for CD34** and consistently **(-)** for CD117

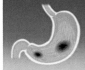

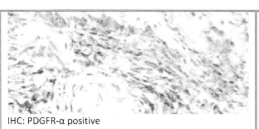

IHC: PDGFR-α positive

- Associated with **mutations in platelet-derived growth factor receptor-α (*PDGFRA*) gene** and PDGFR-α protein expression
- Good prognosis

Path Presenter

Onion skin arrangement

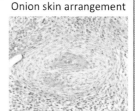

Bland foamy histiocytes in lamina propria

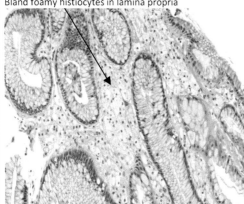

GASTRIC XANTHOMA

MORPHOLOGY

- Collection of bland **foamy histiocytes** in the lamina propria without mitotic activity and background inflammation
- Endoscopy: Single or multiple while/yellow nodule(s)
- IHC: (+) **CD68** and (-) for cytokeratin

OTHER HIGH YIELD POINTS

- Associated with H. Pylori infection, bile reflux, and **hypercholesterolemia**

Path Presenter

CD68

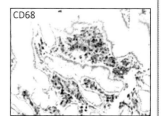

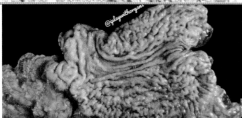

Diffuse-type gastric cancer: Image credit: Cory Nash

GASTRIC ADENOCARCINOMA

MORPHOLOGY

- Malignant epithelial neoplasm with invasion of lamina propria or beyond
- Early gastric carcinoma has three macroscopic subtypes

Type 0-I (Protruding)	Polypoid lesions
Type 0-IIa (Superficial elevated)	Slightly elevated/protruding
Type 0-IIb (Superficial flat)	No elevation or depression
Type 0-IIc (Superficial depressed)	Slightly depressed lesions
Type 0-III (Excavated)	Deeply depressed lesions

- Advanced gastric carcinoma is subtyped according to Borrmann classification
  - As localized growth with a fungating or ulcerated appearance or
  - As infiltrative growth with or without ulceration
- Linitis plastica or scirrhous carcinoma: Infiltrative growth with abundant fibrous stroma reaction resulting in thickened and rigid stomach wall
- Among the several histopathological classifications, Laurén and WHO classification are the widely accepted ones
- **Five main WHO histological subtypes** include: tubular, papillary, poorly cohesive (including signet-ring cell and other subtypes), mucinous, and mixed adenocarcinomas
- **Tubular adenocarcinoma:** Most common subtype, composed of dilated or slit-like branching tubules of variable diameter
  - Tumors with solid structures and barely recognizable tubules are classified as poorly differentiated tubular (solid) carcinoma
- **Poorly cohesive carcinoma (including signet-ring cell carcinoma and non-signet ring cell type):** Second most common type, composed of neoplastic cells that are isolated or arranged in small aggregates without well-formed glands
  - **Signet-ring cell type:** Composed predominantly or exclusively of signet-ring cells, which are characterized by a central, optically clear, globoid droplet of cytoplasmic mucin with an eccentric nucleus

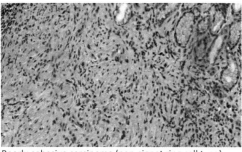

Poorly cohesive carcinoma (non-signet ring cell type)

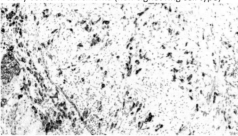

Cytokeratin IHC highlights tumor cells

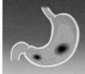

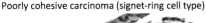
Poorly cohesive carcinoma (signet-ring cell type)

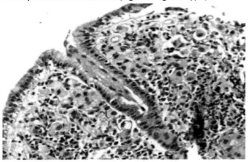
Tubular adenocarcinoma (gland-forming)

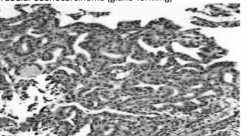
Mucinous adenocarcinoma

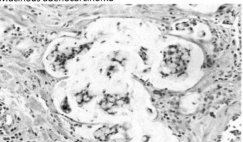
Adenocarcinoma with lymphoid stroma (EBER ISH)

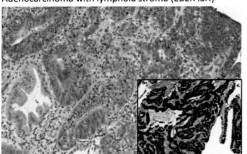
Micropapillary carcinoma

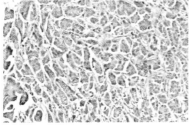
Path Presenter

- ➢ **Non-signet ring cell type:** Composed of neoplastic cells resembling histiocytes or lymphocytes with deeply eosinophilic cytoplasm and pleomorphic nuclei
- **Mucinous adenocarcinoma:** Composed of malignant epithelium in extracellular mucin pools, with the latter accounting for > 50% of the tumor area; tumor cells may be in glands/tubules or single cells
- **Papillary adenocarcinoma:** Relatively rare subtype; shows an exophytic growth pattern with elongated finger-like processes lined by cuboidal or columnar cells supported by fibrovascular cores
  - ➢ Well-differentiated tumor with a pushing invasion and frequent infiltration by inflammatory cells
  - ➢ Associated with a higher frequency of liver metastasis and poor prognosis
- **Mixed adenocarcinoma:** Contains two or more distinct histological subtypes; often have a poorer prognosis than those with only one component
- **(Adeno)carcinoma with lymphoid stroma:** Also known as lymphoepithelioma-like carcinoma or medullary carcinoma
  - ➢ Characterized by irregular sheets, or ill-defined tubules, or syncytia of polygonal cells embedded in prominent lymphocytic infiltrate
  - ➢ Predilection for proximal stomach or gastric stump and often **EBV-associated** (better prognosis)
  - ➢ A subset of gastric carcinomas with **microsatellite instability (MSI)** have similar histological phenotype (better prognosis)
- **Hepatoid adenocarcinoma and related entities:** Composed of large polygonal eosinophilic hepatocyte-like neoplastic cells
  - ➢ Bile and PAS-D positive intracytoplasmic eosinophilic globules can be seen; **(+)** for AFP and HepPar-1
  - ➢ Other alpha-fetoprotein producing adenocarcinomas include papillary or tubular-type with clear cytoplasm, adenocarcinoma with enteroblastic differentiation, and yolk-sac tumor-like carcinoma
- **Micropapillary adenocarcinoma:** small clusters of tumor cells without fibrovascular cores protruding into clear spaces
  - ➢ Worse prognosis like micropapillary carcinomas in other organs
  - ➢ Proportion of micropapillary component required for the classification is not established
- **Gastric adenocarcinoma of fundic-gland type:** Very rare and assumed to develop from oxyntic gland adenoma
  - ➢ Three subcategories: chief cell-predominant (~99% of reported cases), parietal cell-predominant, and mixed phenotype
- By **Laurén classification:** Tumors are categorized as intestinal (tubular and papillary type in WHO), diffuse (poorly cohesive signet-ring cell and other type in WHO), and mixed type

OTHER HIGH YIELD POINTS

- Environmental risk factors include *H. pylori* (a strong risk factor which follows Correa's cascade: chronic infection→ chronic inflammation → intestinal metaplasia → dysplasia → carcinoma), EBV infection, tobacco smoking, and dietary factors
- Carcinoma involving the gastroesophageal junction with center ≤2 cm into the proximal stomach should be staged as esophageal cancer
- Predictive biomarkers: **Anti-ERBB2 (HER2) therapy** benefits patients with unresectable or metastatic/recurrent ERBB2-positive carcinomas and **PD-L1 expression** is a biomarker of response to immune checkpoint inhibitor therapy

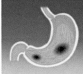

GASTRIC ADENOCARCINOMA

- Familial/hereditary setting includes **CDH1 mutations in hereditary diffuse gastric cancer** and **APC exon 1B mutations in gastric adenocarcinoma and proximal polyposis of the stomach (GAPPS)**
- Four molecular subtypes are proposed by The Cancer Genome Atlas (TCGA):

EBV (~9%)	Microsatellite Unstable (~22%)	Genomically Stable (~20%)	Chromosomally Unstable (~50%)
Gastric carcinoma with lymphoid stroma Associated with CpG island (CIMP) and *CDKN2A* promoter hypermethylation pathway Frequent *PIK3CA* and *ARID1A* mutations PD-L1 and PD-L2 amplified Better prognosis	Associated with MLH1, CpG island (CIMP), and *CDKN2A* promoter hypermethylation pathway Better prognosis	Poorly cohesive (diffuse) morphology Overall fewer copy number alterations, however, frequent *CDH1* and *RHOA* alterations/mutations Poor prognosis	Predominantly intestinal type morphology Frequent *TP53* mutations and amplifications of receptor tyrosine kinase (RTK) Extensive DNA copy number variations

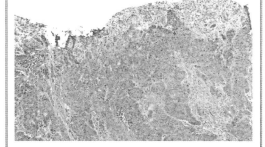

GASTRIC SQUAMOUS CELL CARCINOMA
MORPHOLOGY
- Malignant epithelial neoplasm with squamous cell differentiation, characterized by keratinocyte cells with intercellular bridges and/or keratinization

OTHER HIGH YIELD POINTS
- Very rare; **extension from lower esophageal squamous cell carcinoma needs to be ruled out**
- Frequently presents at an advanced stage and is associated with poor outcome

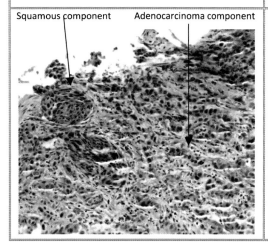

Squamous component   Adenocarcinoma component

GASTRIC ADENOSQUAMOUS CARCINOMA
MORPHOLOGY
- Primary gastric carcinoma composed of both **glandular and squamous cell components, with the squamous component constituting ≥ 25% of the tumor**
- Mucins stain: highlights glandular differentiation, p63/p40 stain helps determine the presence and extent of squamous cell component

OTHER HIGH YIELD POINTS
- Very rare tumor
- Males more commonly affected (>60 years of age)
- Generally aggressive; tumor metastasis to regional lymph nodes, liver, and peritoneum is common

Path Presenter

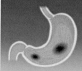

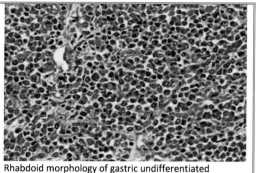

Rhabdoid morphology of gastric undifferentiated carcinoma

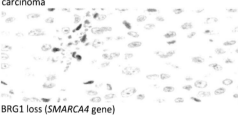

BRG1 loss (*SMARCA4* gene)

GASTRIC UNDIFFERENTIATED CARCINOMA
MORPHOLOGY
- Primary gastric carcinoma composed of anaplastic cells without specific cytological or architectural type of differentiation
- Diffuse sheets of anaplastic cells with variable cytology including polygonal, rhabdoid, spindled, sarcomatoid, carcinoma with osteoclast-like giant cells or carcinoma with lymphoepithelioma-like features
  - A glandular component may be observed and can vary from minimal to prominent; this suggests an origin via dedifferentiation
- IHC: **Variable** expression of pan-cytokeratin and consistent expression of vimentin; EMA may be helpful in keratin-poor tumor

OTHER HIGH YIELD POINTS
- Probably driven by various components of the **SWI/SNF chromatin-remodeling complex**
- Aggressive tumors; must rule out EBV-associated carcinoma with lymphoid stroma, aggressive lymphomas, melanoma, germ cell neoplasms, and sarcomas with epithelioid pattern

<u>Path Presenter</u>

Well-differentiated NET-Type 1

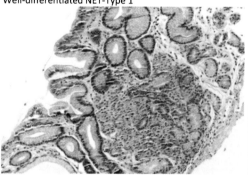

Well-differentiated NET-Type 3

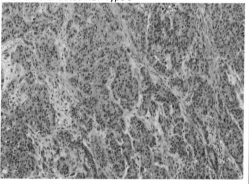

GRADING OF NEUROENDOCRINE TUMORS		
NET Grade (G)	Mitotic rate (per 2mm²)	Ki-67 index (%)
G1	<2	<3
G2	2-20	3-20
G3	>20	>20

GASTRIC NEUROENDOCRINE NEOPLASMS
MORPHOLOGY
- Epithelial neoplasms with neuroendocrine differentiation, including well-differentiated neuroendocrine tumor (NET), poorly differentiated neuroendocrine carcinoma (NEC), and mixed neuroendocrine-non-neuroendocrine neoplasm (MiNEN)
- NET: Composed of well-differentiated cells arranged in nests, acini, trabeculae, and ribbons, with abundant eosinophilic cytoplasm and monomorphic round nuclei (stippled/salt and pepper chromatin)
- Three main types of Enterochromaffin-like-cell (ECL-cell) NETs include
- **Type 1:** Associated with hypergastrinemia due to **chronic autoimmune atrophic gastritis**; autoantibody mediated destruction of parietal cells → achlorhydria → compensatory hyperplasia of antral G-cells (to try to signal to make more acid) → secrete gastrin → ECL cell hyperplasia and NET formation
  - **Most cases are grade 1 or 2 (G1 or G2),** with very rare incidence of G3 tumors
- **Type 2:** Associated with **Zollinger-Ellison syndrome** (hypergastrinemia) due to duodenal or pancreatic gastrinoma
- **Type 3:** Sporadic, grade ranges from G1-G3, however, often with **higher metastasis rate and tumor stage**
- Serotonin-producing EC-cell NET: Rare subtype and usually nonfunctional
- Gastrin-producing G-cell NET: Usually non-functioning, but may cause Zollinger–Ellison syndrome and those functional tumors are referred as "gastric gastrinoma"
- Somatostatin-producing D-cell NET: Positive for somatostatin
- NEC: Composed of poorly formed trabeculae or sheets of poorly differentiated cells, and are subtyped as small cell and large cell NEC
  - Small cell NEC: Cells with scant cytoplasm, hyperchromatic nuclei with molding and absent nucleoli
  - Large cell NEC: Large cells with abundant eosinophilic cytoplasm and vesicular nuclei showing prominent nucleoli
- NECs typically feature mitotic count of >20/mm² and Ki-67 proliferation index frequently >60-70%

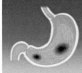

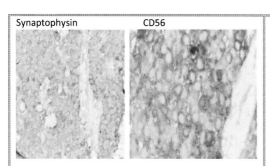
Synaptophysin   CD56

- Mixed neuroendocrine-non-neuroendocrine neoplasm (MiNEN): Mixed adenocarcinoma-NEC (MANEC), mixed adenocarcinoma-NET, and mixed adenoma-NET are seen

OTHER HIGH YIELD POINTS
- *TP53* and *RB1* mutations can help distinguish NEC from G3 NET (wild type in NET)
- Prognosis of NENs depends on tumor type, grade, and stage

Path Presenter

	Type 1	Type 2	Type 3
Cause	Autoimmune gastritis	Zollinger-Ellison syndrome, often MEN1 syndrome	Sporadic
Demographic	More frequent in females	No sex predilection	More frequent in males
Focality	Multifocal	Multifocal	Solitary
Arises from	ECL-cell (body/fundus)	ECL-cell (body/fundus)	ECL, EC, G & D-cells (anywhere)
Frequency	80-90%	5-7%	10-15%
Hypergastrinemia	Yes (secondary)	Yes (Primary)	No
ECL-cell proliferation	Yes	Yes	No
Acid secretion	Low or absent	High	Normal
Background mucosa	Atrophic gastritis	Parietal cell hyperplasia	Normal
Stage at diagnosis	Most are low stage	Usually, low stage	Often advanced
5-year survival	~100%	60-90%	<50%

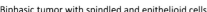

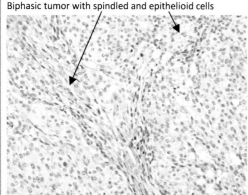
Biphasic tumor with spindled and epithelioid cells

GASTROBLASTOMA
MORPHOLOGY
- Biphasic tumor consisting of uniform spindle cells and epithelial cells arranged in nests, arising in the gastric muscularis propria
- IHC: Epithelial component expresses pan-cytokeratins, focal CD56, and CD10; spindle cell component is (-) for keratins but (+) for CD56 and CD10; (-) for C-KIT, DOG1, CD34, SMA, desmin, synaptophysin, chromogranin, and S100

OTHER HIGH YIELD POINTS
- Characteristic gene fusion: *MALAT1-GL1*

Path Presenter

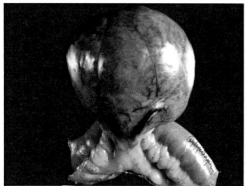
GIST in the small bowel in this image: Well-circumscribed lesion

GASTROINTESTINAL STROMAL TUMOR (GIST)
MORPHOLOGY
- Mesenchymal neoplasm characterized by differentiation towards **interstitial cells of Cajal** and can occur anywhere in the gastrointestinal tract
- Gross: Usually well circumscribed mass of variable size, centered within muscularis propria
- Microscopy: Most gastric GISTs are spindle cell type, epithelioid morphology in 20-25% cases, and some feature mixed phenotype

- **Spindle cell type:** Usually arranged in diffuse sheets or vague storiform pattern, cells with eosinophilic cytoplasm (can have cytoplasmic vacuoles), and rare nuclear pleomorphism
  ➤ Distinct histologic patterns include sclerosing, palisaded-vacuolated (most common type), diffuse hypercellular, and sarcomatous type (with nuclear atypia and high mitosis)

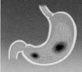

GIST- Spindle cell type

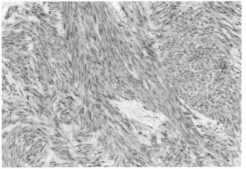

CKIT Positive

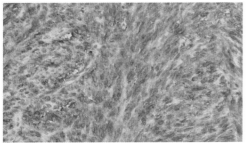

GIST: Epithelioid type

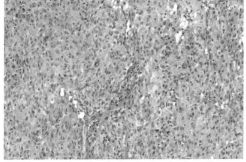

SDHB immunohistochemical stain showing loss of expression in epithelioid GIST

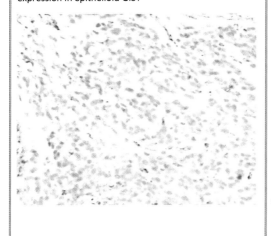

- Small intestinal and colonic GISTs are usually spindle cell type, and those with low biological potential often contain skenoid fibers (extracellular collagen globules)

- **Epithelioid GIST:** Clear to eosinophilic cytoplasm, may show sclerosing, discohesive, hypercellular or sarcomatous morphology with substantial atypia and mitotic activity
  - **SDH-deficient GISTs characteristically show epithelioid morphology,** gastric location, multinodularity, increased chance of lymphovascular invasion, and lymph node metastasis

- **Dedifferentiated GIST:** Progression to high-grade (KIT-negative) sarcomatous morphology observed either de novo or after therapy with imatinib
  - Can be associated with heterologous epithelial, myogenic, or angiosarcomatous differentiation
- IHC: Most tumors are diffusely **(+)** for **C-KIT (CD117)**; **DOG1/ANO1**- equally sensitive and specific as C-KIT, reactive in ~50% of C-KIT negative GISTs; most spindle cell type GISTs (especially gastric) are positive for **CD34**
- SDH-deficient GISTs exhibit loss of SDHB protein expression irrespective of which SDH gene is mutated

OTHER HIGH YIELD POINTS
- ~54% GISTs arise in the stomach, ~30% in the small intestine, ~5% in the colon and rectum, and about ~1% in the esophagus
- About 75% of GISTs harbor gain-of-function mutations in *KIT* (most often in exon 11 or exon 9) and 10% harbor *PDGFRA* activating mutations
  - Both oncogenes are located on chromosome 4, encoding for type III receptor tyrosine kinases
  - The mutations are mutually exclusive and result in the constitutive activation of either KIT or PDGFRA
- Many GISTs that are wildtype for *KIT* and *PDGFRA* harbor alterations in SDH subunit genes, leading to SDH dysfunction
  - SDH-deficient GISTs usually occur in younger patients and nearly all pediatric GISTs are SDH-deficient
- Majority are sporadic and 5-10% GISTs arise in the setting of various syndromes
- Most syndromic GISTs are SDH-deficient which includes
  - **Carney triad** (GIST, pulmonary chondroma, paraganglioma); non-hereditary disorder and usually show *SDHC* promoter methylation
  - **Carney–Stratakis syndrome** (GIST and paraganglioma); autosomal dominant disorder with SDH germline mutation
- Neurofibromatosis type 1 (NF1) patients rarely develop GISTs; often multifocal and most are in small intestine
- Familial GISTs (extremely rare) are caused by germline mutations of *KIT* or *PDGFRA*, and usually are multifocal with aggressive behavior
- Most important prognostic parameters for GIST are mitotic activity, tumor size, and anatomical location
  - Tumor rupture is an adverse factor

Path Presenter

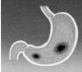

SMALL BOWEL: NORMAL

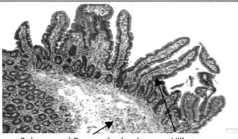

Submucosal Brunner's glands   Villus

SMALL INTESTINE ASSOCIATIONS	
Villi	Blunt with Celiac Disease
Goblet cells/Paneth cells	Missing in autoimmune enteropathy
Intraepithelial lymphocytes	Increased in Celiac, peptic injury, infections, small bowel overgrowth
Plasma cells	Absent in immunodeficiency
Critters	Look in between villi and surface
Vessels	Look for amyloid and vasculitis
Endocrine cells	Absent in endocrine dysgenesis

• **Duodenum:** Villi and submucosal Brunner mucus glands are identifiable features

• Duodenum is 25-30 cm long, C-shaped, and located in the upper abdomen

• Head of the pancreas lies in the C-loop

• Duodenum is divided into four sections: superior, descending, horizontal, and ascending

• Villus to crypt ratio: 3-5:1

• **Jejunum and Ileum:** Tallest villi in the jejunum; ileum can appear nodular due to Peyer's patches; no Brunner glands in the jejunum and ileum

• Entire small bowel has the following layers: Mucosa (includes lamina propria, epithelium, and muscularis mucosae), submucosa (blood vessels and fibroadipose tissues), muscularis propria (inner circular and outer longitudinal smooth muscle), subserosa, and serosa

Path Presenter

SMALL BOWEL: NON-NEOPLASTIC

Acute duodenitis with neutrophils in the epithelium

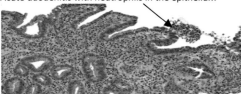

Peptic injury with foveolar metaplasia

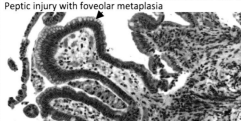

ACUTE DUODENITIS

MORPHOLOGY

• **Neutrophils in the duodenal epithelium**

OTHER HIGH YIELD POINTS

ETIOLOGIES

• **Infection:** Most common with *Helicobacter pylori*; can lead to ulcers; other etiologies include adenovirus, cytomegalovirus

• **Peptic duodenitis:** Acute inflammation + gastric foveolar metaplasia + Brunner gland hyperplasia; seen with excess gastric acid and/or *Helicobacter pylori*

• **Medications:** NSAIDs commonly

• **Inflammatory bowel disease:** Crohn disease can affect the duodenum

Path Presenter

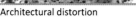

Architectural distortion

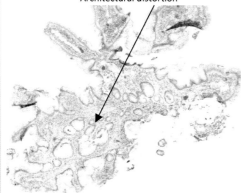

CHRONIC INJURY IN INFLAMMATORY BOWEL DISEASE

MORPHOLOGY

• **Architectural distortion** - Crypt branching and drop-out

• **Pyloric metaplasia**

• Often with villous blunting and basal plasmacytosis

• Also see acute inflammation (cryptitis and crypt abscesses)

• Look for granulomas and transmural inflammation in resection specimens

OTHER HIGH YIELD POINTS

• Particularly in Crohn disease in the terminal ileum   Pyloric metaplasia

Path Presenter

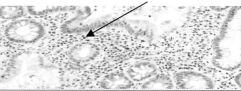

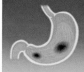
INFECTIONS

Giardia "falling leaves"

GIARDIA

MORPHOLOGY

- Characteristic trophozoites are **pear-shaped, binucleate, faintly basophilic organisms** seen in between villi with no associated inflammation
- Sometimes mild villous blunting and intraepithelial lymphocytes can be seen
- Look like **"falling leaves"** in the bowel lumen   Path Presenter

OTHER HIGH YIELD POINTS

- **Most common protozoa infection in the United States**
- Usually acquired from contaminated water; can be fecal-oral and sexually transmitted
- More common in children, with travel, and immunocompromised
- Causes diarrhea (unclear pathogenesis), often watery and foul-smelling
- Infection can be chronic in immunocompromised

Organisms are located at the apex of epithelial cells along the luminal border

CRYPTOSPORIDIA   Path Presenter

MORPHOLOGY

- Protozoal parasite-Cryptosporidium species, most common *C. hominis and C. parvum*
- Organisms are **2-5 µm** in diameter and **located at apex of epithelial cells along the luminal border**, basophilic on H&E
- Villous blunting with mixed inflammatory infiltrate may be seen
- Positive for modified AFB

OTHER HIGH YIELD POINTS

- Small bowel is the most common site
- Other organs: colon, stomach, biliary tree, respiratory tract
- Clinical presentation: In immunocompetent hosts, self-limited profuse diarrhea (1-2 days); in immunocompromised, debilitating symptoms

Image credit: Dr. Megan Smith, Twitter @megothelioma

Round forms of Cyclospora, perinuclear and intracellular

CYCLOSPORA

MORPHOLOGY

- *Cyclospora cayetanensis* is the only species that infects humans
- Round forms: **2-3 µm**; crescentic merozoites: 5-6 µm
- **Intracellular, within the upper 1/3rd of the epithelium**; parasitophorous vacuoles

OTHER HIGH YIELD POINTS

- Foodborne and waterborne intestinal parasite
- Infection is mild to asymptomatic; treated with Bactrim
- Endemic in tropics and subtropical regions of Latin America, Central and Southeast Asia, Middle East, and North Africa

Path Presenter

Tiny dots in the supranuclear cytoplasm

MICROSPORIDIA   Path Presenter

MORPHOLOGY

- Caused by *Enterocytozoon bieneusi* and *Encephalitozoon intestinalis*
- Small spores **(2-3 µm) in the supranuclear cytoplasm in epithelial cells** and lamina propria macrophages
- Minimal to no changes in the mucosa

OTHER HIGH YIELD POINTS

- Causes chronic diarrhea in immunocompromised patients
- Diagnosis by stool examination, polymerase chain reaction (PCR)

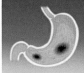

Intestinal cell with varying protozoan infections: Size, location, and morphology

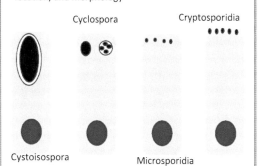

Cyclospora

Cryptosporidia

Cystoisospora

Microsporidia

CYTOISOSPORA (ISOSPORA)

MORPHOLOGY

- Opportunistic infection by protozoan parasite *Cystoisospora belli* (formerly known as *Isospora belli*)
- Large, **20-33 μm in length and 10-19 μm in width**, perinuclear/subnuclear
- Intraepithelial inclusions that infect epithelial cells and macrophages
- Schizonts and merozoites are crescent-shaped
- Sexual forms are round with prominent nucleus and nucleolus
- Parasitophorous vacuoles

OTHER HIGH YIELD POINTS

- Causes diarrhea and weight loss

Foamy macrophages in duodenal lamina propria (PAS)

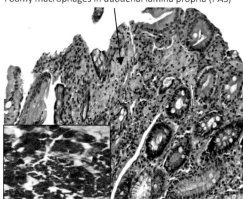

WHIPPLE DISEASE

MORPHOLOGY

- Rare bacterial infection caused by *Tropherma whipplei* often diagnosed on small bowel biopsies
- Lamina propria expanded by a **foamy macrophage infiltrate**, diffuse or patchy
- **PAS/PAS-D positive**: granular particles that appear sickle-shaped

OTHER HIGH YIELD POINTS

- Affects small intestine>esophagus>stomach> appendix>colon
- Symptoms of malabsorption, diarrhea, arthralgias, pain, and neurological symptoms
- Differential diagnosis: *Mycobacterium avium intracellulare complex* (PAS negative, AFB positive)

Path Presenter

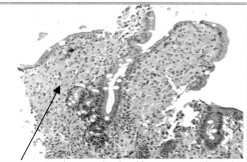

Foamy macrophages in duodenal lamina propria (AFB +)

MYCOBACTERIUM AVIUM COMPLEX (MAC)

MORPHOLOGY

- Expansion of lamina propria by **foamy macrophages** containing MAC (**FITE and AFB positive, PAS negative**)

OTHER HIGH YIELD POINTS

- Seen in immunocompromised patients
- Differential diagnosis: Whipple disease (PAS positive, FITE/AFB negative); mycobacterium tuberculosis causes necrotizing granulomatous inflammation

Path Presenter

Inflammation rich in eosinophils   Adult worm

STRONGYLOIDES

MORPHOLOGY

Path Presenter

- Nematode infection that affects **immunocompromised people**
- **Adult worms, larvae, and eggs** can be found in crypts
- Inflammation with neutrophils and **often eosinophils**, may resemble inflammatory bowel disease

OTHER HIGH YIELD POINTS

- Worldwide distribution; very common in the tropics and the southeast United States
- Often get through the skin when barefoot on contaminated soil
- Skin→Lung→GI tract→Feces→Next host (or autoinfect)
- Female lives and lays eggs in the small intestine
- Can be asymptomatic; when symptomatic- diarrhea, pain, and bleeding

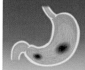

SMALL BOWEL: NON-NEOPLASTIC

Ectopic gastric-oxyntic type glands

ECTOPIC/HETEROTOPIC TISSUE Path Presenter

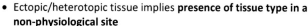

MORPHOLOGY
- Ectopic/heterotopic tissue implies **presence of tissue type in a non-physiological site**
- **Gastric and pancreatic heterotopic tissue** can be found in the small bowel
- In gastric tissue, one can see foveolar epithelium with antral glands or oxyntic glands with parietal and chief cells
- In pancreatic tissue, one can see acini, duct, and/or islet cells

OTHER HIGH YIELD POINTS
- **Can form a mass lesion/polyp**; symptoms can range from abdominal pain, obstruction, intussusception, and perforation to asymptomatic

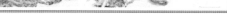

Dilated mucosal and submucosal lymphatic channels

LYMPHANGIECTASIA/LYMPHANGIOMA Path Presenter

MORPHOLOGY
- **Lymphangiectasia:** Dilated mucosal and submucosal lymphatic vessels without mass formation; can be primary or secondary
- **Lymphangioma:** Mass forming lesion of dilated lymphatic channels in loose connective tissue stroma; may have smooth muscle wall and lymphoid aggregates
- Positive for CD34, CD31, D2-40, and Factor 8

OTHER HIGH YIELD POINTS
- Lymphagiectasia can be primary or secondary; primary more common in children; can lead to diarrhea and protein-losing enteropathy if extensive; secondary due to obstruction, tumor, adhesions, stricture, prior surgery; need to exclude malignancy
- Lymphangioma is a benign lesion

Smooth muscle wall

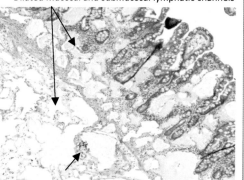

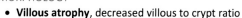

CELIAC SPRUE/GLUTEN-SENSITIVE ENTEROPATHY Path Presenter

MORPHOLOGY
- **Villous atrophy**, decreased villous to crypt ratio
- **Increased intraepithelial lymphocytes (IELs)**, typically >20 lymphocytes/100 enterocytes; "Crescendo" at tip of villi
- Scalloped villi may be seen endoscopically
- CD3 immunohistochemical stain can highlight IELs if needed

OTHER HIGH YIELD POINTS
- **Gluten exposure** triggers inflammation, primarily in the duodenum; causes diarrhea and weight loss
- Positive serology for **Antigliaden, Tissue Transglutaminase (TTG), and Antiendomysial (EMA) antibody** (if not IgA deficient)
- Associated with haplotypes **HLA-DQ2 or DQ8**; absence of both essentially excludes the diagnosis
- **Increased risk of malignancy** (small intestinal T-cell lymphoma and adenocarcinoma)
- May be associated with lymphocytic colitis/gastritis
- Differential diagnosis for increased intraepithelial lymphocyte with/without blunting: Tropical sprue, collagenous sprue, peptic injury, infection, medications, autoimmune enteropathy, and bacterial overgrowth
- **Tropical sprue:** post-infectious; after traveling to Africa, Asia, or South America; similar histology to Celiac
- **Collagenous sprue:** May be a component of refractory sprue; lacks auto-antibodies and may not respond to gluten-free diet; similar histology to Celiac
- **Bacterial overgrowth:** Diagnosis >100,000 colony-forming units/mL in culture (small bowel fluid aspirate)

Blunted villi

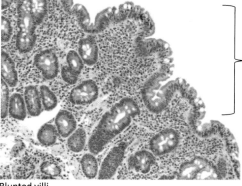

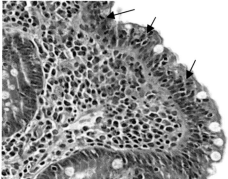

Increased intraepithelial lymphocytes

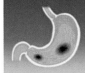

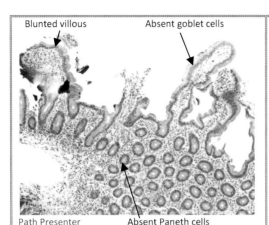

Blunted villous

Absent goblet cells

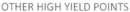

Path Presenter

Absent Paneth cells

AUTOIMMUNE ENTEROPATHY

MORPHOLOGY

- **Diminished/absent goblet cells and Paneth cells** (not required for diagnosis)
- Villous blunting, increased intraepithelial lymphocytes, increased crypt apoptosis

OTHER HIGH YIELD POINTS

- Intractable diarrhea
- Presents at **infancy and early age**
- Multifactoral; associated with Immune dysregulation, polyendocrinopathy, Enteropathy, X-linked (IPEX syndrome); Autoimmune Polyendocrinopathy Candidiasis Ectodermal Dystrophy (APECED) syndrome; IPEX-like syndrome
- Extraintestinal manifestations: diabetes, autoimmune hepatitis, alopecia, ectodermal dystrophy, candidiasis, hypothyroidism
- Exact pathogenesis is unclear: **anti-enterocyte and anti-goblet cell antibodies**

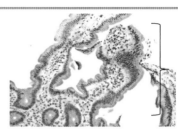

Absent goblet cells

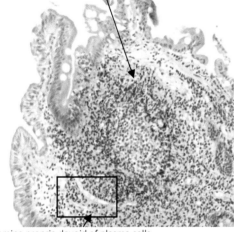

Lymphoid aggregates

Lamina propria devoid of plasma cells

COMMON VARIABLE IMMUNODEFICIENCY   Path Presenter

MORPHOLOGY

- Immunodeficiency disorder with characteristic histologic feature of **absence of plasma cells in the lamina propria** (not required for diagnosis as they can be present in some cases)
- Lymphoid aggregates, mild villous blunting, increased intraepithelial lymphocytes
- Often find other infectious agents such as Giardia

OTHER HIGH YIELD POINTS

- **Second most common immunodeficiency disorder** after selective IgA deficiency
- Age of onset varies from childhood to adulthood with a bimodal peak age in the first and third decades
- B-cell impairment causing **hypogammaglobulinemia** with IgA or IgM deficiency and reduced immunoglobulins lead to **increased susceptibility to infections** especially sinopulmonary and gastrointestinal infections

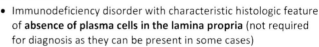
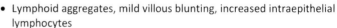
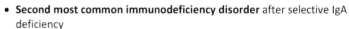

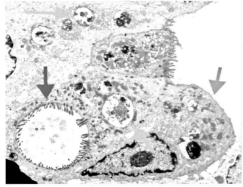

Electron microscopy (EM): Loss of surface microvilli (blue arrow), cytoplasmic inclusions with immature microvilli (red arrow), and abnormal vacuoles (green arrow)

MICROVILLOUS INCLUSION DISEASE (MVID)

MORPHOLOGY

- Accumulation of PAS-positive granules at the apical pole of immature enterocytes, together with atrophic band indicating microvillous atrophy
- **CD10 and PAS stain positive within the enterocytes (cytoplasmic staining) versus just linear brush border staining in normal controls** (see pictorial depiction below)

OTHER HIGH YIELD POINTS

- **Congenital intestinal disorder** characterized by **severe, watery diarrhea** and an inability of the intestine to absorb nutrients
- No treatment exists for MVID; rarely live beyond two years of age

EM image courtesy of Dr. Vighnesh Walavalkar, Twitter @vighnesh_w, used with permission

Control   MVID

PAS

CD10

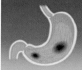

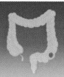

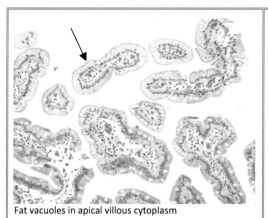

Fat vacuoles in apical villous cytoplasm

ABETALIPOPROTEINEMIA
MORPHOLOGY

- Mutation in **MTP gene** encoding Microsomal Triglyceride Transfer Protein (MTTP); autosomal recessive
- Causes defect in synthesis and export of apoprotein B from intestinal mucosal cells; leads to **fat vacuoles in the villous epithelium**

OTHER HIGH YIELD POINTS

- Symptoms: failure to thrive, diarrhea, steatorrhea
- Free fatty acids and monoglycerides cannot assemble in chylomicrons and becomes triglycerides in cells causing cytoplasm vacuolization
- CBC with **acantholytic cells (burr cells)** and **lipid profile shows no chylomicrons, no VLDL, and no LDL**   Path Presenter

Image courtesy of Dr. Juan Putra @path_putra

Thin circumferential membrane composed of mucosa, submucosa, and fibrosis

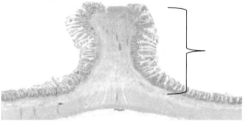

Gross image courtesy of Dr. Trupti Mandalia, @Pathmath1, used with permission

DIAPHRAGM DISEASE
MORPHOLOGY

- **Thin circumferential membranes** similar to plicae circularis, composed of **mucosa and submucosa with fibrosis**
- Causes **strictures**; also see ulcers and even perforation

OTHER HIGH YIELD POINTS.

- **Related to NSAIDs use**
- Involves the small bowel

Path Presenter

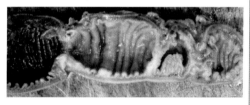

Thickened subepithelial collagen band

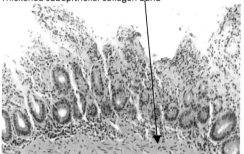

Image courtesy of Dr. Anju Pandey @anjuthevirgo

OLMESARTAN ENTEROPATHY
MORPHOLOGY

- A sprue-like enteropathy associated with **Olmesartan** and to a lesser degree another angiotensin II receptor antagonists
- Variable morphology from **increased intraepithelial lymphocytes and villous blunting to thickened subepithelial collagen**   Path Presenter

OTHER HIGH YIELD POINTS

- Mainly **affects the duodenum**
- **Negative celiac serologies**
- Clinical symptoms of diarrhea that resolve with discontinuation of medication
- Differential diagnosis: Rule out celiac disease

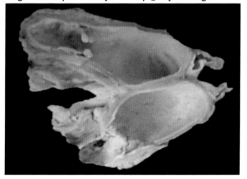

ENTERIC DUPLICATION CYST
MORPHOLOGY

- **Cystic outpouching that looks similar histologically to the normal bowel wall and has a shared muscle layer**
- Can occur anywhere throughout the GI tract, **most common in the ileum** in the small bowel
- Can be associated with gastric heterotopia

OTHER HIGH YIELD POINTS

- Pathogenesis: Developmental abnormality with abnormal luminal recanalization
- Can present with symptoms of pain, nausea/vomiting, and gastrointestinal bleeding

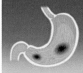

SMALL BOWEL: NEOPLASTIC

Intestinal type: Pencillate hyperchromatic nuclei
Apical mucin (foveolar)   Pyloric gland adenoma

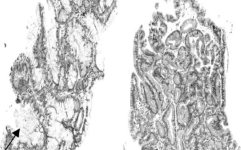

ADENOMA
MORPHOLOGY

- **Intestinal type:** Similar to tubular adenoma of colon with "picket-fence nuclei:" elongate, pseudostratified, and hyperchromatic
- Nuclei remain in basal location in low grade dysplasia while high grade dysplasia shows cytologic pleomorphism, prominent nucleoli, architectural complexity, intraluminal necrosis, and no breach of basement membrane
- **Foveolar adenoma:** Tubulovillous architecture, tall columnar epithelium that resembles gastric foveolar cells and has a characteristic mucinous cap; prone to harbor high-grade dysplasia
- **Pyloric gland adenoma:** Tightly packed tubules that are lined by a monolayer of cuboidal cells that have granular eosinophilic to ground glass cytoplasm; no apical mucin cap

OTHER HIGH YIELD POINTS

- Within the small intestine, duodenum is predisposed to developing adenomas
- Mean age of diagnosis is 65 years, with a slight male predilection
- Non-ampullary duodenal adenomas (~60%) are associated with Familial Adenomatous Polyposis (FAP) or MUTYH- Associated Polyposis

Path Presenter

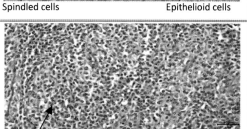

Spindled cells   Epithelioid cells

GANGLIOCYTIC PARAGANGLIOMA
MORPHOLOGY

- Three characteristic cell types: **epithelioid, spindle-shaped, and ganglion-like**
- IHC: Epithelioid cells: **(+)** CD56, synaptophysin, chromogranin-A, somatostatin, progesterone receptor, pancreatic polypeptide
- Ganglion cells: **(+)** S100, CD56, synaptophysin, chromogranin-A, somatostatin, pancreatic polypeptide
- Spindled cells: **(+)** S100, BCL2

OTHER HIGH YIELD POINTS

- **Rare tumor of the periampullary region and the second part of the duodenum**
- **Usually benign,** however, ~7% can metastasize
- Unencapsulated submucosal lesion

Path Presenter

Images courtesy of Dr. Phoenix Bell, Twitter
@PhoenixBell, used with permission

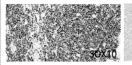

Monotonous tumor cells with prominent nucleoli

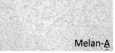
SOX10   Melan-A

MALIGNANT GASTROINTESTINAL (GI) NEUROECTODERMAL TUMOR/CLEAR CELL SARCOMA-LIKE TUMOR OF THE GI TRACT
MORPHOLOGY

- Malignancy with **sheets** of **monotonous tumor cells, macronucleoli,** scanty cytoplasm, and conspicuous mitoses
- Nested, solid, pseudopapillary, pseudoalveolar, microcystic, rosette-like architecture; osteoclast-like giant cells can be seen   Path Presenter
- IHC: **(+)** for **S100, SOX10, synaptophysin,** and vimentin while **(-)** for **HMB45, Melan-A,** CD117, DOG1, **cytokeratin**

OTHER HIGH YIELD POINTS

- Small bowel is the most common site in GI tract; Median age: 35 years; M=F
- Translocation has **EWSR1 rearrangement (EWSR1- ATF1[t(12;22)] or EWSR1-CREB1)**

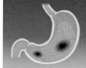

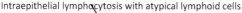
Intraepithelial lymphocytosis with atypical lymphoid cells

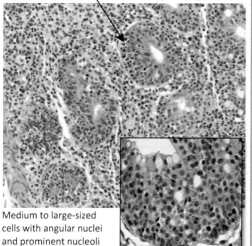

Medium to large-sized cells with angular nuclei and prominent nucleoli

ENTEROPATHY-ASSOCIATED T-CELL LYMPHOMA
MORPHOLOGY
- Features of celiac disease with **increased intraepithelial lymphocytes**, crypt hyperplasia, and villous atrophy
- Lesion with **pleomorphic infiltrate of medium to large sized neoplastic cells** with prominent nucleoli, angulated nuclei, anaplasia, mitotic figures, and necrosis
- IHC: **(+)** for CD3, CD7, TIA, Perforin, granzyme B, CD103, and CD30; **(-)** for CD20, EBER; **loss of some T cell markers such as CD2, CD4, CD5, and CD8**

OTHER HIGH YIELD POINTS
- **T-cell lymphoma that occurs in Celiac disease** and affects the intestine; jejunum >ileum/duodenum
- Stronger association with refractory disease
- Rare bone marrow, other viscera, and large intestine involvement
- Clonal *TCR* gene rearrangement
- Aggressive clinical course

Path Presenter

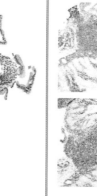

Many lymphoid aggregates

Neoplastic follicles lack tangible body macrophages and mantle zones

FOLLICULAR LYMPHOMA, DUODENAL TYPE
MORPHOLOGY
- **Lymphoma confined to the mucosa and/or submucosa of the duodenum**
- Almost always low grade (grade 1-2) unlike systemic follicular lymphoma; lamina propria is also infiltrated
- Neoplastic follicles lack tingible body macrophages and mantle zones
- IHC: **(+)** CD20, CD10, BCL2, **low** Ki-67

OTHER HIGH YIELD POINTS
- Lymphoma derived from follicular B lymphocytes
- Usually affects the second part of the duodenum but may involve jejunum and ileum; no systemic involvement
- **t (14;18)**
- **Excellent prognosis, local treatment, and indolent course**
- A small percentage of patients progress to nodal disease (<10%)

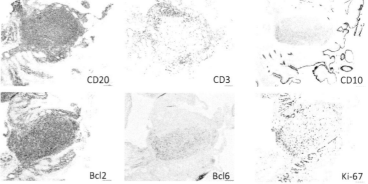
CD20   CD3   CD10
Bcl2   Bcl6   Ki-67

Path Presenter

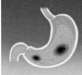

Nested architecture of NET with stippled chromatin

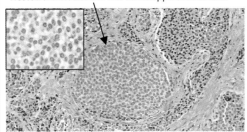

Somatostatinoma
Psuedoglandular architecture   Psammoma bodies

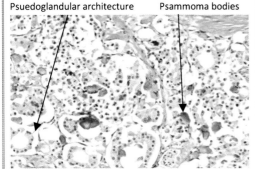

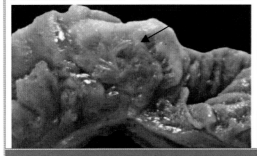

WELL-DIFFERENTIATED NEUROENDOCRINE TUMOR
MORPHOLOGY
- Monotonous tumor cells with round/oval nuclei and **stippled (salt and pepper) chromatin**
- Architecture can be trabecular, nested, corded, ribbons, acinar, and/or pseudoglandular
- IHC: **(+)** AE1/3, Cam5.2, Chromogranin-A, Synaptophysin; **(-)** CK7, CK20

GRADING

Grade	Mitoses	Ki-67
1	<2 mitoses/2 mm^2	<3%
2	2-20 mitoses/2 mm^2	3-20%
3	>20 mitoses/2 mm^2	>20%

OTHER HIGH YIELD POINTS
- Majority of tumors are non-functioning; functional ones include
- **Gastrinoma:** Gastrin expressing NET in the duodenum; **causes Zollinger Ellison syndrome** (hypergastrinemia, peptic ulcer disease, diarrhea)
- **Somatostatinoma:** Somatostatin expressing NET in the ampulla; causes diabetes, stones, diarrhea; **psammoma bodies** is a characteristic feature
- **Carcinoid syndrome:** Diarrhea, bronchospasms, flushing, tricuspid valve fibrosis; occurs when liver metastasis present
- May be associated with syndromic conditions: **Multiple Endocrine Neoplasia (MEN) type 1** is associated with duodenal gastrinomas; ampullary somatostatinoma can arise in the setting of **Neurofibromatosis 1**
- Differential diagnosis: Poorly differentiated neuroendocrine carcinoma- large cell or small cell carcinoma; these lose well-differentiated NET architecture and cytology; instead, they have necrosis and prominent mitoses

Path Presenter

Gross image courtesy of Dr. José G. Bellassai, @BellassaiJb, used with permission

APPENDIX: NON-NEOPLASTIC

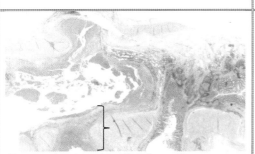

NORMAL HISTOLOGY
- Colonic-type epithelium with irregular glands/crypts and lamina propria
- **Prominent lymphoid aggregates in the mucosa/submucosa**
- Muscularis mucosae and submucosa may be attenuated but usually present
- Muscularis propria with longitudinal and circular smooth muscle

OTHER HIGH YIELD POINTS   Path Presenter
- Located in the retrocecal region commonly
- May have an immunological role

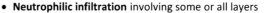

ACUTE APPENDICITIS   Path Presenter
MORPHOLOGY
- **Neutrophilic infiltration** involving some or all layers
- Can be described as acute focal, suppurative, gangrenous, and perforated; can be associated with periappendicitis

OTHER HIGH YIELD POINTS
- Disease of the **young/adolescents** most commonly; Males > Females
- Pathogenesis: **obstruction** due to fecalith, lesions, hypertrophic lymphoid aggregates, diverticulosis, and/or vascular compromise leading to infection
- **Most common emergency abdominal surgery**

Transmural acute neutrophilic inflammation

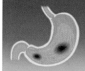

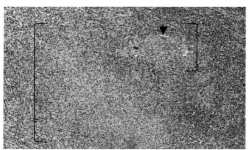

Granulomatous inflammation with a collection of histiocytes including giant cells(arrowhead)

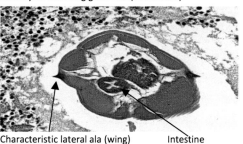

Characteristic lateral ala (wing)   Intestine

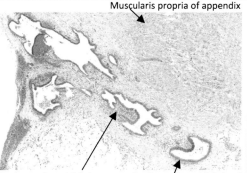

Muscularis propria of appendix

Benign endometrial stroma   Benign endometrial gland

GRANULOMATOUS APPENDICITIS

MORPHOLOGY

- **Granulomatous or xanthogranulomatous inflammation** in addition to neutrophilic inflammation

OTHER HIGH YIELD POINTS

- Clinically resembles acute appendicitis
- Rare; seen in less than 2% of appendectomies
- Etiologies: **Idiopathic, *Yersinia*, interval appendicitis, *Mycobacterium tuberculosis* infection, pinworm (*Enterobius vermicularis*), sarcoidosis, Crohn disease**

Path Presenter

[QR code]

ENTEROBIUS VERMICULARIS/PINWORM:

- Granulomatous inflammation + **nematode with characteristic lateral alae**
- Pinworm is common in children and presents with **pruritis ani** (nocturnal pruritis) as female migrates to the anus and lays eggs
- Transmission occurs via the fecal-oral route and inhalation of dust-containing eggs
- Humans are the only natural host

ENDOMETRIOSIS

MORPHOLOGY

- **Ectopic benign endometrial glandular and stromal tissue**
- Sometimes stroma can be difficult to identify; in place, macrophages and hemosiderin pigment may be present (evidence of chronic hemorrhage)
- If cytologic atypia is present, atypical endometriosis is a consideration
- IHC: **CD10** highlights the stroma; glands are **(+) for** ER and PR

OTHER HIGH YIELD POINTS

- Appendix is an uncommon site; more common sites are ovary, fallopian tubes, cul de sac, and broad ligaments

Path Presenter

[QR code]

APPENDIX: NEOPLASTIC

Appendiceal serrated lesions and polyps
Appendiceal neuroendocrine neoplasms
Appendiceal mucinous neoplasms
Appendiceal adenocarcinoma
Appendiceal goblet cell adenocarcinoma

SERRATED LESIONS AND POLYPS

MORPHOLOGY

- Mucosal epithelial polyps with serrations (saw-tooth) architecture
- **Hyperplastic polyp:** Luminal part shows serrations, bland cytology (no dysplasia) and the base is non-dilated
- **Serrated lesion without dysplasia:** The abnormal serrations extend to the crypt base with abnormal shapes (L-shaped, inverted T) and unequivocal basal dilatation; epithelium shows no dysplasia
- **Serrated lesion with dysplasia:** Epithelial atypia is also present and can be adenoma-like, serrated, or traditional serrated adenoma-like

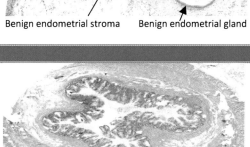

Serrated lesion: L-shaped crypt   T-shaped crypt

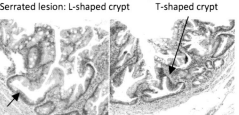

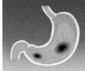
Serrated lesion with low-grade serrated-type dysplasia

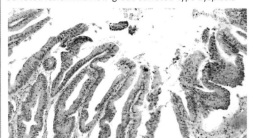

- Tubular adenoma/tubulovillous adenoma/villous adenoma and traditional serrated adenoma (rarely) can also occur in the appendix (see Colon section for details)

OTHER HIGH YIELD POINTS
- Males = females
- Hyperplastic polyps are usually seen in post-inflammatory conditions
- Serrated polyps have more *KRAS* than *BRAF* mutations

Path Presenter

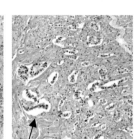

GI Neuroendocrine Neoplasms

Well-differentiated neuroendocrine tumor
1. G1
2. G2
3. G3

Poorly differentiated neuroendocrine carcinoma
1. Small cell carcinoma
2. Large cell carcinoma

EC-NET

Tubular NET

APPENDICEAL NEUROENDOCRINE TUMORS (NETs)
MORPHOLOGY
- Neuroendocrine tumors of the appendix are morphologically similar to other areas in the GI tract
- Enterochromaffin (EC)-cell NETs most common: polygonal monotonous tumor cells arranged in large nests with peripheral palisading
- L-cell NETs have a distinct trabecular or glandular growth pattern
- Tubular NET has stromal retraction and mimics adenocarcinoma
- Poorly differentiated neuroendocrine carcinoma of the appendix is extremely rare but morphologically like other organs
- IHC: **(+)** Chromogranin-A and synaptophysin; EC-NET **(+)** for serotonin
- For grading, please see the small bowel section

OTHER HIGH YIELD POINTS
- **Most common appendiceal tumor** by far
- Found incidentally or with acute appendicitis
- NETs mainly occur at the tip
- Slight female predominance and majority <40 years
- **Good prognosis (>95%)** if confined to the appendix

Path Presenter

Mucinous adenocarcinoma

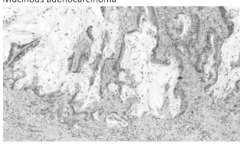

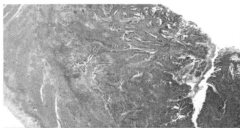

Non-mucinous adenocarcinoma

APPENDICEAL ADENOCARCINOMA
MORPHOLOGY
- Malignant glandular neoplasm with infiltrative edges and morphology similar to that seen in colon cancer
- **Mucinous adenocarcinoma:** Extracellular mucin comprising >50% of tumor with floating strips/glands/clusters of malignant epithelial cells
- **Non-mucinous adenocarcinoma:** Irregular glands infiltrating the wall of the appendix with desmoplastic stroma
- **Signet-ring cell carcinoma:** >50% of tumor composed of signet-ring cells which may sometimes be in pools of mucin
- **Undifferentiated carcinoma:** Rare

OTHER HIGH YIELD POINTS
- 5-6th decade; can occur anywhere in the appendix
- Presentation can be of appendicitis, abdominal pain, mass, GI bleed, and/or obstruction
- *KRAS* and *GNAS* mutations in mucinous carcinomas; microsatellite instability in non-mucinous adenocarcinomas
- Patients with mucinous carcinoma have a better outcome than ones with non-mucinous carcinoma
- Differential diagnosis: LAMN (LAMN lacks infiltrating invasion)

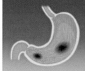

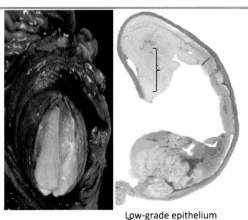

Low-grade epithelium

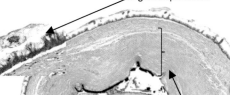

Lamina propria/submucosa replaced by fibrosis

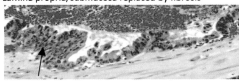

High-grade appendiceal mucinous neoplasm

Grade 1 Clusters of goblet-like cells and endocrine cells

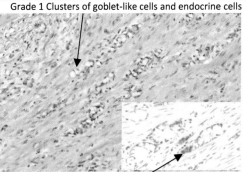

Synaptophysin highlighting neuroendocrine cells

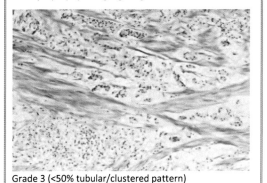

Grade 3 (<50% tubular/clustered pattern)

APPENDICEAL MUCINOUS LESIONS

- Low-grade Mucinous Neoplasm (LAMN)
- High-grade Mucinous Neoplasm (HAMN)

MORPHOLOGY

- LAMN has **hypermucinous epithelium** with villous/serrated architecture, low-grade columnar to cuboidal epithelium resembling **low-grade dysplasia**
- Has broad borders with **pushing-type invasion with fibrosis** of lamina propria and submucosa, and very attenuated to non-existent submucosal lymphoid aggregates
- Mucin may dissect through the wall of the appendix (with or without epithelium) and disseminate into the peritoneum (pseudomyxoma peritonei)
- HAMNs are rare; **high-grade cytology**, complex architecture with similar growth pattern as LAMN (such as pushing borders, subepithelial fibrosis, pushing invasion, rupture)

OTHER HIGH YIELD POINTS

- Males = females; wide-age range, most common in the sixth decade
- LAMN shows **KRAS and GNAS** mutations; higher grade tumors less commonly have GNAS mutations; GNAS mutation associated with mucin production
- Prognosis depends on stage with great prognosis in tumors limited to the appendix and variable prognosis if peritoneal dissemination present
- Hyperthermic intraperitoneal chemotherapy with cytoreduction has increased survival
- Differential diagnosis: Diverticula can rupture and extrude mucin and mimic LAMN

Path Presenter

APPENDICEAL GOBLET CELL ADENOCARCINOMA (GCA)

MORPHOLOGY

- **Amphicrine (having both endocrine and exocrine features) tumor with goblet-like mucinous cells, endocrine cells, and Paneth-like cells**
- Low-grade pattern: Tubules and clusters of goblet-like mucinous cells; endocrine and Paneth-like cells with granular eosinophilic cytoplasm, mild nuclear atypia, and no stromal reaction
- High-grade pattern: Tumor cells infiltrating as single cells, complex anastomosing tubules, cribriform masses, sheets or signet-ring cells (areas of classic low-grade morphology are still present even if focally)
- IHC: Chromogranin-A and synaptophysin highlight variable cells; not required

TUMOR GRADING

Path Presenter

Grade	Tubular/Clustered (Low-grade Pattern)	High-grade pattern
G1	>75%	<25%
G2	50-75%	25-50%
G3	<50%	>50%

OTHER HIGH YIELD POINTS

- Previously known as **"Goblet cell carcinoid"** or **"Adenocarcinoma ex Goblet cell carcinoid"**
- Often involves distal appendix; males= females; mean age: 50-60 years
- Usual affects the distal appendix
- Mutations in the **WNT signaling pathway** (CTNNA1, CTNNB1) and chromatin remodeling genes (ARID1, ARID2); **TP53** mutations in high-grade tumor

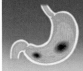

COLON: NORMAL

MORPHOLOGY
- In the colonic mucosa, crypts should be oriented parallel to one another, perpendicular to the surface (like test tubes in a rack), resting on the muscularis mucosae
- Muciphages in the rectum are considered normal
- Colon layers: Mucosa, submucosa, muscularis propria, subserosa, and serosa

OTHER HIGH YIELD POINTS

REGIONAL VARIATION	
Right colon	**Left colon**
More lymphocytes	Less lymphocytes
Paneth cells normal	Paneth cells abnormal
Fewer goblet cells	More goblet cells

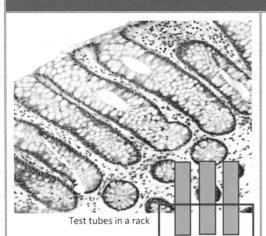
Test tubes in a rack

INFLAMMATORY/NON-NEOPLASTIC CONDITIONS OF THE COLORECTUM

Focal active colitis	Microscopic colitis: lymphocytic and collagenous
Acute colitis	Granulomatous colitis
Chronic active colitis	Mucosal prolapse/solitary rectal ulcer syndrome
Ischemic colitis	Pigments and inorganic material
Pseudomembranous colitis	Radiation colitis/proctitis
Eosinophilic colitis	Diverticular disease
Graft Versus Host Disease	

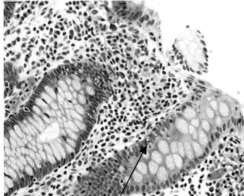
Focal active colitis: Rare neutrophils in crypts
Crypt abscess (neutrophils in the lumen of the gland)

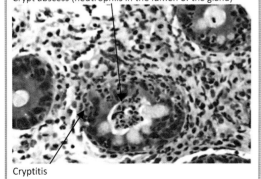
Cryptitis

FOCAL ACTIVE COLITIS
MORPHOLOGY
- Terminology used when **rare collections of neutrophils** are identified in crypt epithelium (otherwise normal)

OTHER HIGH YIELD POINTS
- **Etiology:** Bowel preparation artifact (most commonly); other etiologies are medications (especially NSAIDs), acute self-limited colitis (resolves in <4 weeks; commonly implicated organisms are *Campylobacter*, *Salmonella*, *Shigella* or *Yersinia*; with abrupt onset of fever), ischemic colitis, and inflammatory bowel disease (more insidious onset)

ACUTE COLITIS
MORPHOLOGY
- Terminology used when there is **easily visible cryptitis (neutrophils in the crypts) and crypt abscesses, WITHOUT features of chronicity**

OTHER HIGH YIELD POINTS
- **Etiology considerations:**
  - **Infections:** Usually acute bacterial or viral infections (e.g. *Cytomegalovirus, Salmonella, Shigella, Campylobacter, Yersinia, Aeromonas, Clostridium Difficile, E.coli*), so make sure this has been evaluated clinically; often food contamination (fecal-oral); may see pseudomembranes
  - **Medications:** Especially NSAIDS; others include Kayexalate, Sevelamer, Ipilimumab (immune checkpoint inhibitors)
  - **Inflammatory bowel disease:** Usually has features of chronicity; however, emerging or partially treated cases can show acute colitis only

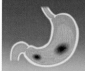

Crypt branching and shortening

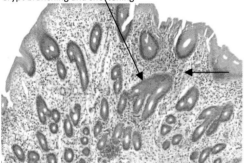

Basal lymphoplasmacytosis

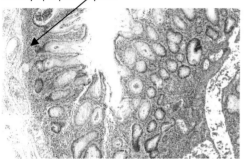

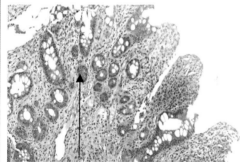

Paneth cell metaplasia

Path Presenter

CHRONIC ACTIVE COLITIS
MORPHOLOGY

- Acute inflammation, cryptitis, crypt abscesses, ulcers/erosions and

FEATURES OF CHRONICITY
Architectural distortion (crypt branching, loss, and shortening)
Basal lymphoplasmacytosis
Paneth cell or pyloric gland metaplasia

OTHER HIGH YIELD POINTS
ETIOLOGIES

- **Inflammatory bowel disease (IBD):** Chronic systemic autoimmune inflammatory disease; on a mucosal biopsy, it can be impossible to distinguish Crohn from Ulcerative colitis; the purpose of biopsies is to assess activity and dysplasia
- **Infection**: Always rule out cytomegalovirus in refractory inflammatory bowel disease
- **Diverticular disease:** Most common in older patients in sigmoid colon; can mimic IBD with diverticulitis and Segmental Colitis Associated with Diverticulosis (SCAD)
- **Diversion-associated colitis**: In bowel diverted from fecal stream (causes short chain fatty acid deficiency); microscopic finding is **florid lymphoid hyperplasia with prominent germinal centers**
- **Sexually Transmitted Diseases (STD) proctocolitis**: Usually biopsies show abundant plasma cells; common culprits- *Syphilis* and *Chlamydia* (lymphogranuloma venereum)
- **Cord Colitis Syndrome:** Chronic active colitis with granulomas; seen in the setting of umbilical cord transplantation
- **Medications:** NSAIDs, Ipilimumab, resins.

Path Presenter

PSEUDOMEMBRANOUS COLITIS
MORPHOLOGY

- **Acute colitis with adherent inflammatory exudate (pseudomembrane)** overlying sites of mucosal injury
- Crypts show superficial necrosis and dilatation; later crypts can be necrotic and mimic ischemic colitis
- **Pseudomembranes:** Mucopurulent exudate erupts out of crypts in a mushroom-like cloud with debris, neutrophils, and extracellular mucin

OTHER HIGH YIELD POINTS

- **Usually occurs after broad-spectrum antibiotics**
- 25% caused by *Clostridium difficile*; other organisms include *Clostridium perfringens, Staphylococcus, Klebsiella oxytoca, Candida, Salmonella*
- Differential diagnosis: **Ischemia and other infections** (such as *E. coli*)

Path Presenter

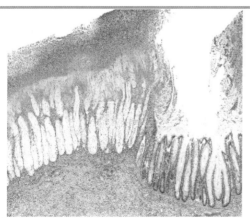

Mushroom-like exudate with neutrohils, mucin, and debris

[]

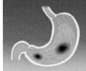

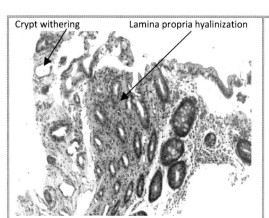

Crypt withering | Lamina propria hyalinization

Path Presenter

ISCHEMIC COLITIS
MORPHOLOGY
- Superficial epithelial damage, crypt withering, lamina propria hyalinization and hemorrhage, and mild acute inflammation; Deeper crypts near the muscularis mucosae may appear more viable with reactive changes

OTHER HIGH YIELD POINTS
ETIOLOGIES
- **Ischemia:** Due to poor perfusion; **most common in "watershed" areas** (splenic flexure, rectosigmoid, and ileocecal regions) in older patients with vascular occlusion or low-flow states
- **Infections:**
  - **_E. coli_ O157:H7 (EHEC)-** Endothelial damage from toxin→ fibrin thrombi often seen; associated with Hemolytic Uremic Syndrome (anemia, low platelets, renal failure)
  - **_C. Difficile_-** Pseudomembranes, less hyalinization and crypt withering
- **Medications:** NSAIDs, kayexalate, sevelamer, ipilimumab

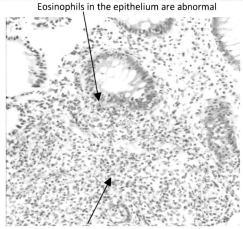

Eosinophils in the epithelium are abnormal

Increased lamina propria eosinophils

EOSINOPHILIC COLITIS
MORPHOLOGY
- Increased intraepithelial and lamina propria eosinophils; any in the submucosa or muscle are abnormal
- No strict cut-off, **>60 eosinophils is likely too many**

OTHER HIGH YIELD POINTS   Path Presenter

ETIOLOGIES
- Parasites
- Connective tissue disease/vasculitis
- Food allergies
- Medications
- Systemic mastocytosis
- Inflammatory bowel disease (particularly Crohn)
- Eosinophilic colitis/gastroenteritis: Diagnosis of exclusion; can be associated with eosinophil-rich inflammation in other organs (e.g., esophagus and/or small bowel); layer of bowel involved determines symptoms

---

Increased intraepithelial lymphocytes

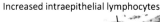

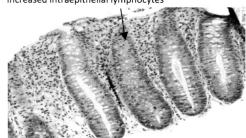

Thickened subepithelial collagen table-collagenous colitis

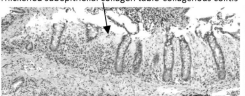

MICROSCOPIC COLITIS
- **Chronic watery non-bloody diarrhea**; **normal endoscopic** findings
- Etiologies: Idiopathic, viral infections, medications (NSAIDs, Olmesartan, antidepressants)

MORPHOLOGY
- **Lymphocytic colitis:** Increased intraepithelial lymphocytes (>20 lymphocytes/100 epithelial cells) and surface epithelial damage
- **Collagenous colitis:** Increased subepithelial collagen layer (irregular thickening, trapped inflammatory cells, blood vessels, and fibroblasts) and increased intraepithelial lymphocytes; trichrome stain highlights the collagen layer

OTHER HIGH YIELD POINTS
- Classically affects the **right colon** more than left; **females > males**
- Mild cases can be treated with loperamide, mesalazine, bismuth while moderate to severe cases with steroids   Path Presenter   Path Presenter

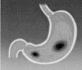
Granulomatous inflammation

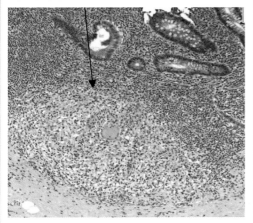

GRANULOMATOUS COLITIS
MORPHOLOGY
- **Granulomas are collections of histiocytes with surrounding lymphocytic cuff**; they can be necrotizing, non-necrotizing, well-formed, ill-defined (vague)
- **Granulomatous** inflammation warrants **AFB/FITE and GMS/PAS-D** stains to rule out infectious etiologies   Path Presenter

OTHER HIGH YIELD POINTS
ETIOLOGIES
- **Crohn disease:** Loose, non-necrotizing granulomas; seen in less than half of the cases; of note, ulcerative colitis can have granulomatous reaction to crypt rupture
- **Infections:** Especially if necrotizing, rule out fungi and mycobacteria; look for parasites (such as schistosomiasis); *Yersinia*
- **Sarcoidosis:** Well-formed epithelioid granulomas that sometime coalesce
- **Other etiologies:** Medications, cord-colitis syndrome, diverticular disease, common variable immunodeficiency, non-specific mucosal injury

Dilated mucosal vessels

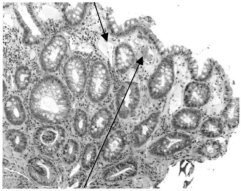

Fibrinoid vascular necrosis

RADIATION COLITIS/PROCTITIS
MORPHOLOGY
- Acute changes (1-2 months): **Lamina propria edema, fibrinoid vascular necrosis,** ulcer, epithelial atypia, increased epithelial apoptoses, mucosal neutrophil inflammation with **increased eosinophils**
- Late changes (months or years later): mucosal atrophy with crypt loss, fibrosis, **dilated telangiectatic vessels, vessel hyalinization and intimal thickening**; may see crypt architectural distortion, Paneth cell metaplasia, and fibrosis   Path Presenter

OTHER HIGH YIELD POINTS
- History of radiation to pelvic or abdominal malignancy
- **Rectosigmoid** is most commonly affected
- Symptoms can be within 1-2 months of therapy or months or years later
- Differential diagnosis: Ischemia, IBD

Segmental colitis associated with diverticulosis (SCAD)

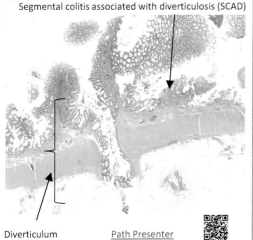

Diverticulum   Path Presenter

DIVERTICULAR DISEASE
MORPHOLOGY
- **Outpouching of colonic mucosa** and submucosa through the muscularis propria covered by subserosa/serosa (most are false diverticula); true diverticula are uncommon and involve outpouching of all layers of the intestinal wall
- Diverticulosis can be **complicated by acute/chronic diverticulitis** (4-15%), hemorrhage, and segmental colitis associated with diverticulosis (SCAD)

OTHER HIGH YIELD POINTS
- **Sigmoid and descending colon are the most common sites**; right-sided diverticular disease and ismore common in Asia
- Highest incidence in the western world; prevalence increases with age
- Etiology: Abnormal colonic motility leads to increased segmental contractions, increased intraluminal pressure, and diverticula formation
- SCAD can mimic IBD; however, changes are limited to vicinity of diverticula

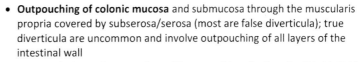

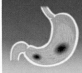

Crypt drop-out/loss

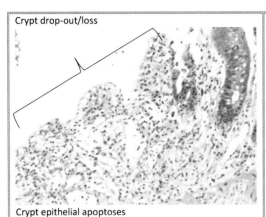

Crypt epithelial apoptoses

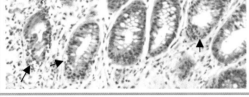

GRAFT VERSUS HOST DISEASE (GVHD)
MORPHOLOGY

- **Complication of stem cell transplantation**
- Characteristic features are **crypt apoptosis**, crypt dropout, and ulceration
- Inflammation tends to be sparse
- Architectural distortion and fibrosis are markers of long-standing GVHD

LERNER SYSTEM FOR GRADING GVHD	
Grade	Findings
1	Isolated apoptotic bodies
2	Loss or damage of isolated crypts, w/ or w/o crypt abscesses
3	Loss of two or more contiguous crypts
4	Extensive crypt loss with epithelial destruction

OTHER HIGH YIELD POINTS

- Donor T-cells recognize host tissue antigens as foreign leading to T-cell activation→ cytokine storm→ end organ damage
- **Skin > gastrointestinal tract > liver** affected

Path Presenter

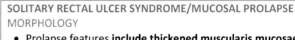

Muscle fibers splaying into the lamina propria

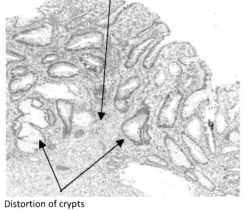

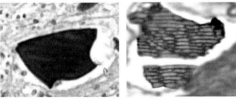

Distortion of crypts

SOLITARY RECTAL ULCER SYNDROME/MUCOSAL PROLAPSE
MORPHOLOGY

- Prolapse features **include thickened muscularis mucosae fibers with splayed fibers extending into the lamina propria**
- Other features include superficial mucosal ulceration, villiform change, crypt hyperplasia and distortion, ectatic vessels
- Late changes may mimic colitis cystica profunda

OTHER HIGH YIELD POINTS

- Solitary or multiple ulcerated or polypoid lesions, 4-10 cm from anal margin
- 3-4th decade; more common in women
- Etiology: **abnormal function of anal/pelvic floor muscles during defecation**

Path Presenter

Kayexalate: Purple+fish scales Sevelamer: Pink to yellow

Cholestyramine: Bright pink to orange

Image courtesy of Dr. Monika Vyas Twitter @Mvgs1706, used with permission

PIGMENTS AND INORGANIC MATERIAL
MEDICATION RESINS

- **Kayexalate: Used to treat hyperkalemia** in renal failure; it causes ischemic and ulcerative changes; linked to fatalities, so can be a critical diagnosis; **Purple** on H&E with narrow **fish-scale** pattern
- **Sevelamer: Used to treat hyperphosphatemia** in renal failure; can be associated with mucosal injury; **bright pink to rusty yellow** on H&E with an irregular fish-scale pattern
- **Bile acid sequestrants (cholestyramine):** Binds bile acids (lowers cholesterol); not associated with injury; bright pink to orange on H&E with classically smooth, glassy texture (scales may be present as an artifact of knife cutting)

Path Presenter

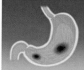

Brown pigment-laden macrophages in lamina propria

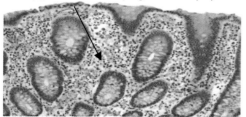

Tattoo pigment

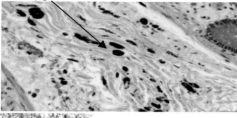

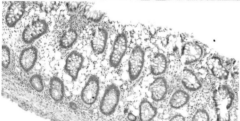

Pseudolipomatosis
Empty spaces (gas-filled) with foreign body giant cells

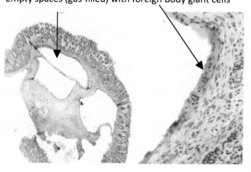

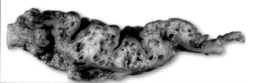

MELANOSIS COLI
- **Fine brown-black pigment in the cytoplasm of macrophages** commonly found in the lamina propria
- **Consists of lipofuscin**; although classically associated with **laxative use**, it can be seen with any other disorder with increased epithelial turnover, including constipation
- Differential diagnosis: Hemosiderosis (pigment is bright-brown and coarse)- iron stain positive

Path Presenter

TATTOO PIGMENT
- **Black coarse granules in macrophages** often with foreign-body giant cell reaction
- Used to **mark lesions endoscopically for later identification**

PSEUDOLIPOMATOSIS/AIR
- Empty spaces without associated foreign body giant cell reaction seen in colorectal biopsies commonly
- **Attributed to insufflation artifact;** no associated nuclei; tend to be variable in size
- Differential diagnosis: Mucosal lipoma (associated with Cowden syndrome)
- IHC: S100 negative

PNEUMATOSIS CYSTOIDES INTESTINALIS
- **Empty spaces (gas-filled) with foreign body giant cell reaction** (the reaction implies it happened in vivo)
- May occur in children and adults
- Can be incidental or associated with severe disease
- In adults, can be idiopathic or due to infection with gas-producing bacteria such as *Clostridia,* drugs, chemotherapy, obstruction, pulmonary disease or connective tissue disease

Path Presenter

Gross image courtesy of Dr. Brian Cox @Dr_Brian_Cox, used with permission

MEDICATION INDUCED INJURY	
Pattern of colitis	**Associated drug**
Eosinophilic colitis	NSAIDs, gold, carbamazepine, antiplatelet agents, estrogens
Lymphocytic or collagenous colitis	NSAIDs, lansoprazole, ticlopidine, ranitidine, simvastatin, flutamide, carbamazepine, sertraline, penicillin, checkpoint inhibitors, Idelalisib
Focal active colitis	NSAIDs, Bowel preparation (esp. oral sodium phosphate), checkpoint inhibitors, Idelalisib
Ischemic colitis	NSAIDs, antibiotics, amphetamines, digitalis, diuretics, chemotherapy, nasal decongestants, constipation-inducing medications, laxatives, vasopressor agents, cocaine, ergotamine, serotonin agonists/antagonists including sumatriptan,

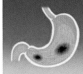
	estrogen, progesterone, glutaraldehyde, and immunomodulators such as interleukin
Apoptotic colitis	Bowel preparation (esp. oral sodium phosphate), mycophenolate mofetil, laxatives, chemotherapeutic agents (esp. 5-fluorouracil), NSAIDs, cyclosporine, checkpoint inhibitors, Idelalisib, TNF-alpha inhibitors
Pseudomembranous colitis	NSAIDs, antibiotic-associated Clostridium difficile colitis
Neutropenic colitis	Chemotherapy
Mucosal ulcers, erosions, and strictures	NSAIDs, methotrexate, nonabsorbable drugs: Kayexalate, sevelamer, colesevelam

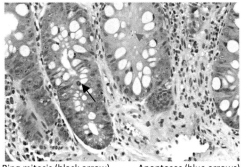

Ring mitosis (black arrow)   Apoptoses (blue arrows)

Regenerative crypt with atypia after injury

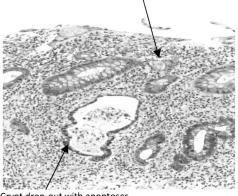

Crypt drop-out with apoptoses

Mycophenolate mofetil injury: Apoptotic bodies

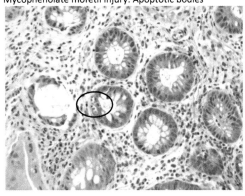

CHARACTERISTIC INJURY PATTERNS AND MEDICATIONS
CHOLCHICINE
- Multiple arrested metaphase mitoses, particularly "rings;" increased apoptotic bodies and reactive changes
- Used in the treatment of gout
- Inhibits microtubule polymerization→ interferes with mitosis, chemotaxis, and neutrophil degranulation
Path Presenter

CHEMOTHERAPY-RELATED INJURY
- Epithelial atypia, sometimes mimics dysplasia
- Taxol causes ring mitoses similar to colchicine
- Severe neutropenia can cause "neutropenic colitis" where after mucosal damage opportunistic bacteria invade and cause necrosis and pneumatosis leading often to septic shock
Path Presenter

MYCOPHENOLATE MOFETIL INJURY
- Immunosuppressive drug usually used after solid organ transplantation
- GI toxicity often limits the use
- Increased crypt apoptoses, patchy neutrophilic infiltration, degenerated damaged crypts, scattered eosinophils
- Differential diagnosis: GVHD (less eosinophils)
Path Presenter

CHECKPOINT INHIBITOR INJURY
- Anti-PD1, anti PD-L1, and anti-CTLA therapies
- Activate immune tumor destruction, but can also cause autoimmune "immune-related adverse events"
- Responds to steroids
- Microscopic findings include all or some of the findings of lymphocytic colitis, collagenous colitis, acute self-limited colitis, and apoptotic colitis
Path Presenter

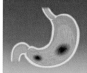

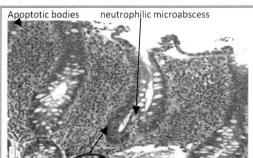
Apoptotic bodies   neutrophilic microabscess

Intraepithelial lymphocytes

IDELALISIB
- Specific small molecule drug used to treat chronic lymphocytic leukemia/small lymphocytic lymphoma and follicular lymphoma
- Causes severe diarrhea
- Overlapping injury morphology as with checkpoint inhibitors such as increased apoptoses, lymphocytic colitis, and active colitis

COLON: INFECTIOUS ETIOLOGIES

CYTOMEGALOVIRUS
MORPHOLOGY
- Cytomegaly with **nuclear "owl's eye (Cowdry-A) pink, nucleolus-like inclusions and cytoplasmic granular and pink to purple hof-like inclusions**
- Cells affected commonly are stromal and endothelial cells
- Background may show ulceration, mixed inflammation infiltrates rich in neutrophils; immunosuppressed patients may show less inflammation

OTHER HIGH YIELD POINTS
- Most common in **immunocompromised hosts** such as Human Immunodeficiency Virus (HIV) patients, inflammatory bowel disease patients on therapy, and graft versus host disease cases

Path Presenter

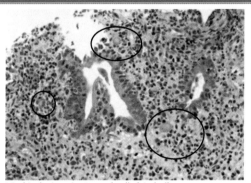
Viral inclusions in stromal cells (circled)
Organisms mimic histiocytes (within the ulcer)

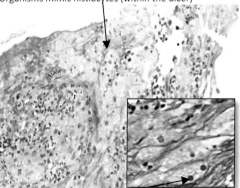

Ingested red blood cells

AMEBIASIS
MORPHOLOGY
- Infection caused by pathogenic species of amebae, mostly *Entamoeba Histolytica*
- Amebae: trophozoites that are 10-60 μ, nucleus 3-5 μ with central condensation of chromatin and peripheral rim of chromatin; numerous fine vacuoles in the cytoplasm give them a **foamy appearance mimicking histiocytes; the clue is to look for ingested red blood cells**
- Discrete **ulcers (flask-shaped)** with intervening normal mucosa
- Stains: Negative for CD68 and positive for PAS and Trichrome

OTHER HIGH YIELD POINTS
- Commonly involves the colon, most commonly cecum and right colon
- Usually asymptomatic but may present as fulminant colitis

Path Presenter

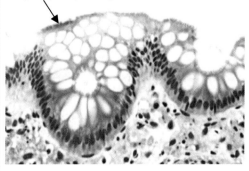

Fuzzy, fringed layer of organisms

SPIROCHETOSIS
MORPHOLOGY
- **Fuzzy, fringed layer of organisms at the surface of epithelium** (non-invasive)
- No associated inflammatory infiltrate
- Stains: Positive for silver stains (Warthin-starry, Steiner) and spirochete immunohistochemical stain

OTHER HIGH YIELD POINTS

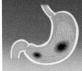

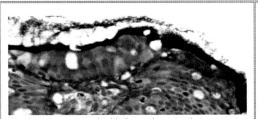

Warthin-starry stain- highlighting the spirochetes
Smudy basophilic inclusions of adenovirus

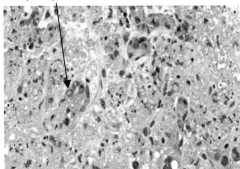

- Variable spirochete species, but most are **Brachyspira aalborgi or Brachispira pilosicoli**
- More common in the developing world, HIV patients, and men
- Most cases are asymptomatic; if associated with diarrhea, can treat with antibiotics   Path Presenter

ADENOVIRUS
MORPHOLOGY
- **Smudgy basophilic inclusions** in the surface epithelium, often in goblet cells → can be round or crescent-shaped
- Colon shows increased apoptosis and epithelial sloughing

OTHER HIGH YIELD POINTS
- **Common cause of childhood diarrhea**; can cause intussusception due to lymphoid hyperplasia
- In immunocompromised hosts, can cause diarrhea and potentially disseminated disease (hepatitis and pneumonitis) and death

COLON: INFLAMMATORY BOWEL DISEASE

Normal colon   Architectural distortion

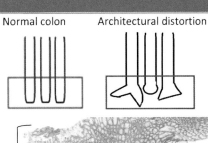

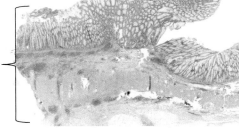

Transmural chronic inflammation in Crohn

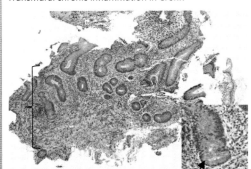

Architectural distortion   Paneth cells

Nomenclature for colitis	Morphologic features
Acute	Neutrophils in the epithelium, glandular lumens
Chronic	Architectural distortion
	Basal lymphoplasmacytosis
	Paneth cell metaplasia (left colon)
	Pyloric metaplasia (mostly in small bowel)

CROHN DISEASE
MORPHOLOGY
- Patchy **transmural** chronic active inflammation involving upper and lower gastrointestinal tract
- Characteristic features are **transmural inflammation, skip lesions, granulomas, ulcers (superficial aphthous type to fissuring), muscle and nerve hypertrophy, pyloric gland metaplasia, fibrosis/strictures, and fistulas including perianal fistulas, pseudo-polyps, creeping fat**

OTHER HIGH YIELD POINTS
- Onset of disease at 20-40 years with a second peak in 50-60 years
- Small bowel involvement in 80%, ileocolonic involvement in 30-40%
- Extraintestinal manifestations: arthritis, uveitis, pyoderma gangrenosum, primary sclerosing cholangitis, and pulmonary processes
- Increased risk of dysplasia and carcinoma

Path Presenter

ULCERATIVE COLITIS
MORPHOLOGY
- Chronic active inflammation in **the rectum** proceeding proximally in a continuous **diffuse** pattern (pan-colitis)
- Changes are limited to the **mucosa and superficial submucosa** with ulceration

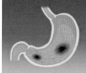

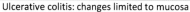
Ulcerative colitis: changes limited to mucosa

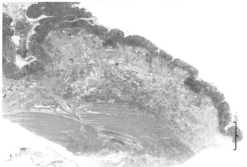

Normal colon   Involved by inflammatory bowel disease

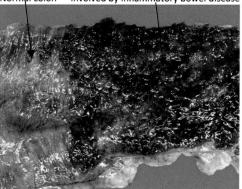

Indefinite for dysplasia (surface still shows maturation)

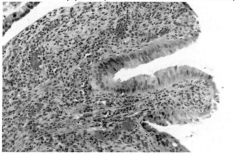

Low grade dysplasia: Atypical cells extend to the surface

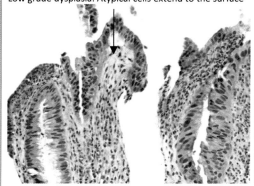

- Small bowel usually not involved but can see mild inflammation in terminal ileum in 20% ("backwash ileitis"); absence of granulomas; no fistulas or fissures; toxic megacolon; pseudopolyps

OTHER HIGH YIELD POINTS
- Onset of disease at 15-30 years with a second peak in 50-70 years
- Extraintestinal manifestations similar to Crohn disease
- Increased risk of dysplasia and carcinoma

Path Presenter

INDETERMINATE COLITIS
- 10% of inflammatory bowel disease patients are unclassifiable, often due to pathologic and clinical overlap between Ulcerative colitis and Crohn disease

DYSPLASIA IN INFLAMMATORY BOWEL DISEASE
- Inflammation→ DNA oxidative damage→ Cancer
- Risk proportion to severity and duration of inflammation
- Risk proportion to severity and duration of inflammation
- Cancer risk in inflammatory bowel disease (~2% risk)
- Screening recommendations:
  - First 8-10 years after diagnosis→ no increased screening
  - Years 10-20→ Every 1-3 years (shorter interval with worse disease, especially if primary sclerosing cholangitis present)
  - Years 20 onwards→1-2 years
- Treatment of dysplasia: With modern techniques, including high-definition and chromoendoscopy, most dysplasia is visible. As such, it can be completely resected endoscopically. Once a dysplastic lesion has been resected, in the absence of surrounding dysplasia, ongoing meticulous colonoscopic surveillance is appropriate. Proctocolectomy is only recommended for dysplasia if endoscopic resection is not possible, or if nonvisible high-grade dysplasia or adenocarcinoma is found

INDEFINITE FOR DYSPLASIA
- Epithelial atypia that cannot be classified as either reactive or dysplastic
- Two causes: atypia in the setting of inflammation or ulceration or surface is not present for evaluation
- Management: Treat active disease and repeat biopsy in 3-12 months

LOW-GRADE DYSPLASIA
- Enlarged, hyperchromatic, smooth, "pencillate" nuclei with nuclear stratification but maintained basal orientation (similar to sporadic adenoma), higher nuclear to cytoplasmic ratio, little to no surface maturation, abruption transition, prominent apoptoses
- Molecular: IBD-associated dysplasia shows more copy number aberrations and aneuploidy than sporadic adenomas; TP53 mutations are frequently present early
- Management: Complete endoscopic resection if visible; otherwise proctocolectomy to exclude cancer

Path Presenter

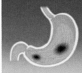

p53 IHC: overexpression in low-grade dysplasia

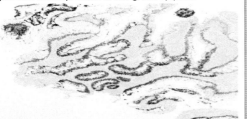

High-grade dysplasia with cribriform architecture

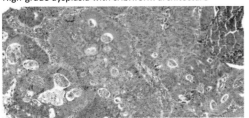

Serrated epithelial change

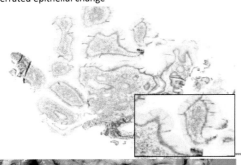

HIGH-GRADE DYSPLASIA

- Enlarged, hyperchromatic, pleomorphic nuclei, often plumper nuclei than low grade; irregular nuclear contours, prominent nucleoli, loss of nuclear polarity, complex architecture such as cribriforming, crypt branching/budding
- Molecular: P53 staining often highlights both grades: Dysplasia→ Strong P53 staining (or null-type) at the surface in atypical areas

NON-CONVENTIONAL LESIONS
SERRATED EPITHELIAL CHANGE

- Distorted crypt architecture with serrations at the top and bottom of crypts
- Nuclei are bland with goblet-rich epithelium
- Controversial risk of cancer; some consider it indefinite for dysplasia
- Emerging genetics, likely *TP53* mutations

Path Presenter

NON-CONVENTIONAL DYSPLASIA

- Hypermucinous, traditional serrated adenoma-like, sessile serrated lesion-like, Paneth cell differentiation, goblet cell-deficient, terminal epithelial differentiation

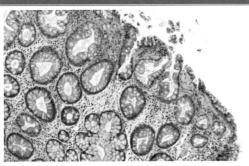
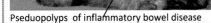

Pseudopolyps of inflammatory bowel disease

DISTINGUISHING FEATURES OF CROHN AND ULCERATIVE COLITIS

CROHN	ULCERATIVE COLITIS
Rectum spared	Rectum affected
Anal lesions in 75%	Anal lesions are rare
Deep fissures and fistulas	Horizontal fissures
Inflamed serosa	Serosa unaffected
Strictures	No strictures
Patchy transmural inflammation	Continuous, diffuse inflammation limited to mucosa/submucosa
Granulomas may be present	No granulomas

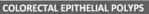

COLORECTAL EPITHELIAL POLYPS

HYPERPLASTIC POLYP   Path Presenter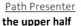

- **Serrated architecture with serrations limited to the upper half of the crypts**; mild nuclear enlargement but not as severe as conventional dysplasia; microvesicular and goblet-cell rich variants
- Soft features: Thickened subepithelial collagen, base has retained neuroendocrine cells
- Very common polyp, particularly in rectum; tend to be numerous, ≤ 5 mm
- **No significant risk of malignant transformation**
- Microvesicular variant may contain *BRAF* mutation; goblet cell rich may show *KRAS* mutation

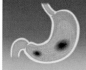

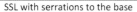
SSL with serrations to the base

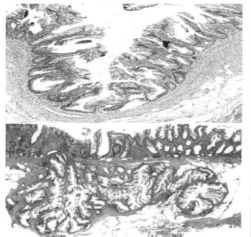

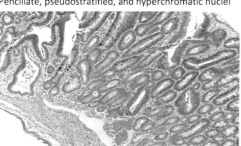

SSL with prolapse into the submucosa

SESSILE SERRATED LESION/POLYP/ADENOMA (SSL)
MORPHOLOGY
- Serrated neoplastic precursor lesion of colorectal cancer
- **Serrations extends to the base with asymmetrical growth such as boot-shaped, inverted-T; only one unequivocal distorted** crypt is required
- May contain fibroblastic/perineuriomatous stroma
- May develop traditional or serrated cytologic dysplasia

OTHER HIGH YIELD POINTS
- Currently referred to as sessile serrated lesion; former names sessile serrated adenoma/polyp
- Usually large (≥ 1 cm), **sessile, right-sided**
- Sporadic microsatellite instability pathway: Normal colon → *BRAF* V600E→ HP→ DNA methylation → SSL → MLH1 promoter methylation/deficiency → Microsatellite instability → Dysplasia → Carcinoma

Path Presenter

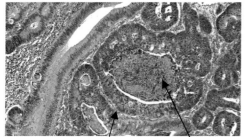

High-grade dysplasia: Cribriforming and necrosis

Pencillate, pseudostratified, and hyperchromatic nuclei

TUBULAR ADENOMA
MORPHOLOGY
- Dysplasia is characterized by "picket fence" nuclei that are elongated, **pencillate, pseudostratified, hyperchromatic**
- **Low-grade dysplasia:** Nuclei remain in basal orientation (in the bottom half of the cell); changes should involve at least the upper half of the crypts and luminal surface
- **High-grade dysplasia:** Cytologic pleomorphism with rounded nuclei, increased nuclear to cytoplasmic ratio, prominent nucleoli, open chromatin, and architectural complexity such as cribriforming, luminal necrosis
- **Intramucosal carcinoma:** Single cell infiltration into lamina propria, small irregular glands in the lamina propria (considered in-situ disease in the colorectum)

OTHER HIGH YIELD POINTS
- Variants: Tubular adenoma- greater than 75% tubules; tubulovillous adenoma- greater than 25% villi; and villous adenoma- greater than 75% villi
- **Chromosomal Instability Pathway (most common):** *APC* → *KRAS*→ *p53* (also often β-Catenin and *SMAD4*)
- **Lynch Microsatellite Instability Pathway:** Germline MMR mutation → Loss of heterozygosity → Microsatellite instability   Path Presenter

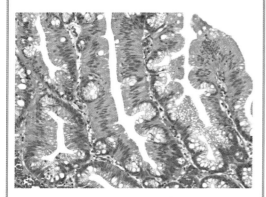

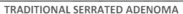

TRADITIONAL SERRATED ADENOMA
MORPHOLOGY
- Columnar cells with mucin depleted, **eosinophilic cytoplasm**
- Nuclei with low grade dysplasia, pencillate; **ectopic crypts** are a unique feature

OTHER HIGH YIELD POINTS
- Uncommon
- Often pedunculated, villous, and **left-sided**
- Contain either *KRAS* or *BRAF* mutations
- Unlike hyperplastic polyps, considered cancerous

Path Presenter

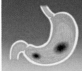

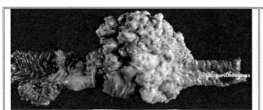

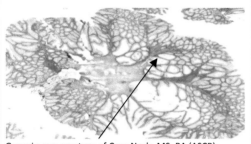

Gross image courtesy of Cory Nash, MS, PA (ASCP)
Arborizing smooth muscle

HAMARTOMATOUS POLYPS
PEUTZ-JEGHERS POLYP
MORPHOLOGY
- Hamartomatous polyp (non-neoplastic) with multilobulated architecture, **arborizing smooth muscle**, and bland (non-dysplastic) epithelium

OTHER HIGH YIELD POINTS
- Seen in **Peutz-Jegher's syndrome** that show germline mutation in **STK11/LKB1** gene (can be sporadic or inherited)
- Most frequent in the small bowel
- Additional findings of mucocutaneous **melanotic macules** (lips and oral mucosa)
- Increased risk of many cancers such as stomach, colon, pancreas, breast etc
- Additional associations- **Ovarian sex cord stromal tumor with annular tubules, sertoli cell tumors, cervical adenoma malignum**

Path Presenter

Smooth, spherical and pedunculated polyp

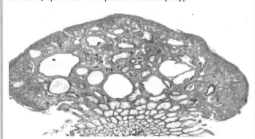

Cystic glands and abundant inflamed stroma

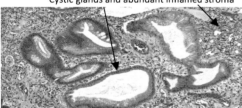

JUVENILE POLYP
MORPHOLOGY
- Hamartomatous polyp (non-neoplastic) that is smoothly spherical and pedunculated; **prominent cystic glands**, **abundant inflamed stroma without dysplasia**; surface may be eroded

OTHER HIGH YIELD POINTS
- **Most common pediatric colon polyp**
- Extremely low risk of malignant transformation unless syndromic
- Majority are solitary; multiple may indicate **Juvenile Polyposis Syndrome (JPS)**
- JPS is autosomal dominant caused by germline defect in **SMAD4 or BMPR1A**
- JPS is defined by ≥5 juvenile polyps or any number if positive family history
- Usually 50-200 polyps
- Can develop dysplasia and colon cancer; age at colon cancer ~35 years

Path Presenter

COLORECTAL MESENCHYMAL POLYPS

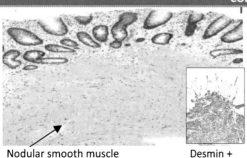

Nodular smooth muscle   Desmin +

LEIOMYOMA
- Often presents as a small submucosal polypoid mass/polyp; M>F; generally <1 cm
- In the colon, majority arise in the rectosigmoid
- Benign **smooth muscle neoplasm comprising of bland spindled cells with intersecting fascicles** and no significant mitotic activity
- IHC: **(+) for desmin** and SMA while **(-)** for CKIT, DOG1, CD34, and S100

Path Presenter

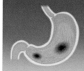

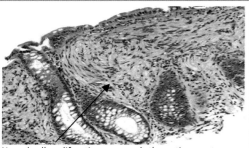

Neural cell proliferation surrounds the native crypts

SCHWANN CELL HAMARTOMA
- Benign poorly circumscribed mucosal **neural cell proliferation** that presents as a polyp; F>M; generally, < 1 cm
- No ganglion cells are present; no syndromic association
- Can arise anywhere but more common in distal colorectum
- IHC: **(+) for S100** and neurofilament while **(-)** for EMA, SMA, CKIT, DOG1, and CD34
- Differential diagnosis: Perineurioma (EMA+) and ganglioneuroma (ganglion cells present)   Path Presenter

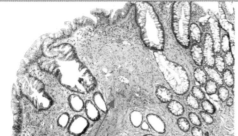

Spindle cell peirneurial proliferation, EMA+

PERINEURIOMA
- Benign polypoid **poorly circumscribed lesion** comprising of a **spindle cell perineurial proliferation,** usually confined to the mucosa
- Overlying epithelium usually shows surface hyperplastic changes or can be associated with another polyp such as a serrated polyp or tubular adenoma
- IHC: **(+) for EMA, claudin 1, CD34, and GLUT1** while **(-)** for CKIT, desmin, and S100   Link

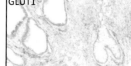
GLUT1

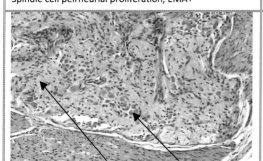

Neoplasm with Schwann cells and ganglion cells

GANGLIONEUROMA
- **Benign** mesenchymal polyp
- Unrelated to a similarly named lesion of the adrenal gland
- Expansion of lamina propria by bland spindled **Schwann cells** with scattered or abundant **ganglion cells**
- Multiple ganglioneuromas raise consideration for **Cowden syndrome**
- IHC: Schwann cells are **(+)** for S100
- Ganglion cells are **(+)** for S100, synaptophysin and NSE

Path Presenter

COLON/RECTUM: ADENOCARCINOMA

Adenocarcinoma, not otherwise specified

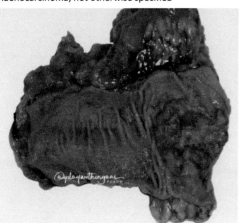

MORPHOLOGY
- Invasive adenocarcinoma is defined by the **infiltration of neoplastic glands into the submucosa**
- Single cells, desmoplastic stroma, complex architecture, and necrosis are some features that can be seen
- Grading based on gland formation: Well-differentiated (>95%), moderately differentiated (50-95% glands), poorly differentiated (<50% gland formation)
- IHC profile: Generally **(+)** for CK20, CDX2, SATB2, and Villin while **(-)** for CK7

OTHER HIGH YIELD POINTS
- Third most common cancer in the United States
- Associated with processed food, obesity, red meat, low fiber diet, and alcohol
- Most arise through the adenoma → carcinoma sequence

Gross image courtesy of Cory Nash, MS, PA (ASCP), Dept of Pathology, University of Chicago; used with permission

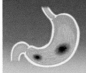

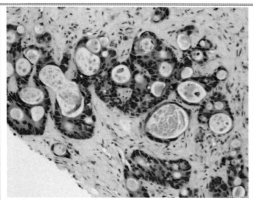

Path Presenter

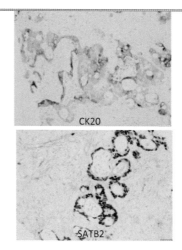

CK20

CDX-2

SATB2

CK7

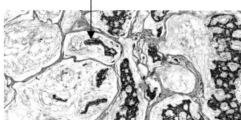

Mucinous carcinoma

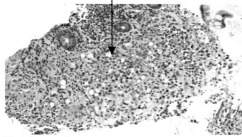

Signet ring cell carcinoma

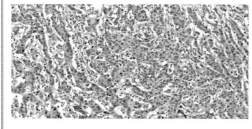

Medullary carcinoma

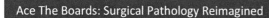

SUBTYPES OF CARCINOMA

- Although most colon cancers are "NOS" (Not Otherwise Specified), some subtypes exist, many of which have distinct morphology, clinical implications, and molecular alterations

MUCINOUS ADENOCARCINOMA

- >50% of tumor composed of pools of extracellular mucin (the **most common** subtype); if <50% mucin →Adenocarcinoma with mucinous features
- No prognosis implications
- Enriched for Microsatellite Instability (MSI)-high tumors

SIGNET-RING CELL ADENOCARCINOMA

- >50% of tumor is composed of signet-ring cells (prominent intracytoplasmic mucin displacing the nucleus)
- Worse outcome
- Associated with Lynch syndrome and MSI-high

MEDULLARY CARCINOMA

- Sheets of malignant cells with vesicular nuclei, prominent nucleoli, abundant eosinophilic cytoplasm, and a prominent inflammatory infiltrate
- Better prognosis
- *BRAF* mutations→ MSI-high

Path Presenter

SERRATED ADENOCARCINOMA

- Morphologically like serrated polyps

MICROPAPILLARY ADENOCARCINOMA

- Small clusters of tumor cells with stromal retraction
- Worse outcome (like in other organs) with early metastasis to lymph nodes

ADENOMA-LIKE ADENOCARCINOMA

- Pushing invasion with minimal desmoplasia
- Difficult to diagnose on biopsy
- Good prognosis

ADENOSQUAMOUS ADENOCARCINOMA

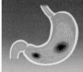
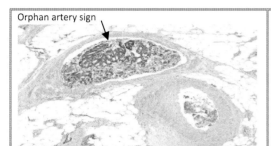
Orphan artery sign

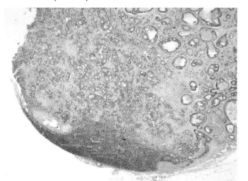
Tumor buds (arrows)

Tumor metastasis in a lymph node

OTHER MORPHOLOGIC FEATURES

LARGE VENOUS INVASION
- Tumor involving endothelium-lined spaces with an identifiable smooth muscle layer or elastic lamina
- Difficult to diagnose on biopsy
- Extramural venous invasion (outside muscularis propria) is a risk factor for liver metastasis
- Orphan artery sign: Artery with a large, rounded tongue of tumor next to it
- EVG can highlight elastic lamina of arteries and veins

TUMOR BUDDING
- Single cells or small clusters of < 5 cells at the advancing front of the tumor
- High tumor budding is a significant risk factor for nodal involvement/poor outcome. Represents "epithelial-mesenchymal transition"

LYMPH NODE VERSUS TUMOR DEPOSITS
- Lymph node metastasis has residual lymphoid tissue surrounding it; usually rounded contour
- Tumor deposit is a focus in fat without identifiable lymph node tissue, nerve or vascular structure

Tumor deposit

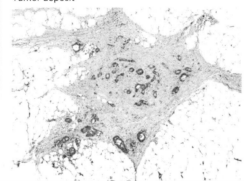

Path Presenter

Anterior peritoneal reflection

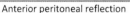
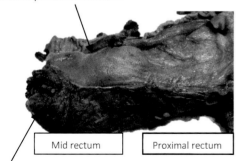

Mid rectum | Proximal rectum

Mesorectal fat/envelope

RECTAL CANCER: UNIQUE ANATOMIC CONSIDERATIONS
- Portion of rectum is not covered by peritoneum/serosa (anterior peritoneal reflection) but rather mesorectal fat (non-peritonealized surface)
- The quality of surgical technique/completeness of mesorectal envelope is the key determinant of local recurrence and long-term survival
- Gross assessment of mesorectal envelope: Complete (good bulk, smooth surface, no visible muscle), nearly complete (moderately bulky, minor irregularities (> 5 mm), versus incomplete (visible muscularis propria)
- Mesorectal fat radial margin/circumferential margin: Considered positive if tumor is <1 mm from inked margin

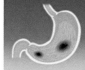

MOLECULAR PATHWAYS OF COLORECTAL CANCER

1) CHROMOSOMAL INSTABILITY PATHWAY (NON-HYPERMUTATED PATHWAY)

- ~85% of colorectal cancers
- Adenoma to carcinoma sequence; large chromosome arm gains and losses
- Common mutations: *APC* (early, starts adenoma →activates the WNT pathway), *KRAS*, and *TP53*
- *RAS* mutations (~50% of tumors)→resistant to anti-EGFR therapy (used to treat metastatic cancer)

2) MICROSATELLITE INSTABILITY PATHWAY (MSI, HYPERMUTATED PATHWAY)

- ~15% of colorectal cancers
- **SPORADIC:** *BRAF* mutation → *MLH1* promoter hypermethylation → Inactivation of mismatch repair (MMR) enzymes → Serrated polyp → Carcinoma
- **LYNCH-ASSOCIATED:** Germline mutations in MMR proteins→ Loss of heterozygosity→ Adenoma → Carcinoma→ Lots of mutations → More immunogenic → More inflammatory response to tumor → Better outcome (responds to checkpoint inhibitors (e.g., anti-PD-L1 drugs))

3) ULTRAMUTATED PATHWAY

- ~3% of colorectal cancers
- *POLE* (DNA replication enzyme) mutation → Lots of mistakes with DNA replication → Ultramutated tumor

TUMOR SYNDROMES

```
              ┌─────────────┐
              │  MMR IHC    │
              └─────────────┘
        ┌───────────┼───────────┐
        ▼           ▼           ▼
  ┌──────────┐ ┌──────────┐ ┌──────────┐
  │MMR intact│ │  MSH2,   │ │  MLH1    │
  │          │ │ MSH6, or │ │deficient │
  │          │ │  PMS2    │ │  (with   │
  │          │ │          │ │  PMS2)   │
  └──────────┘ └──────────┘ └──────────┘
        ▼           ▼           ▼
  ┌──────────┐ ┌──────────┐ ┌──────────┐
  │ Probably │ │ Probably │ │  BRAF    │
  │ NOT Lynch│ │  Lynch   │ │ Testing  │
  │(sporadic)│ │          │ │          │
  └──────────┘ └──────────┘ └──────────┘
                       ┌───────┴───────┐
                       ▼               ▼
                 ┌──────────┐   ┌──────────┐
                 │   BRAF   │   │ No BRAF  │
                 │ mutation │   │          │
                 └──────────┘   └──────────┘
                       ▼               ▼
                 ┌──────────┐   ┌──────────┐
                 │ Sporadic │   │  MLH1    │
                 │          │   │methylation│
                 │          │   │ testing  │
                 └──────────┘   └──────────┘
                       ┌───────┴───────┐
                       ▼               ▼
                 ┌──────────┐   ┌──────────┐
                 │   No     │   │Methylation│
                 │methylation│  │ detected │
                 └──────────┘   └──────────┘
                       ▼               ▼
                 ┌──────────┐   ┌──────────┐
                 │ Probably │   │ Sporadic │
                 │  Lynch   │   │          │
                 └──────────┘   └──────────┘
```

LYNCH SYNDROME (HEREDITARY NON-POLYPOSIS COLORECTAL CANCER)

- Germline mutations with mismatch repair (MMR) genes
- Autosomal Dominant → Defective DNA repair → Many mutations ("hypermutated") → Microsatellite unstable
- **Most common form of heritable colorectal cancer (CRC)**
- CRC usually develops before age 50, often with multiple primaries (~80% lifetime risk)
- Also at risk for endometrial cancer, upper urinary tract and other GI cancers, and sebaceous skin tumors
- Universal screening of all new CRC: Do IHC first (algorithm in the left tab), can also do MSI testing by PCR
- Looking for LOSS of staining. Normal is intact staining of all 4 MMR enzymes
- Lynch-related CRC is more often right-sided and arises from adenomas
- Sporadic MMR-deficient tumors, that come from sessile serrated polyps, and are associated with *BRAF V600E* mutations and then MLH-1 promoter hypermethylation and MLH1 loss of expression
- MMR-deficient CRC: Associated with **high grade, mucinous differentiation, and lymphocytic infiltrates (hypermutated state is immunogenic)**
- Better survival compared to MMR- intact CRC (probably due to host response); automatically approved for PD-L1 therapy

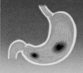

Unicryptal adenoma

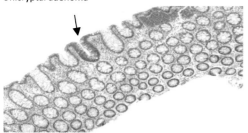

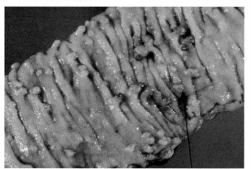

Path Presenter   Innumerable polyps in the colon

Image courtesy of: WebPathology.com, @WebPathology, used with permission

FAMILIAL ADENOMATOUS POLYPOSIS (FAP)

- Germline mutation in **APC** gene; Tumor suppressor → Loss leads to lots of tumors
- **Autosomal Dominant**- almost complete penetrance
- Hundreds of colorectal adenomas carpeting colon, more on left side
- Mean age of colorectal cancer diagnosis: 40 years (so often prophylactic colectomy in 20's)
- Also at risk for duodenal and gastric adenomas (less cancer risk though); need to undergo regular surveillance upper endoscopies also
- First morphologic finding: Single dysplastic crypts ("unicryptal adenoma")

VARIANTS
ATTENUATD FAP

- Less than 100 adenomas, right-sided, older age of presentation and diagnosis of cancer
- Mutation in different part of *APC* gene

GARDNER'S SYNDROME

- **FAP with prominent extraintestinal manifestations** (including desmoid tumors, osteomas, epidermoid cysts, papillary thyroid carcinoma (classically the cribriform-morular variant), and nasopharyngeal angiofibromas)

TURCOT SYNDROME

- "Glioma polyposis syndrome"- **FAP with brain tumor** (usually Medulloblastoma)

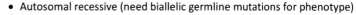

Tubular adenomas

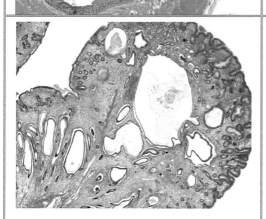

MUTYH (or MYH) -ASSOCIATED POLYPOSIS

- Autosomal recessive (need biallelic germline mutations for phenotype)
- *MYH* gene is involved in base excision repair → defects result in *APC* and *RAS* mutations
- Results in multiple adenomas (usually < 100), may have extraintestinal manifestations of FAP
- Increased risk of colorectal cancer, usually right-sided, even in absence of polyps
- Differential diagnosis: HNPCC/Lynch, attenuated FAP

CRONKHITE-CANADA SYNDROME

- Uncertain etiology (NOT clearly genetic), non-familial
- Often older male (~50 years old)
- **Hamartomatous polyps** and **protein-losing enteropathy**
- Diffusely nodular mucosa throughout GI tract; broad, sessile hamartomatous polyps with edema and cystic dilations in stomach, looks like hyperplastic polyps; in the colon, looks like juvenile polyps
- **"Ectodermal" manifestations:** onychodystrophy, alopecia, cataracts, glossitis, vitiligo
- Increased risk of colon cancer   Path Presenter

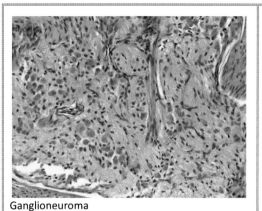
Ganglioneuroma

COWDEN SYNDROME

- *PTEN* **mutation;** tumor suppressor → mutation causes lots of tumors
- Autosomal dominant
- Other *PTEN* syndromes: Bannayan-Riley Ruvalcaba syndrome and Lhermitte-Duclos disease
- Associated tumors: Multiple hamartomas (mouth, GI tract), thyroid carcinoma (usually follicular), breast cancer (high risk), endometrial cancer, trichilemmomas, lipomas, glycogenic acanthosis (esophagus), hyperplastic polyps-look alikes (stomach), stroma rich polyps with cystically dilated glands mimicking juvenile polyps, mucosal lipomas (relatively unique), ganglioneuromas

ANUS

ANATOMY

- Anal canal begins where rectum enter the puborectalis sling at the apex of the anal sphincter complex (1-2 cm proximal to the dentate line)
- Anus encompasses three different mucosa types: glandular, transitional, squamous

- Dentate line is marked by transitional type mucosa and anal glands appear subjacent to the mucosa

ANUS: NON-NEOPLASTIC CONDITIONS

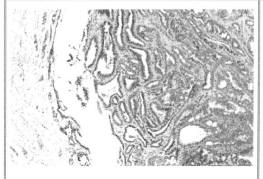
Tailgut cyst

DEVELOPMENTAL AND ACQUIRED CYSTS
DUPLICATION CYST

- Lined by columnar organized gastrointestinal epithelium with a well-formed, double muscular layer and nerve plexus

TAILGUT CYST

- (Retrorectal cystic hamartoma) Cystic mass near sacrum lined by any type of gastrointestinal tract epithelium, including squamous, with disorganized smooth muscle bundles

OTHERS

- Epidermal inclusion cyst
- Median raphe cyst
- Mature cystic teratoma

Path Presenter

ECTOPIC BREAST TISSUE

- The "milk line" extends to the perianal area, so you can have ectopic breast tissue and even breast tumors (e.g., hidradenoma, phyllodes tumors)

HIDRADENOMA PAPILLIFERUM

- **Well-circumscribed nodule** with papillary architecture of ducts lined by a double layer of epithelial cells with decapitation secretion (**essentially the cutaneous counterpart of a breast intraductal papilloma**); apocrine features are common
- Benign neoplasm arising in the anogenital mammary-like glands, found in the vulva or perianal region
- Almost exclusively in **middle-aged women**

Path Presenter

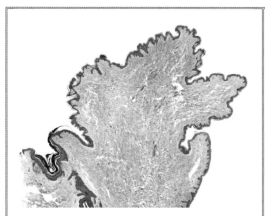

FIBROEPITHELIAL POLYP

MORPHOLOGY

- Non-neoplastic polyp: Benign polypoid projections of anal squamous epithelium with underlying subepithelial hyalinized vascular stroma
- May have multinucleated giant cells or fibroblasts with bizarre nuclei (large, smudged, hyperchromatic), which are thought to be degenerative
- Often CD34+

OTHER HIGH YIELD POINTS

- Synonyms: Hypertrophic anal papillae or skin tag
- Very common; resembles hemorrhoids clinically
- Differential diagnosis: Hemorrhoids (these have large dilated vascular spaces)

Path Presenter

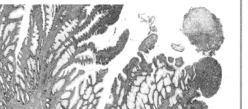

INFLAMMATORY CLOACOGENIC POLYP

MORPHOLOGY

- Surface may include squamous, glandular, or transition zone epithelium, which is often hyperplastic, without dysplasia
- Classic feature- fibromuscular proliferation around glands
- Stromal inflammation, surface ulceration, and granulation tissue are often present

OTHER HIGH YIELD POINTS

- Non-neoplastic polyp arising at the anal transition zone; may involve lower rectum, often anterior
- Thought to be due to prolapse (on a spectrum with solitary rectal ulcer syndrome and rectal prolapse)

Path Presenter

ANUS: NEOPLASTIC

SQUAMOUS INTRAEPITHELIAL LESION

- Anal canal involvement: Anal Intraepithelial Neoplasia (AIN)
- Perianal skin involvement: Perianal Intraepithelial Neoplasia (PAIN)

AIN1: Koilocytes

AIN3: Full thickness cytologic atypia and mitoses

GRADE	MORPHOLOGIC FEATURES
Low-grade, AIN1/PAIN1, Condyloma	Cytologic atypia and mitotic figures limited to the **lower 1/3rd** of epithelium with associated superficial **koilocytic atypia**; atypia meaning hyperchromatic nuclei with irregular nuclear contours Koilocytes= large superficial cells with large hyperchromatic **"raisinoid" nuclei with perinuclear halos**; cells can be multinucleated If papillomatous exophytic growth→ Condyloma; they often have epithelial thickening, parakeratosis, broad rete pegs, koilocytic atypia
High-grade, AIN 2-3/PAIN2-3	Marked cytologic atypia and superficial mitotic figures involving **full thickness (for CIS/AIN3) or up to 2/3rd thickness for AIN2**; nuclei are hyperchromatic with irregular nuclear contours; loss of architectural polarity (top looks like bottom) IHC: **Diffuse block-like p16 staining**

Path Presenter

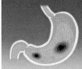
Paget's disease: Primary (no associated neoplasm)

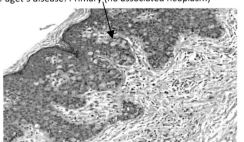

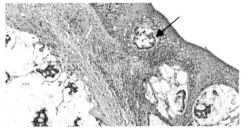

Secondary Paget's disease with underlying anal mucinous carcinoma

PAGET'S DISEASE
MORPHOLOGY
- Pagetoid spread of malignant glandular cells within the squamous epithelium (an in-situ lesion)
- Large pleomorphic cells with abundant pale cytoplasm- may infiltrate singly or form glandular structures in the squamous epithelium
- **Primary or secondary:** Primary is not associated with an underlying neoplasm; derived from adnexal structures, has apocrine phenotype (IHC: CK7+, CK20/CDX2-, GCDFP-15/GATA-3+)
- **Secondary: Derived from an underlying rectal or anal neoplasm** (often rectal adenocarcinoma); phenotype depends on underlying malignancy (often CK20 and CDX2+)
OTHER HIGH YIELD POINTS
- Critical to differentiate primary from secondary; if primary, strong tendency to recur and can become invasive
- Differential diagnosis: Melanoma and squamous cell carcinoma in situ

Path Presenter

Basaloid squamous cell carcinoma: Hyperchromatic cells

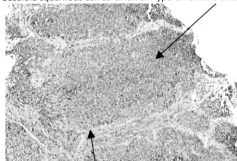

Peripheral palisading

Verrucous carcinoma: Exophytic bulbous growth

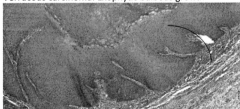

Verrucous carcinoma: pushing endophytic invasion

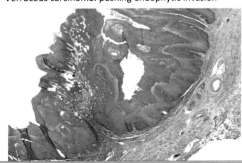

SQUAMOUS CELL CARCINOMA
- If a lesion can be completely visualized with gentle traction of the buttocks, it is considered a perianal lesion (not anal), which is similar to skin lesions on other parts of the body
- Carcinoma above the dentate line → metastasis to perirectal and internal iliac nodes
- Carcinoma below the dentate line → metastasis to inguinal and femoral lymph nodes
MORPHOLOGY
- Malignant epithelial tumor derived from the anal squamous mucosa with **keratin production, intercellular bridges, and frequent Human Papilloma Virus (HPV) infection**; infiltrating squamous cell clusters and strands with malignant nuclei and eosinophilic cytoplasm
- **Basaloid pattern:** Formerly called cloacogenic carcinoma; marked hyperchromasia, scant cytoplasm, and peripheral palisading (reminiscent of basal cell carcinoma)
- Admixed mucin-containing cells
- **Verrucous carcinoma:** Bland, well-differentiated thickened epithelium with bulbous exophytic fronds and endophytic "pushing" invasion; lacks HPV cytopathic effect or significant atypia; difficult to diagnose on biopsy; often associated inflammatory infiltrate; locally destructive but does not metastasize

OTHER HIGH YIELD POINTS
- Most common in older patients and women
- HPV infection in ~90% of cases (most commonly HPV type 16)
- Risk factors: Immunodeficiency (such as HIV), receptive intercourse, smoking

Link   Link

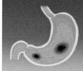

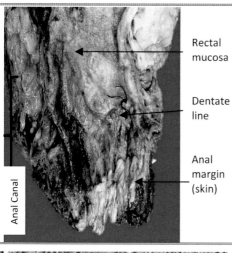

Rectal mucosa

Dentate line

Anal margin (skin)

Anal Canal

ANAL ADENOCARCINOMA

- Adenocarcinoma that arises in the anal canal; can be extramucosal or intramucosal
- **Intramucosal:** arises from luminal mucosa and is intestinal type like other colorectal cancers
- **Extramucosal** arises from anal glands, fistulas, or other structures but not overlying mucosa
- **Anal gland adenocarcinomas** arise from the anal glands/ducts; **(+)** for **CK7** while **(-) CK20 and CDX2**; differential diagnosis - metastasis (such as gynecologic) and intestinal type adenocarcinoma (CK7+/-, CK20 and CDX2+)
- Most **fistula associated adenocarcinomas arise in the setting of Crohn disease and are mucinous**
- All these tumors can be associated with secondary Paget's disease

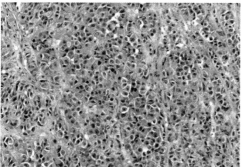

Melanoma with discohesive epithelioid tumor cells showing prominent nucleoli

MELANOMA
MORPHOLOGY

- Malignant transformation of melanocytes in the anal mucosa/ transition zone
- Polypoid mass near dentate line; typically epithelioid morphology; large, malignant cells with frequent macronucleoli, dusky greyish cytoplasm with frequent pigmentation; cells can be discohesive, plasmacytoid
- IHC: **(+)** for SOX10, S100, HMB45, Melan-A; **(-)** for cytokeratins

OTHER HIGH YIELD POINTS

- Very rare; typically affects elderly patients, more commonly women
- Molecular: *BRAF* mutations→ BRAF inhibitors (e.g., vemurafenib) and *CKIT* mutations→ tyrosine kinase inhibitors (e.g., imatinib)   Path Presenter

- Poor prognosis

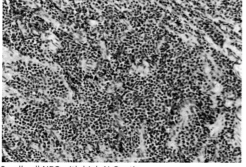

Small cell NEC with high N:C ratio

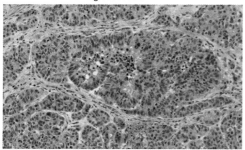

Large cell NEC with more cytoplasm

NEUROENDOCRINE CARCINOMAS (NECs)

- **NECs are much more common in the anus than well-differentiated neuroendocrine tumors**
- NECs often arise from non-neuroendocrine tumors and subsequently develop neuroendocrine differentiation
- Two variants: Small cell type and large cell type
- Not graded as considered high-grade
- IHC: **(+)** for CD56, synaptophysin, chromogranin-A, INSM1; **Ki-67 tends to be >20%, often much higher**
- Molecular: Commonly *p53* and *RB1* mutations among others
- Treatment: Platinum based therapy

MORPHOLOGIC FEATURES	
SMALL CELL NEUROENDOCRINE CARCINOMA	**LARGE CELL NEUROENDOCRINE CARCINOMA**
Fusiform nuclei, finely granular chromatin, scant cytoplasm, and nuclear molding, extensive necrosis, many mitoses	Large round nuclei, with prominent nucleoli, moderate amount of cytoplasm, and sheet-like or nested growth
Ki67 almost 100%	Ki67 often around 55-80%

Path Presenter

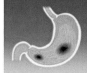

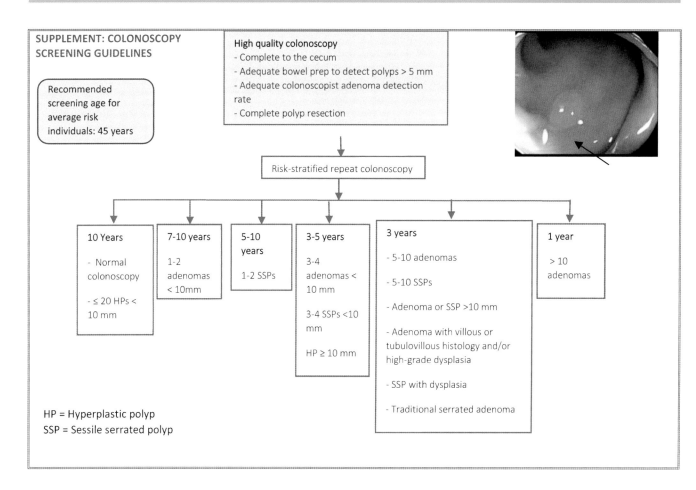

SUPPLEMENT: COLONOSCOPY
SCREENING GUIDELINES

Recommended screening age for average risk individuals: 45 years

High quality colonoscopy
- Complete to the cecum
- Adequate bowel prep to detect polyps > 5 mm
- Adequate colonoscopist adenoma detection rate
- Complete polyp resection

Risk-stratified repeat colonoscopy

10 Years
- Normal colonoscopy
- ≤ 20 HPs < 10 mm

7-10 years
1-2 adenomas < 10mm

5-10 years
1-2 SSPs

3-5 years
3-4 adenomas < 10 mm
3-4 SSPs <10 mm
HP ≥ 10 mm

3 years
- 5-10 adenomas
- 5-10 SSPs
- Adenoma or SSP >10 mm
- Adenoma with villous or tubulovillous histology and/or high-grade dysplasia
- SSP with dysplasia
- Traditional serrated adenoma

1 year
> 10 adenomas

HP = Hyperplastic polyp
SSP = Sessile serrated polyp

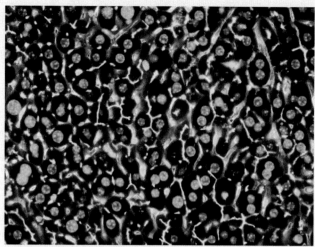

Liver, immunofluorescence microscopy.
Image courtesy: Amy Engevik, MD

CHAPTER 6: LIVER PATHOLOGY

Upasana Joneja, MD
Akanksha Gupta, MD
Manju Ambelil, MD
Binny Khandakar, MD

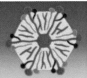
STEATOSIS/STEATOHEPATITIS

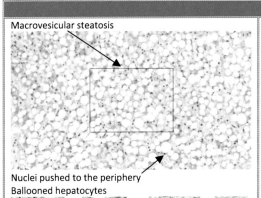

Macrovesicular steatosis

Nuclei pushed to the periphery

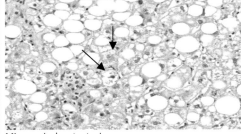

Ballooned hepatocytes

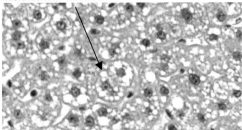

Microvesicular steatosis

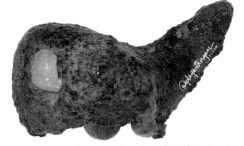

Non-alcohol fatty liver disease (yellow gross appearance) with cirrhosis

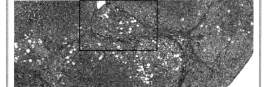

Image courtesy of: Cory Nash, MS, PA (ASCP), University of Chicago; used with permission
Cirrhosis with nodules of fibrosis, Trichrome stain

STEATOSIS/STEATOHEPATITIS

MORPHOLOGY
- **Steatosis** = Abnormal accumulation of fat within hepatocytes
- **Steatohepatitis = Fat + inflammation, acidophil bodies, and ballooning (active lobular injury)**
- These are part of the same disease process, and both lead to fibrosis, but steatohepatitis leads to fibrosis faster (essentially a difference in grading activity)
- Portal infiltrates may be present but are usually mild. If they are severe, consider additional diagnoses
- **Ballooned hepatocytes:** liver cell injury characterized by **cell swelling and enlargement** with no fat and thin, wispy cytoplasm

OTHER HIGH YIELD POINTS

MACROVESICULAR
- Represents a change in lipid metabolism
- Predominant pattern = nucleus pushed to the side by usually a single medium to large sized droplet; smaller droplets may also be mixed in

MICROVESICULAR
- Usually represents mitochondrial injury
- Nucleus remains central with innumerable, fine fat droplets
- **Only use this term if it is a diffuse change (not focal, or in a primarily macrovesicular case)**

QUANTIFYING FAT
- Estimate the % of cells with macrovesicular steatosis in the entire specimen
- Often starts in zone 3

Amount of Fat	Grade
• <5%	• Normal
• 5-33%	• Mild
• 34-66%	• Moderate
• >67%	• Severe

FIBROSIS
- Fatty liver disease causes **pericellular, pericentral fibrosis first** (where the most fat is)
- Progresses to portal and pericentral fibrosis
- Bridging fibrosis
- Cirrhosis (once cirrhotic, there may be relatively little fat)

Pericellular fibrosis   Portal Fibrosis   Bridging fibrosis

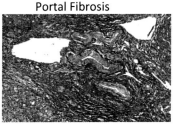
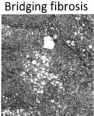

Link   Link

Path Presenter

Macrovesicular Steatosis

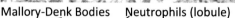

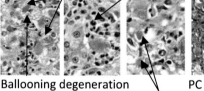

Mallory-Denk Bodies   Neutrophils (lobule)

Ballooning degeneration   PC Fibrosis

Lobular cholestasis

ALCOHOLIC HEPATITIS
MORPHOLOGY

- Hepatocyte injury and inflammation resulting from chronic alcohol consumption
- H&E: Macrovesicular steatosis. **Findings that Favor EtOH**: More hepatocyte **ballooning**, more **neutrophilic** lobular inflammation, more **Mallory-Denk** bodies, lobular **cholestasis**, and more diffuse **pericellular (PC) fibrosis**
- **Mallory-Denk Bodies** = pink, ropey cytoplasmic inclusions = ubiquitinated cytokeratins (positive for p62, ubiquitin, CK18); Ballooned hepatocytes are negative for CK18.
- **But Histology can be identical to NASH!**

OTHER HIGH YIELD POINTS

- AST/ALT ratio typically >2

Path Presenter

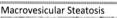

Macrovesicular Steatosis

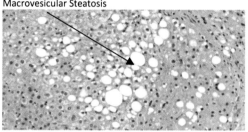

Ballooning   Lobular lymphocytes

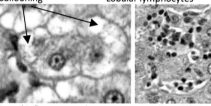

Portal inflammation (sometimes, usually mild)

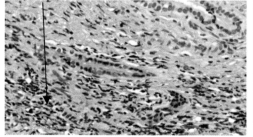

Acidophil body   Cirrhosis

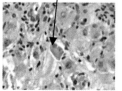

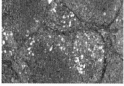

NON-ALCOHOLIC STEATOHEPATITIS (NASH)
MORPHOLOGY

- H&E: **Steatosis, ballooning,** lobular lymphocytes and neutrophils (exception in pediatric patients, where the inflammation is more portal), acidophil bodies, **pericellular fibrosis**
- Sometimes adults have mild portal inflammation, mainly lymphocytes

OTHER HIGH YIELD POINTS

Staging of fibrosis using NASH-CRN system

FIBROSIS	
0	None
1a	Mild zone 3 sinusoidal fibrosis
1b	Moderate zone 3 sinusoidal fibrosis
1c	Portal fibrosis only
2	Zone 3 sinusoidal fibrosis and portal fibrosis
3	Bridging fibrosis
4	Cirrhosis

Grading using the NASH-CRN system

Steatosis	Lobular Inflammation	Hepatocellular Ballooning
0: <5%	0: None	0: None
1: 5-33%	1: <2 foci/20x field	1: Mild, few
2: 34-66%	2: 2-4 foci/20x field	2: Moderate-marked, many
3: >66%	3: >4 foci/20x field	

- Sum the individual components for a total grade (maximum of 8)

Path Presenter

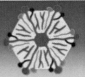

Glycogenated nucleus

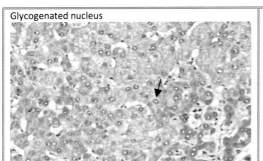

Mild portal based chronic inflammation

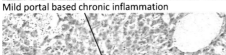

Cirrhosis   Interface activity

WILSON'S DISEASE
MORPHOLOGY
- Variable
- Can present as acute hepatitis, fulminant hepatitis, chronic hepatitis, or cirrhosis
- **Steatohepatitis, possible Mallory-Denk bodies and glycogenated nuclei**
- Later chronic hepatitis with mild chronic portal inflammation (predominantly lymphocytic with some plasma cells) with interface activity and cirrhosis

OTHER HIGH YIELD POINTS
- Mutations of **copper transport protein (*ATP7B* gene)** results in the inability to excrete copper in bile → copper accumulation in the liver and other tissues
- Variable presentation: **Acute or chronic liver disease, neurologic/ psychiatric findings, hemolytic anemia, ± Kayser-Fleischer rings**
- Labs: **Low ceruloplasmin**, Increased urine copper, AST/ALT ratio >2.2, Alk Phos/T. Bili <4
- When considering diagnosis, send tissue block for copper quantification

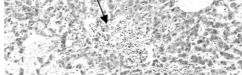

Infant   Kids   Adult

Steatosis/Steatohepatitis

Cholestasis

TOTAL PARENTAL NUTRITION (TPN)
- Long-term TPN can lead to liver injury
- Etiology: Unclear, multifactorial
- Histology is variable: Steatosis/steatohepatitis or cholestasis depending on age; cholestasis is more common in neonates than adults; steatosis/steatohepatitis more common in adults
- Can lead to significant fibrosis if TPN is continued
- Severe cases may require liver/small bowel transplant

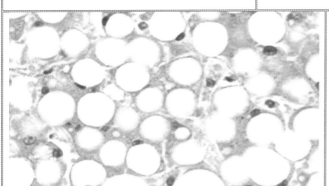

OTHER CAUSES OF MACROVESICULAR STEATOSIS
- Drugs including **amiodarone**, glucocorticoids, **methotrexate**, tamoxifen, and certain chemotherapeutic agents
- Other conditions, including malnutrition (marasmus or kwashiorkor) (e.g., hypothyroidism, elevated cortisol, growth hormone deficiency), cystic fibrosis

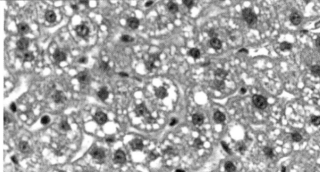

OTHER CAUSES OF MICROVESICULAR STEATOSIS
- **Reye's syndrome**, inborn errors of metabolism, Drugs, Toxins, **Acute fatty liver of pregnancy**

Link   Link   Link   Path Presenter

PORTAL TRACT CHRONIC INFLAMMATION

Portal infiltrates and interface activity

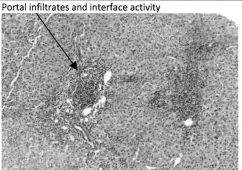

Higher magnification: Portal lymphoid aggregates

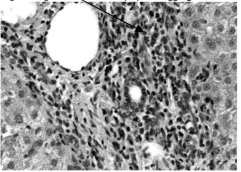

Scattered lobular inflammation

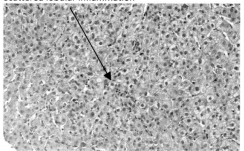

Hepatitis B: Sanded nuclei   Ground glass hepatocytes

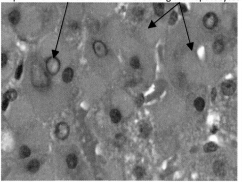

Link   Link   Link

CHRONIC HEPATITIS C
MORPHOLOGY
- Variably **dense portal lymphocytic infiltrates**; few plasma cells can be seen
- **Periportal interface activity**
- Scattered lobular collections of inflammatory cells ± acidophil bodies

OTHER HIGH YIELD POINTS
- **~90% develop chronic infection; blood borne**
- Antibodies (anti-HCV) indicate exposure
- Detection of HCV RNA indicates virus persistence
- Slow, silent, progressive disease (over decades) → cirrhosis (**risk of HCC**)
- Newer medications: Ledipasvir/sofosbuvir(Harvoni) →highly effective

VIRAL HEPATITIS: DISTINGUISHING ACUTE VS CHRONIC
- Often use clinical definition = elevated liver enzymes for ≥6 months
- Fibrosis also indicates chronic damage
- Diffuse moderate lobulitis means acute or acute-on-chronic
- Stage viral hepatitis using Batts-Ludwig, Ishak, Scheuer, or METAVR systems (reasonably similar)

CHRONIC HEPATITIS B
MORPHOLOGY
- Portal chronic inflammatory infiltrates with interface activity and lobular inflammation
- **Ground glass hepatocytes** (eosinophilic cytoplasm due to HBsAg) and **sanded nuclei** (HBcAg excess in nuclei)
- HBsAg= infected, HBcAg= actively replicating

OTHER HIGH YIELD POINTS
- **~10% develop chronic** disease; **blood borne**

FIBROSING CHOLESTATIC HEPATITIS B
- Variant with more progressive/worse disease
- **Usually immunosuppressed state** (e.g. post-transplant)
- Bile ductular reaction, extensive cholestasis, cell swelling, and fibrosis

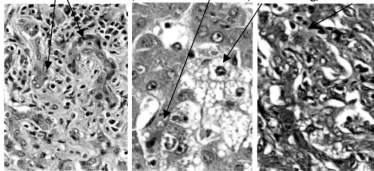

HEPATITIS D
Requires Hep B infection →acute-on-chronic hepatitis

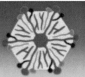

Centrivenular chronic inflammation

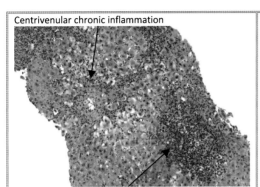

Dense portal infiltrates
Plasma cells are conspicuous

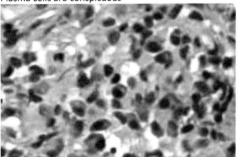

Hepatocyte apoptosis

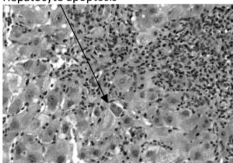

Regenerative rosette

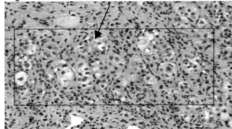

Emperipolesis

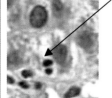

Path Presenter

AUTOIMMUNE HEPATITIS

MORPHOLOGY

- **Dense portal infiltrates** with marked interface activity → **lymphocytes and plasma cells**
- Lobular injury including **centrivenular inflammation** and apoptotic hepatocytes
- Regenerative rosette formation
- Can have "Overlap" with primary biliary cholangitis

OTHER HIGH YIELD POINTS

- Strong **female** predominance
- Elevated AST/ALT (often marked)
- Serology: (+) **Anti-Smooth Muscle Antibody, ANA,** LKM-1, Elevated IgG

Finding	Cutoff	Points
Autoantibodies (maximum 2 points!)		
ANA or SMA	≥ 1:40	1
ANA or SMA	≥ 1:80	2
LKM-1	≥ 1:40	2
SLA	Positive	2
Serum IgG		
	> Upper limit of normal	1
	> 1.10 times the upper limit of normal	2
Histology		
	No evidence of hepatitis	Disqualifying (Not AIH!)
	Atypical for AIH	0
	Compatible with AIH	1
	Typical of AIH	2
Absence of viral hepatitis		
Viral serology all negative		2

Histology:

Typical:
1) Lymphoplasmacytic interface hepatitis extending into the lobule
2) Regenerative rosette formation
3) Emperipolesis

Compatible: Chronic hepatitis with lymphocytic infiltration without all the features considered typical

Atypical: Signs of another diagnosis, such as steatohepatitis

Scoring: ≥6: Probable AIH ≥7: Definite

Modified from Hennes EM et al. Simplified criteria for the diagnosis of autoimmune hepatitis. Hepatology. 2008 Jul;48(1):169-76.

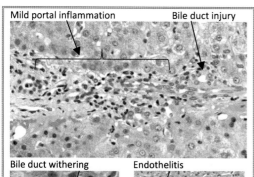

Mild portal inflammation — Bile duct injury

Bile duct withering — Endothelitis

GRAFT-VS-HOST DISEASE (GVHD)
MORPHOLOGY
Early phase
- **Damage to bile duct epithelium:** cytoplasmic swelling and vacuolation, withering, drop out; enlarged, overlapping nuclei and apoptosis
- Mild portal chronic inflammation
- **Possible endothelitis**

Late phase
- **Loss of bile ducts**, increased fibrosis

OTHER HIGH YIELD POINTS
- Usually post-stem cell transplant (transplanted immunocompetent T-cells attack new host)
- Involves skin, liver, GI tract → rash, ↑liver function enzymes, diarrhea and vomiting

Path Presenter

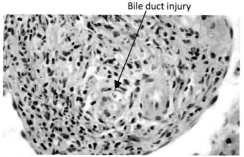

Bile duct injury

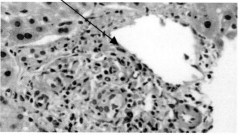

Endothelitis

Images courtesy of Dr. Ronald Miick, Cooper University Hospital, NJ

Chronic rejection: Foam cell arteriopathy

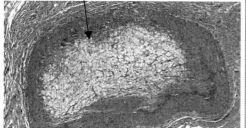

Image courtesy of Dr. Moghimi Ali, New South Wales

REJECTION
- Immune-mediated inflammation/damage in transplanted liver; usually targets bile ducts and vessels

T cell-mediated rejection
- Formerly called acute cellular rejection
- Mixed portal inflammation (lymphocytes, eosinophils), **bile duct injury**, and **endotheliitis**

Plasma cell-rich rejection
- Formerly called de novo autoimmune hepatitis
- **Portal and/or central plasma rich (>30%) infiltrates and lymphocytic cholangitis**
- Difficult to diagnose if patient carries a diagnosis of autoimmune hepatitis previously

Chronic rejection
- Bile duct injury →**eventual loss/paucity**; also lose hepatic arterioles
- Chronic vascular damage **with foam cell arteriopathy and luminal narrowing**

Antibody-mediated rejection
- **Positive serum Donor Specific Antibody (DSA)**
- Portal vascular dilatation, endothelial hypertrophy, **arteritis,** edematous portal tract and cholestasis
- (+) **C4d IHC** showing staining in >50% veins and capillaries

Path Presenter

Chronic rejection: Portal tract with absent bile duct

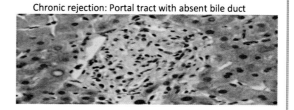

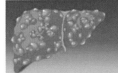 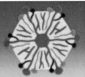

LOBULAR INJURY

- Indicates an **acute process** (too injurious to be chronic!) and often patient has very high transaminases
- Features: Lobular disarray (normal plate structure disrupted), **lobulitis** (lymphocytes attacking hepatocytes in lobule), conspicuous **acidophil bodies** (apoptotic hepatocytes)

Acute viral hepatitis

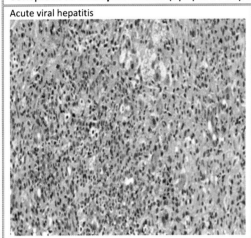

Acetaminophen toxicity

ACUTE VIRAL HEPATITIS
MORPHOLOGY
- Lobular damage and disarray, **diffuse lobular inflammation** rich in lymphocytes, plasma cells, histiocytes, hepatocyte swelling and necrosis
- May see **mild** portal and periportal inflammation
- **No fibrosis**

OTHER HIGH YIELD POINTS
- Largely a clinical term used with elevation in liver associated enzymes of <6 months duration
- **Most common cause is hepatotropic viruses** such as hepatitis A, B, E (acute infections are subclinical in hepatitis C); hepatitis A and E are spread by fecal-oral ("**the vowels hit the bowels**")
- **Drugs/toxins, Wilson disease, and early autoimmune hepatitis** can present with this pattern
- Diagnosis for viruses confirmed by serology or serum PCR

DRUG REACTION
- Two chief mechanisms: **Intrinsic** (predictable, dose-dependent, less inflammation, more necrosis) vs. **idiosyncratic** (majority of cases, not dose-dependent, more inflammation)
- **Tylenol causes intrinsic injury with extensive zone 3 necrosis and minimal inflammation due to N-acetyl-p-benzoquinone imine (NAPQI) accumulation**; treatment: **N-acetylcysteine**
- Very diverse findings that can **mimic** other disorders such as **autoimmune hepatitis**; clinical context is key
- Herbal and botanical drugs are an important but often overlooked cause of hepatotoxicity

Link   Link

Prominent giant cell transformation

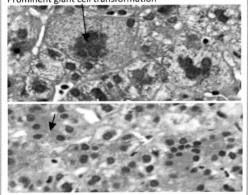

Canalicular cholestasis

IDIOPATHIC NEONATAL HEPATITIS
(AKA NEONATAL GIANT CELL HEPATITIS)
MORPHOLOGY
- Lobular disarray with prominent giant cell transformation
- Absent to mild lobular inflammation (despite name); canalicular and hepatocellular cholestasis; minimal portal tract changes and preserved bile ducts

OTHER HIGH YIELD POINTS   Path Presenter

- Neonatal jaundice with hepatomegaly
- Elevated total bilirubin and conjugated bilirubin
- Variable AST/ALT
- Diagnosis of exclusion (must exclude biliary atresia)
- Loose association with hypopituitarism

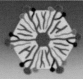
BILIARY DISEASES

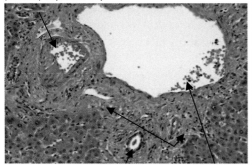

(Normal) Hepatic artery

Bile duct   Portal vein

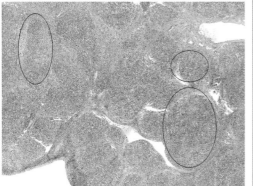

Regenerative nodules with jig-saw fibrosis of variable size (irregular)

BILIARY/CHOLESTATIC PROCESSES

- Laboratory findings: Elevated Alkaline Phosphatase (ALP), Gamma-glutamyl Transferase (GGT) and Bilirubin
- Bile ducts highlighted with **CK7** and **CK19**
- Increased copper deposition in periportal hepatocytes
- Chronic biliary injury leads to CK7-positive staining in periportal hepatocytes that are usually negative
- Chronic biliary injury can lead to biliary-type cirrhosis
- Biliary-type cirrhosis: Jig-saw pattern of fibrosis with irregularly sized regenerative nodules
- Additional clues to biliary type cirrhosis: Cholate stasis, ductopenia, periductal fibrosis, bile infarcts

BILIARY FIBROSIS STAGING (LUDWIG'S)	
I	Inflammation restricted to portal areas and non-suppurative destruction of bile ducts
II	Ductular proliferation, an inflammatory process extending to the interface with hepatic parenchyma
III	Septal and bridging fibrosis
IV	Cirrhosis

Path Presenter

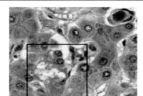
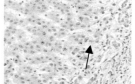

Cholate stasis   Cooper staining in periportal hepatocytes

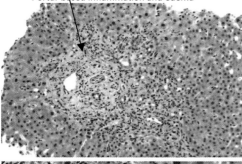

Portal-based inflammation and edema

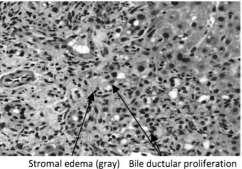

Stromal edema (gray)   Bile ductular proliferation

LARGE DUCT OBSTRUCTION
MORPHOLOGY

- H&E: **Portal tract edema, portal-based mixed inflammation with prominent neutrophils, bile ductular reaction**
- Canalicular and/or ductular cholestasis
- No lobular injury/hepatocyte apoptosis
- No fibrosis in acute biliary flow obstruction; chronic obstruction can lead to fibrosis (more fibrotic portal tract and less edema in chronic cases)

OTHER HIGH YIELD POINTS

- Etiology: **Mechanical blockage of bile ducts** due to gallstones, strictures, tumors
- Usually diagnosed using imaging

Differential diagnosis:

- Ascending cholangitis (requires prominent neutrophils in the bile duct epithelium and/or lumen)
- Marked hepatitis/extensive necrosis can be associated with bile ductular reaction as part of lobular regeneration

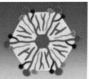

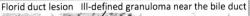
Florid duct lesion   Ill-defined granuloma near the bile duct

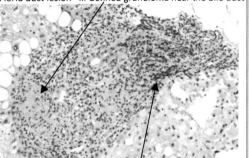
Moderate portal-based chronic inflammation

Bile duct injury with intraepithelial lymphocytes
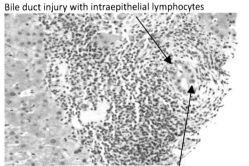

Epithelial injury with vacuolization (space in the cytoplasm)

PRIMARY BILIARY CHOLANGITIS/PRIMARY BILIARY CIRRHOSIS (PBC)
MORPHOLOGY
- H&E: Moderate portal-based chronic inflammation with **lymphocytes injuring the bile duct epithelium (lymphocytic cholangitis), vague non-necrotizing granulomas near the bile duct**
- May be associated with bile ductular reaction, scattered portal eosinophils; **late-stage disease has bile duct loss**
- **Florid duct lesion:** Lymphocytic cholangitis, bile duct injury ± granulomas
- Can develop cirrhosis with increased risk of hepatocellular carcinoma

OTHER HIGH YIELD POINTS
- Autoimmune disease with inflammatory destruction of intrahepatic bile ducts
- **Associated with other autoimmune conditions**: Sjögren, thyroiditis, scleroderma, rheumatoid arthritis, lupus, celiac disease
- Symptoms can be insidious: **pruritis**, malaise, **dark urine, light stools**
- Demographic: **Middle-aged females** of Northern European ancestry
- Laboratory abnormalities: Elevated Anti-Mitochondrial Antibody **(AMA)-M2 fraction (in 95% of patients)** and elevated IgM

Path Presenter

Fibrous obliteration of the bile duct
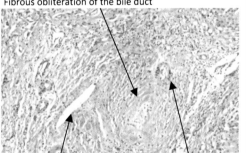
Native portal vein   Native hepatic artery
Periductal fibrosis   ERCP shows strictures

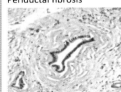 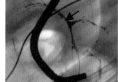

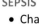

PRIMARY SCLEROSING CHOLANGITIS (PSC)
MORPHOLOGY
- Characteristic feature- **stricturing of bile ducts (concentric periductal fibrosis aka "onion skin fibrosis")**
- Disease commonly affects **large extrahepatic bile ducts**; therefore, on biopsy, changes are similar to large bile duct obstruction, such as portal edema, mixed inflammation, and bile ductular proliferation
- End stage: **Fibrous obliteration of the duct lumen and ductopenia**

OTHER HIGH YIELD POINTS
- Usually diagnosed using imaging: **Cholangiography shows multiple biliary strictures (extrahepatic)**
- Associated with **increased risk of cholangiocarcinoma**
- **Strong association with ulcerative colitis**; frequently in young to middle-aged men   Path Presenter

ERCP image courtesy of Dr. Alexander Towbin, @CincykidsRad; used with permission

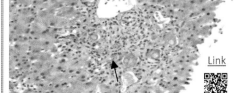
Link
Ductular cholestasis

SEPSIS
- Characteristic feature-**Ductular cholestasis ("cholangitis lenta")**
- Ductular reaction with inspissated bile and flattened, atrophic epithelium
- This pattern is not specific to sepsis; clinical context is critical
- Affects **systemically ill patients with sepsis, bacteremia, or jaundice**

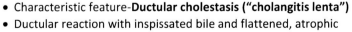

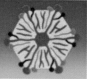
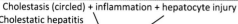
Cholestasis (circled) + inflammation + hepatocyte injury = Cholestatic hepatitis

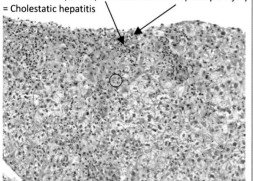

DRUG REACTION

- Most common histologic pattern of drug-induced liver injury is cholestasis
- **Bland/pure cholestasis:** Cholestasis with minimal inflammation
- **Cholestatic hepatitis:** Cholestasis with inflammation and hepatocellular injury
- **Prolonged cholestasis/ductopenia:** Greater than three months
- **Sclerosing duct injury:** Fibrosis affecting large bile ducts (similar to PSC)
- Drugs and patterns of injury can be found at http://livertox.nih.gov/

Path Presenter

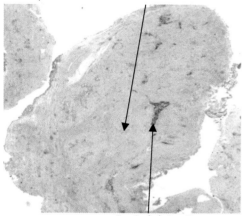
Extrahepatic bile duct with fibrosis

Luminal obstruction

Path Presenter

BILIARY ATRESIA
MORPHOLOGY

- Large bile duct obstruction type findings in liver biopsies: non-specific requires clinical and radiographic correlation
- Affects extrahepatic ducts with fibrosis and luminal obstruction

OTHER HIGH YIELD POINTS

- Idiopathic **prenatal destruction/fibrosis of extrahepatic bile ducts**
- **Most common cause of pathologic infant jaundice**
- Usually present in the first few weeks of life with jaundice and failure to thrive; 10% have mutation in *Jagged1* (JAG1) gene
- Hepatobiliary (HIDA) scan demonstrates the failure of excretion of radiotracer into the duodenum
- **Surgical intervention with Kasai procedure and/or liver transplantation required**

DIFFERENTIAL DIAGNOSIS

- Bile salt deficiencies (previously called Progressive Familial Intrahepatic Cholestasis (PFIC)) and inherent defects in bilirubin metabolism

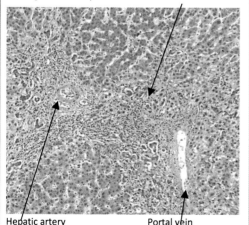
Missing bile duct in portal tract   Ductular reaction

Hepatic artery   Portal vein

NEONATAL PAUCITY OF INTRAHEPATIC BILE DUCTS
MORPHOLOGY

- **Absence of >50% of the bile ducts in portal tracts**
- Ductular reaction and cholestasis may be present
- Eventually can lead to cirrhosis
- **CK7** can be helpful in assessment of missing bile ducts
- Increased copper in periportal hepatocytes

OTHER HIGH YIELD POINTS

- Can be **syndromic or non-syndromic**
- In non-syndromic cases, bile duct loss is present at birth
- Syndromic: **Alagille syndrome** due to *JAG1/NOTCH2* mutations; **associated with cardiac and skeletal abnormalities**

Path Presenter

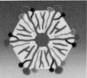

NEONATAL CHOLESTASIS DIAGNOSTIC ALGORITHM

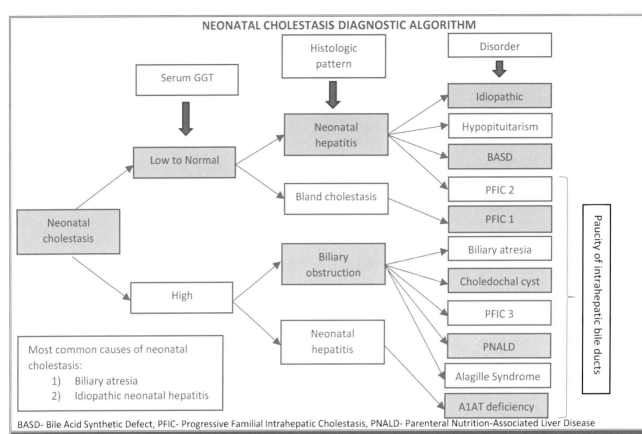

Most common causes of neonatal cholestasis:
1) Biliary atresia
2) Idiopathic neonatal hepatitis

BASD- Bile Acid Synthetic Defect, PFIC- Progressive Familial Intrahepatic Cholestasis, PNALD- Parenteral Nutrition-Associated Liver Disease

VASCULAR PROCESSES

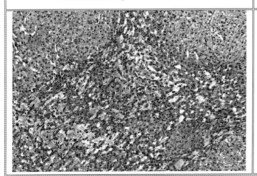

Centrizonal coagulative necrosis

SHOCK LIVER
MORPHOLOGY
- **Central (zone 3) coagulative necrosis** without inflammation
- Collapse of reticulin plate

OTHER HIGH YIELD POINTS
- Pattern is seen with **liver hypoperfusion** of any cause
- Massive elevation in AST and ALT (usually in the 1000s)
- Differential diagnosis: **Acetaminophen (Tylenol) toxicity**

Path Presenter

SINUSOIDAL OBSTRUCTION SYNDROME
MORPHOLOGY
- **Central vein obliteration** by fibrosis (best seen on the trichrome stain)
- Also see sinusoidal dilatation, congestion, and endothelial edema

OTHER HIGH YIELD POINTS
- **Due to injury to the sinusoidal endothelium**
- Etiology: **Chemotherapy or stem cell transplantation**

Figure: Sinusoidal dilatation in sinusoidal obstruction syndrome, image courtesy Dr. Haeryoung Kim, MD.

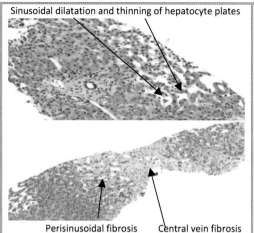

Sinusoidal dilatation and thinning of hepatocyte plates

Perisinusoidal fibrosis   Central vein fibrosis

VENOUS OUTFLOW OBSTRUCTION
MORPHOLOGY
- Acute cases **show sinusoidal dilatation, congestion, and hepatic plate atrophy**
- **Chronicity causes central vein fibrosis and sinusoidal fibrosis** and can lead to cirrhosis

OTHER HIGH YIELD POINTS
- Common etiologies: **Right-sided heart failure, Budd-Chiari**
- Gross liver appearance: **Nutmeg liver**

Image courtesy of Dr. Michal Kunc, Poland

Path Presenter

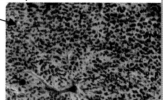

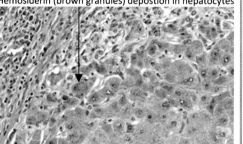

Hemosiderin (brown granules) depostion in hepatocytes

Hepatocellular hemosiderin deposition

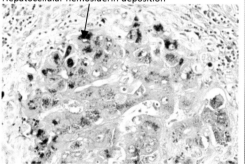

HEREDITARY HEMOCHROMATOSIS
MORPHOLOGY
- Group of inherited disorders of iron metabolism; **Type 1 is due to *HFE* gene mutations** resulting in decreased hepcidin synthesis→ increased iron absorption and storage; **C282Y** is the most common pathogenic allele and accounts for clinically significant iron overload
- **Iron accumulates first within zone 1 (periportal) hepatocytes** with a distinctive pericanalicular pattern and progressively involves all zones
- Iron can also be deposited in the bile duct epithelium and Kupffer cells
- Variable degree of fibrosis and cirrhosis develop over time
- Iron special stain demonstrates iron deposition which is graded semi quantitatively   Path Presenter

OTHER HIGH YIELD POINTS
- Genetic testing and hepatic iron quantification tests are other confirmatory methods
- Differential diagnosis includes **transfusion** and **oral** supplementation-related iron overload, anemias with **ineffective erythropoiesis**, chronic liver diseases including **alcoholic and nonalcoholic fatty liver diseases, chronic hepatitis C and cirrhosis**
- In secondary iron overload: **accumulation predominantly seen in Kupffer cells first,** but substantial hepatocellular deposition occurs when Kupffer cells are saturated

---

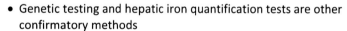

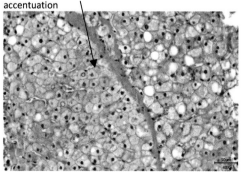

Abundant pale cytoplasm with hepatocyte membrane accentuation

GLYCOGENIC HEPATOPATHY
- Poorly controlled blood sugar levels→ disrupt balance between glycogenesis and glycogenolysis→ abundant glycogen stores →hepatomegaly and elevated LFTs
- Classic clinical setting is **type 1 diabetes mellitus**; also seen in **Mauriac syndrome** (with growth retardation, delayed puberty, cushingoid features and hypercholesterolemia)
- **Diffuse glycogenation of hepatocytes characterized by abundant pale cytoplasm,** often with hepatocyte membrane accentuation; no inflammation; **positive on PAS-D stain**   Path Presenter

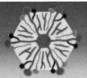
PAS-D positive globules   α1-AT IHC

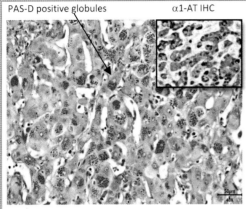

Path Presenter

α1-ANTITRYPSIN DEFICIENCY (α1-AT)
MORPHOLOGY
- Autosomal recessive genetic disorder characterized by decreased α1-AT level
- α1-AT gene is codominant with each allele contributing 50% of total protein; **PiM is the normal**/wild-type allele whereas PiS and PiZ are the most common disease-causing alleles; **PiZZ phenotype accounts for most cases with liver disease**
- Histology shows deposition of **eosinophilic, PAS-D positive globules within periportal hepatocytes;** positive by α1-AT IHC
- Neonatal hepatitis features cholestasis and hepatocyte injury (too early for globule formation)
OTHER HIGH YIELD POINTS
- Bimodal clinical presentation: first is neonates and infants with cholestatic liver disease and second is adults with chronic liver disease

Clusters of ceroid-laden macrophages

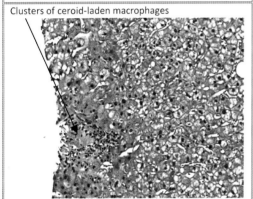

Path Presenter

RESOLVING HEPATITIS
MORPHOLOGY
- **Almost normal appearing liver** with minimal to mild portal inflammation and absent to minimal lobular inflammation
- Mild lobular disarray and lobules often have **scattered clusters of pigmented/ceroid-laden macrophages**
- The Kupffer cell hyperplasia is a clean-up effort in a site of prior injury; Positive with PAS-D stain
- Most common causes are **idiosyncratic drug reaction and acute self-limited viral infections**
OTHER HIGH YIELD POINTS
- Mild cholestasis can also be seen with some drug effects
- Hepatitic injury will resolve after stopping the drug, however liver enzymes may take months to normalize completely

HSV intranuclear inclusions with marginated chromatin

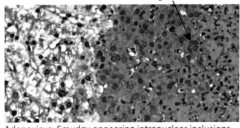

Adenovirus: Smudgy appearing intranuclear inclusions

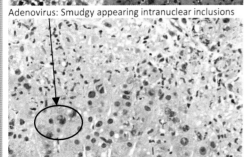

HERPES SIMPLEX VIRUS (HSV) AND ADENOVIRUS INFECTION
MORPHOLOGY
- **Extensive non-zonal hepatocyte necrosis**
- Characteristic intranuclear inclusions are seen adjacent to areas of necrosis
- HSV: Intranuclear inclusions with a rim of marginated chromatin with or without multinucleated hepatocytes
- Adenovirus: Intranuclear inclusions with smudgy nuclear appearance and mild lymphocytic lobular and portal inflammation
- HSV and adenovirus immunohistochemistry confirms the diagnosis
OTHER HIGH YIELD POINTS
- Usually seen in immunocompromised individuals
- Poor prognosis, often fatal

Link Link
  Path Presenter

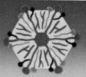
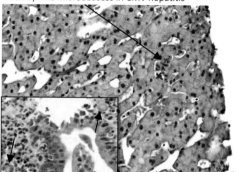
Neutrophilic microabscess in CMV hepatitis

CMV inclusions   Path Presenter

CYTOMEGALOVIRUS (CMV) HEPATITIS
MORPHOLOGY

- Histologic findings are subtle; mild portal or lobular inflammation maybe seen
- Presence of lobular **neutrophilic microabscesses** in some cases is a helpful clue to the diagnosis
- Characteristic viral cytopathic effects (nuclear and cytoplasmic enlargement) with viral inclusions when present, can be seen in hepatocytes, bile duct epithelium, endothelial cells and Kupffer cells

OTHER HIGH YIELD POINTS

- Typically seen in the setting of immunosuppression, however clinically silent infections can occur in immunocompetent individuals
- Variable clinical presentation (asymptomatic to severe infection) is seen in congenital infection

---

Activated lymphocytes in sinusoids giving a string of beads appearance
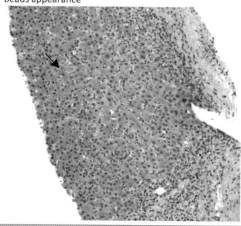

EPSTEIN-BARR VIRUS (EBV) HEPATITIS
MORPHOLOGY

- Often looks like a nondescript hepatitis with mild to moderate portal and lobular inflammation (so often keep in differential diagnosis, especially if young adults or immunocompromised)
- Classically: **lots of activated lymphocytes in sinusoids, giving an appearance of string of beads**
- The degree of hepatocyte injury is usually disproportionately low

OTHER HIGH YIELD POINTS

- Apart from hepatitis, EBV can also cause post-transplant lymphoproliferative disorder (PTLD) and smooth muscle tumors in the liver in immunosuppressed individuals

Path Presenter

Sinusoidal deposition of amyloid (acellular amorphous pink material)
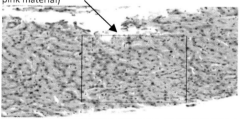
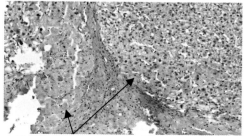
Globular pattern deposition of LECT2 amyloidosis

AMYLOIDOSIS
MORPHOLOGY

- **Amyloidosis of the liver most frequently occurs secondary to systemic diseases** such as multiple myeloma
- Familial/primary amyloidosis is rare and results from mutations in genes that produce amyloidogenic proteins
- Amyloid deposition appears as amorphous, acellular, eosinophilic deposits in vessels and sinusoids leading to hepatocyte atrophy
- Different types of amyloid seen in the liver including **primary, AL, AA, and Leukocyte chemotactic factor 2 (LECT2) amyloidosis**
- A **distinct globular pattern deposition** is seen in LECT2 amyloidosis (also involves kidney)

OTHER HIGH YIELD POINTS

- **Congo red stain** highlights amyloid as brick-red in bright-field microscopy and demonstrates **apple-green birefringence under polarized light**

 Path Presenter

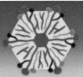
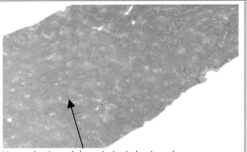

Hyperplastic nodules mimic cirrhosis on low-power; however, trichrome does not confirm cirrhosis

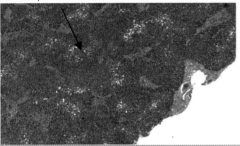

NODULAR REGENERATIVE HYPERPLASIA
MORPHOLOGY

- **Cirrhotic-appearing nodules on gross and radiologic examination; however, histologically no evidence of cirrhosis or fibrosis**
- Results from **changes in hepatic blood flow** from obliteration of small portal veins which leads to localized atrophy→other areas grow to compensate
- Multiple hyperplastic parenchymal nodules (with normal to enlarged hepatocytes) with intervening compressed/atrophied parenchyma
- Findings are best seen on reticulin stain: **Reticulin stain highlights compressed hepatocytes between the nodules**

OTHER HIGH YIELD POINTS

- **Can cause portal hypertension** and mimics cirrhosis

Path Presenter

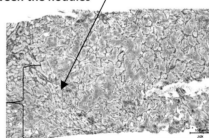

Portal fibrosis with branching abnormal ductal structures

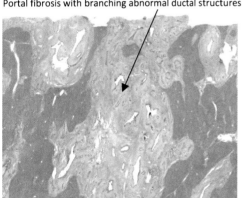

CONGENITAL HEPATIC FIBROSIS
MORPHOLOGY

- Embryologic ductal plate malformation that leads to **bridging fibrosis with prominent malformed ducts**
- Anastomosing irregularly shaped and branching abnormal ductal structures circumferentially arranged around a portal tract
- Varying degrees of portal fibrosis without significant inflammation
- Abnormal/hypoplastic portal veins → leads to portal hypertension

OTHER HIGH YIELD POINTS

- **Associated with autosomal recessive polycystic kidney disease**
- Associated with mutations in **PKHD1 gene**, that codes for fibrocystin

Path Presenter

Images courtesy of Dr. Adam L. Booth, @ALBoothMD; used with permission

Dense secretions in bile ducts   Steatosis   PAS-D

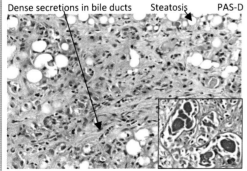

CYSTIC FIBROSIS

- **Autosomal recessive**; mutation in the **CFTR gene** results in impaired chloride transport in various organs; **presents with respiratory problems, meconium ileus, or pancreatic insufficiency**
- **Steatosis is the most common finding** in hepatic lobules, however steatohepatitis is uncommon
- **T**hick abnormal secretions are present in bile ducts (similar to lungs and pancreas) → biliary obstruction → epithelial atrophy, bile ductular proliferation, inflammation → fibrosis → biliary cirrhosis
- **Secretions stain with PAS-D**   Path Presenter
- Portal hypertension due to obliterative portal venopathy and nodular regenerative hyperplasia

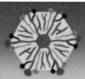
LABORATORY CORRELATION

ACUTE HEPATITIS
Marked transaminitis (AST & ALT >5x normal)

- **Non**-hepatotropic **viruses** (CMV, HSV)
- Hepatitis **A & E**; only acute
- Hepatitis B: **Ground glass** inclusions
- Autoimmune hepatitis: **Plasma cells**
- Massive altered hepatic blood flow (such as **shock**)

CHOLESTATIC HEPATITIS
Elevated Alkaline Phosphatase & GGT; +/- Bili; Jaundice

- **Large** duct obstruction
- PBC: **Female**, + AMA, IgM, lymphocytic cholangitis, and florid duct lesion
- PSC: **Male**, inflammatory bowel disease, concentric fibrosis around ducts; risk of **cholangiocarcinoma**
- Drug reaction

CHRONIC HEPATITIS
Mild transaminitis (AST & ALT <5x normal)

- Hepatitis B: 5% develop chronic hepatitis
- Autoimmune hepatitis: +ANA, ASMA, Elevated IgG: interface **necroinflammatory lymphoplasmacytic infiltrate**
- Hepatitis C: 80% develop **chronic** hepatitis; **nodular aggregates** of lymphocytes
- Hereditary hemochromatosis: **+HFE** gene mutation; elevated transferrin saturation and serum ferritin
- Wilson's disease: Increased liver copper quantitation; mutation in **ATP7B** gene; AST/ALT ratio>2.2; Alkaline Phosphate/total bilirubin <4
- A1AT deficiency: PiZZ phenotype; **hyaline globules** in hepatocytes stain with **PAS-D** stain
- Alcohol-related: Clinical history of alcohol use: AST:ALT >; more likely to show **neutrophils** and **Mallory's hyaline**
- Non-alcoholic steatohepatitis: Diabetes or metabolic syndrome, obesity
- Drug reaction

Based on a presentation by Dr. Max Smith, Mayo Clinic

CIRRHOSIS/ LIVER FAILURE: Synthetic dysfunction such as elevated INR, low albumin, and low platelets

LIVER LESIONS: BENIGN

No portal tracts in the lesion

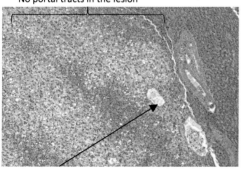

Unpaired artery   Steatosis (yellow gross appearance)

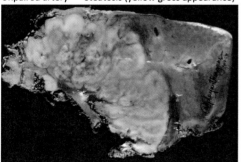

Image courtesy of Cory Nash, MS, PA (ASCP); used with permission

Path Presenter

HEPATOCELLULAR ADENOMA
MORPHOLOGY

- Benign liver neoplasm **associated with use of oral contraceptives/ steroids**
- Composed of benign-appearing hepatocytes with normal plate thickness (1-2 plates) and no cytologic atypia or mitoses
- Key to diagnosis is **absence of true portal tracts; finding of unpaired arteries also helpful**

Four subtypes of hepatocellular adenoma		
Subtype	Phenotype	IHC
Inflammatory/ Telangiectatic (~45%)	Associated with inflammatory infiltrate, sinusoidal dilatation, bile ductular reaction; transformation to HCC can occur	Positive for Serum Amyloid A (SAA) and CRP
ß-catenin activated (~15%)	May have cellular atypia; **highest risk of malignant transformation**	**Nuclear ß-catenin positive**; diffuse strong glutamine synthetase
HNF1alpha-inactivated (~30%)	Have steatosis; associated with adenomatosis (>10 adenomas); low risk of malignant transformation	Loss of LFABP staining
Unclassified (~10%)	Does not fit other categories	

OTHER HIGH YIELD POINTS

- Risk of transformation to hepatocellular carcinoma and or bleeding/rupture

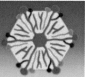

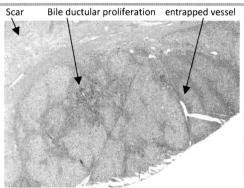

Scar | Bile ductular proliferation | entrapped vessel

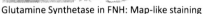

Glutamine Synthetase in FNH: Map-like staining

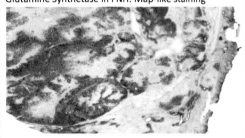

FOCAL NODULAR HYPERPLASIA (FNH)
MORPHOLOGY
- **Regenerative hyperplastic response of hepatocytes due to vascular abnormalities**; not a true neoplasm
- Mimics focal cirrhosis; well-circumscribed with **central stellate scar**, fibrous septa, entrapped vessels, bile ductular reaction, and inflammatory cells
- No true portal tracts
- **"Map-like" staining with glutamine-synthetase**

OTHER HIGH YIELD POINTS
- No association with oral contraceptives; usually asymptomatic
- Most nodules measure **< 5 cm**
- Most common in young women

Gross image courtesy of Cory Nash, MS, PA (ASCP); used with permission
IHC image courtesy of Dr. Matthew Gosse, @MattGosseMD; used with permission
Path Presenter

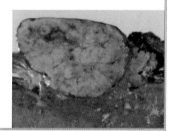

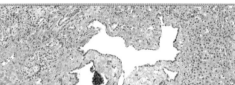

Irregular ducts | Path Presenter

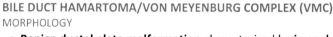

BILE DUCT HAMARTOMA/VON MEYENBURG COMPLEX (VMC)
MORPHOLOGY
- **Benign ductal plate malformation** characterized by **irregular to round dilated bile ducts within fibrous/hyalinized stroma**
- Lumen **may contain bile** or proteinaceous material

OTHER HIGH YIELD POINTS
- Usually **incidental, clinically insignificant, and small (<0.5 cm)**
- If numerous, consideration for ductal malformation-associated diseases such as Caroli disease, Caroli Syndrome, polycystic kidney disease, and congenital hepatic fibrosis should be given

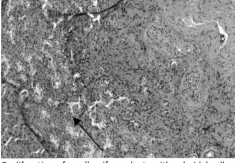

Proliferation of small uniform ducts with cuboidal cells and round regular nuclei

BILE DUCT ADENOMA AND ADENOFIBROMA
MORPHOLOGY
- Bile duct adenoma is a benign lesion characterized by **proliferation of small uniform ducts with cuboidal cells and round regular nuclei**
- Lumen usually **does not contain bile**

OTHER HIGH YIELD POINTS
- Clinically can be mistaken for metastasis intraoperatively
- Usually <1 cm, subcapsular, and well-circumscribed
- ~50% of bile duct adenomas show *BRAF* **V600E mutations**
Path Presenter

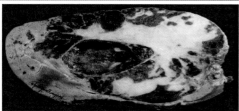

Dilated vascular channels lined by endothelial cells

CAVERNOUS HEMANGIOMA

MORPHOLOGY

- Benign vascular lesion composed of dilated vascular channels lined by single layer of flat endothelial cells separated by fibrous septa
- **(+)** for endothelial markers: ERG, CD31, CD34, FLI1, Factor 8

OTHER HIGH YIELD POINTS

- **Most common benign tumor of the liver**
- Thought to be a malformation and non-neoplastic; diagnosed radiologically
- Often asymptomatic; >5 cm lesions more susceptible to hemorrhage, rupture; they can thrombose and calcify
- More common in females   Path Presenter

Gross image courtesy of Cory Nash, MS, PA (ASCP); used with permission

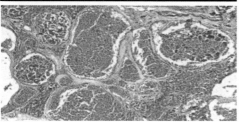

Fat   thick-walled vessels   Smooth muscle

HMB-45   SMA

ANGIOMYOLIPOMA/PECOMA

MORPHOLOGY

- Mesenchymal tumor, like in the kidney
- Well-circumscribed; consists of variable admixture of fat, smooth muscle, and thick-wall blood vessels
- Smooth muscle may appear epithelioid with eosinophilic cytoplasm; cytologic atypia may be present
- Generally benign, however, very rarely malignant behavior has been reported
- **(+)** for HMB-45, SMA, Melan-A, and CKIT

OTHER HIGH YIELD POINTS

- Usually, asymptomatic
- F>M; mean age: 56 years
- Usually sporadic but **~5-10% associated with tuberous sclerosis**
- *TSC1* or *TSC2* mutations

Path Presenter

LIVER LESIONS: MALIGNANT

Fetal epithelial component characterized by thin cells resembing hepatocytes of developing liver

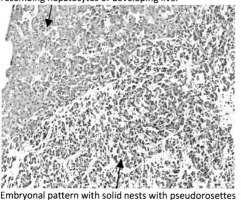

Embryonal pattern with solid nests with pseudorosettes

HEPATOBLASTOMA

MORPHOLOGY

- Malignant tumor recapitulating hepatic ontogenesis
- Shows a variety of epithelial (e.g. fetal and embryonal) and mesenchymal cell types ("teratoid")
- **Frequent ß-catenin mutations;** nuclear localization with immunohistochemistry→ worse prognosis

OTHER HIGH YIELD POINTS

- **Most common liver tumor in children**
- Majority of cases between 5 months and 6 years of age
- Majority are sporadic, however some associated with **Beckwith-Wiedemann, familial adenomatous polyposis, or trisomy 18**
- Serum AFP elevated in ~90% cases   Path Presenter

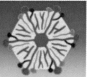

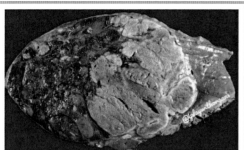

HCC: Green discoloration due to bile production
Image courtesy of Cory Nash, MS, PA (ASCP); used with permission

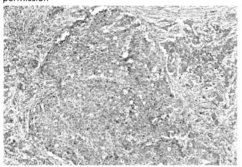

HCC: Loss of normal trabecular architecture

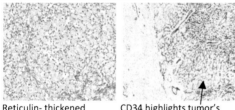

Reticulin- thickened hepatic plates

CD34 highlights tumor's sinuoidal "capillarization"

HEPATOCELLULAR CARCINOMA (HCC)
MORPHOLOGY
- Malignant tumor of hepatocellular differentiation
- **Widening of hepatocellular plates (>2 cells thick); absent portal tracts and unpaired arterioles**
- Other features include cytologic and architectural atypia such as **pseudo-acini/pseudo-gland formation**
- Stains: **Reticulin highlights widened hepatocyte plates**; CD34 shows sinusoidal **"capillarization;" (+)** for Hep-Par1, Arginase, and Glypican-3; glypican-3 is negative in benign liver but positive in moderately-poorly differentiated HCCs

VARIANTS
- **Fibrolamellar HCC** → see section below
- **Steatohepatitic HCC** → Associated with hepatitis C and NASH; macrovesicular steatosis, ballooning degeneration, and Mallory's hyaline present; can be difficult to recognize as carcinoma especially on biopsies
- **Macrovesicular-massive HCC** → Thick trabeculae (>10 cells thick) covered by endothelial cells; aggressive subtype with **high AFP, TP53 mutations or FGF19 amplification**

OTHER HIGH YIELD POINTS
- HCC often occurs in the setting of cirrhosis (associated with chronic liver injury such as viral hepatitis, alcohol, NASH, hereditary hemochromatosis)
- Usually diagnosed clinically with imaging findings and elevated Alpha Fetoprotein (AFP)
- Treated with resection, embolization, or transplant

Path Presenter

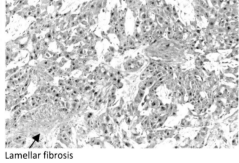

Lamellar fibrosis

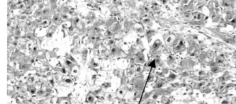

Oncocytic tumor cells with prominent nucleoli

FIBROLAMELLAR CARCINOMA
MORPHOLOGY
- **Malignant tumor comprising of large oncocytic cells with prominent nucleoli, lamellar fibrosis, and cytoplasmic pale bodies**
- **(+)** for CD68 and CK7

OTHER HIGH YIELD POINTS
- Large, solitary tumor; normal AFP
- **Young, non-cirrhotic patients**
- Classically thought to be better prognosis, but this is most likely due to demographics
- Recurrent **DNAJB1-PRKACA fusion**

Path Presenter

Image courtesy of Dr. Kevin Kuan @kkuanMD; used with permission

Small duct type

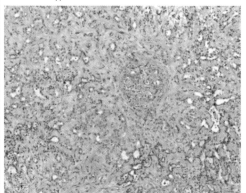

Large duct type

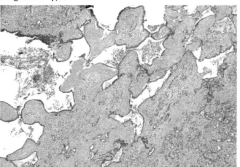

Path Presenter

INTRAHEPATIC CHOLANGIOCARCINOMA
MORPHOLOGY
- **Adenocarcinoma arising in the liver proximal to the left and right hepatic ducts**
- Glands show varying degrees of atypia and differentiation and infiltrate dense fibrous stroma
- **Two variants:**
  - ➤ **Small duct type:** Peripheral, large liver masses, risk factors similar to hepatocellular carcinomas
  - ➤ **Large duct type:** Hilar, obstructive cholestasis, risk factors similar to extrahepatic bile duct carcinomas (see below); precursors include biliary intraepithelial neoplasia and intratubular papillary neoplasms
- **Growth patterns**: mass-forming, periductal infiltrative, intraductal, and mixed
- Need to exclude metastatic carcinoma
- Non-specific immunoprofile: CK7+ CK20-; **(+)** CK19, CEA; Albumin in-situ hybridization supports intrahepatic origin

OTHER HIGH YIELD POINTS
- **Second most common primary malignancy of liver**
- M>F; 55-75 years of age
- Inflammatory disorders such as PSC, liver fluke, Caroli disease, hepatolithiasis, and choledochal cysts can predispose to development of large duct type cholangiocarcinomas
- Intrahepatic tumors show *IDH, EPHA2,* and *BAP1* mutations and *FGFR2* fusions; different from extrahepatic tumors
- Aggressive carcinomas with poor survival rates

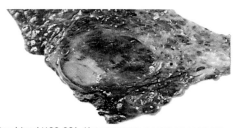

Combined HCC-CCA: Heterogeneous gross appearance

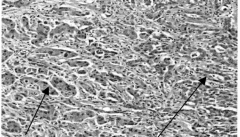

HCC area   CCA area

COMBINED HEPATOCELLULAR (HCC)-CHOLANGIOCARCINOMA (CCA)
MORPHOLOGY
- A single tumor with two morphologically distinct areas of hepatocellular carcinoma and cholangiocarcinoma
- HCC areas of **(+)** heppar1, arginase, and glypican3 while cholangiocarcinoma areas are **(+)** for CK7

OTHER HIGH YIELD POINTS
- **Treatment and prognosis are similar to cholangiocarcinoma;** worse prognosis than HCC
- Transarterial chemoembolization (TACE) has been associated with higher frequency of combined tumors
- Mutations of HCC (such as *CTNNB1*) and CCA (such as *KRAS, IDH1*) have been found

Path Presenter

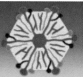
Eosinophilic cells in dense fibrous stroma with signet ring-like features containing RBC (circled)

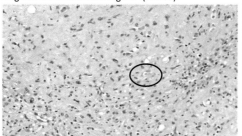

Edge of lesion with infiltrating tumor cells

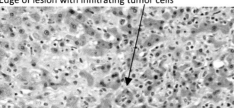

EPITHELIOID HEMANGIOENDOTHELIOMA
MORPHOLOGY
- **Malignant endothelial neoplasm that can be locally aggressive and has metastatic potential**
- Composed of **eosinophilic, slightly epithelioid cells with signet ring-like features representing intracytoplasmic lumina (often containing red blood cells);** associated with dense fibrous stroma
- Can show intravascular papillary growth and infiltrate sinusoidal spaces at the edge of the lesion
- **(+)** for ERG, CD31, CD34, D2-40, FLI1, CAMTA1, TFE3; keratin positive in ~40%

OTHER HIGH YIELD POINTS
- Can affect soft tissue, bone, lung, skin and liver
- ***WWTR1-CAMTA1* or *YAP1-TFE3* fusion**

Path Presenter

CAMTA1 IHC
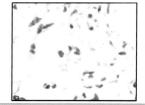

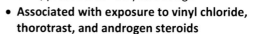

ANGIOSARCOMA
MORPHOLOGY
- Malignant endothelial tumor; **most common liver sarcoma**
- Spindled to epithelioid tumor cells, variably atypical, with mitoses and anastomosing spaces; tumor cells grow along pre-existing vascular spaces; usually large and **multifocal**
- **(+)** for vascular markers: CD31, CD34, ERG, D2-40; keratins **(+)** in up to 35% of cases

OTHER HIGH YIELD POINTS
- M>F; presents at >50 years of age
- **Associated with exposure to vinyl chloride, thorotrast, and androgen steroids**
- Poor prognosis

Path Presenter
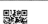

Epithelioid to spindled malignant cells associated with vessels/red blood cells

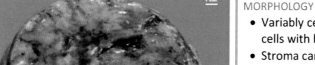

Images courtesy of Dr. Raul Perret, @kells108; used with permission

UNDIFFERENTIATED EMBRYONAL SARCOMA
MORPHOLOGY
- Variably cellular tumor with spindled, oval, and pleomorphic/anaplastic cells with hyaline globules
- Stroma can show myxoid changes
- Hyaline globules are PAS-D positive; high Ki-67

OTHER HIGH YIELD POINTS
- Large tumors, 10-30 cm
- Well-demarcated, solitary, with cystic, gelatinous, and hemorrhagic foci
- 9-15% of pediatric hepatic tumors; usually present 6-10 years
- Presents with abdominal pain, fever, and normal AFP levels
- Often associated with mesenchymal hamartoma; thus also called mesenchymal sarcoma
- Treatment usually involves complete resection and chemotherapy

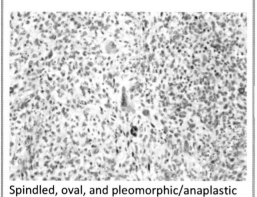

Spindled, oval, and pleomorphic/anaplastic cells

- Cases show **MALAT1** gene rearrangement: **t (11:19)** and mutations in **TP53**

Path Presenter

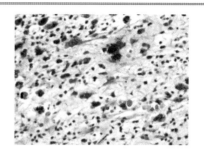

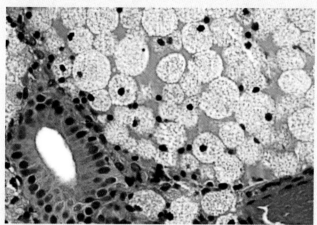

Cholesterol polyp, Gall Bladder (H&E stain). Image courtesy: Akanksha Gupta, MD

CHAPTER 7: PANCREATOBILIARY PATHOLOGY

Manju Ambelil, MD
Snehal Sonawane, MD
Akanksha Gupta, MD

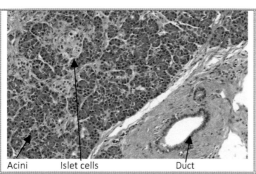

Acini   Islet cells   Duct

PANCREAS NORMAL HISTOLOGY
- **Lobular** architecture with two glandular components and the duct system
- Exocrine glands: composed of **secretory acini**
- Acinus contains columnar to pyramidal cells with a granular appearance
- Endocrine glands/islets of Langerhans: Composed of **4 major cell types** - Beta cells, alpha cells, delta cells, and pancreatic polypeptide cells
- Fine duct channels drain acini and converge into the main duct system
- **Small ducts** lined by **flattened to cuboidal** epithelium and **large ducts** lined by **simple columnar** epithelium
- Lobules are separated by connective tissue containing vessels and nerves

Central stellate scar

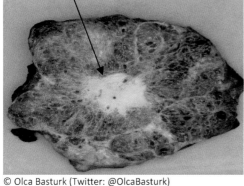

© Olca Basturk (Twitter: @OlcaBasturk)

Multiloculated cysts

SEROUS CYSTADENOMA
MORPHOLOGY
- Gross: Multilocular, sponge-like, or **honeycomb** appearance with a central **stellate fibrous scar**
- Microscopy: Cysts lined by a single layer of cells with defined cell borders
- Composed of bland, uniform, **cuboidal** cells with **clear, glycogen-rich cytoplasm** and **small round nuclei**
- Glycogen→ stains with **PAS** (and digested by diastase)
- IHC: **(+)** for **inhibin, cytokeratin, GLUT-1, and MUC6**
OTHER HIGH YIELD POINTS
- F: M ratio 3:1, usually seen in older women (>60 years of age)
- Associated with von Hippel Lindau Syndrome **(VHL)**
- Most are **benign with excellent prognosis** and low incidence of metastasis→ Serous cystadenocarcinoma

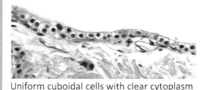

Uniform cuboidal cells with clear cytoplasm   Inhibin

 Path Presenter

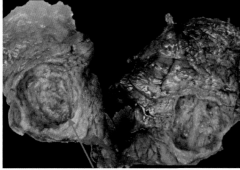

Cyst with fibrous capsule © Upasana Joneja

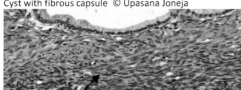

Ovarian type subepithelial stroma © Upasana Joneja

MUCINOUS CYSTIC NEOPLASM (MCN)
MORPHOLOGY
- Gross: **Multilocular** cyst surrounded by a **thick fibrotic capsule**
- Microscopy: Cyst-forming, mucin-producing neoplasm with a distinct **ovarian-type subepithelial stroma** in the wall
- The lining epithelium is predominantly columnar, mucinous epithelium
- Ovarian stroma: densely packed spindled cells
- IHC: **Ovarian** stroma stains **(+) ER, PR, Inhibin, and Smooth muscle actin**; Lining **epithelium stains (+) cytokeratin, CEA and MUC5AC**
OTHER HIGH YIELD POINTS
- Almost exclusively in **women**
- Typically located in the **pancreatic body or tail**
- **Does not** connect to the ductal system (unlike IPMN)
- Must be **thoroughly sampled** to exclude invasive component
- **KRAS** mutations are more common
- Other mutations identified include *TP53* and *SMAD4*

Path Presenter

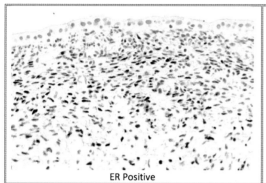

ER Positive

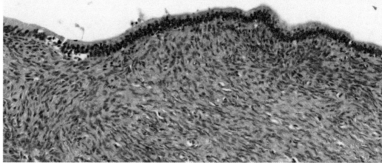

Ovarian type stroma

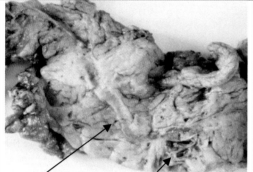

Dilated main duct with multiloculated IPMN
Credit: Upasana Joneja @Ujoneja
Gastric type

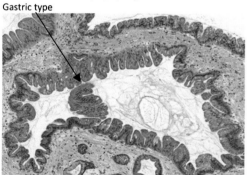

Intestinal type

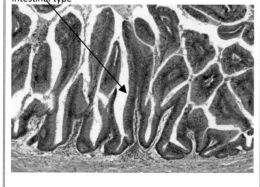

INTRADUCTAL PAPILLARY MUCINOUS NEOPLASM (IPMN)
MORPHOLOGY
- Grossly visible (typically >5 mm) intraductal proliferation of mucinous epithelial cells
- Most often in the **head** of the pancreas, but multi centric disease or involvement of the entire ductal system is possible
- Lesions can involve the main pancreatic duct (main-duct IPMN), branches (branch-duct IPMN), or mixed duct types.
- Microscopy: **Dilated ducts lined with mucinous epithelium**
- Flat or variable numbers of papillae are seen, **no ovarian-type stroma**
- 3 Subtypes
  - ➤ **Gastric type:** Most common, resembles foveolar cells, usually with low-grade dysplasia and branch-duct involvement
  - ➤ **Intestinal type:** Long papillae, tall, columnar epithelium, usually with low- or high-grade dysplasia and main-duct involvement
  - ➤ **Pancreatobiliary type:** Complex branching papillae lined by low cuboidal epithelium with amphophilic cytoplasm resembling biliary epithelium. Usually contains high-grade dysplasia and involves the main duct
- IHC: **(+)** ductal markers: **CK7, CK 19, CEA, CA19-9**. Mucin glycoprotein (MUC) expression and CDX2 are useful to distinguish between subtypes Gastric type: MUC5AC+, MUC6±
- Intestinal type: **(+)** MUC2, CK20, CDX2, MUC5AC
- Pancreatobiliary type: **(+)** MUC1, MUC5AC, MUC6
OTHER HIGH YIELD POINTS
- **KRAS** mutations are the most common. **GNAS** mutations are also common and seem to be relatively unique to **IPMNs**
- **RNF43** is the next common mutation seen
- **TP53 and SMAD4** mutations are seen in those with **invasive** carcinoma
- Invasive carcinoma arising in IPMNs are of two types: tubular or colloid
- **Tubular** carcinomas are similar to pancreatic ductal adenocarcinomas (PDAC) and usually arise in **pancreatobiliary-type** IPMNs
- **Colloid** carcinomas are associated with **intestinal-type** IPMNs and have a better prognosis than PDAC
- Invasive focus of **<5 mm** has a better prognosis

Path Presenter

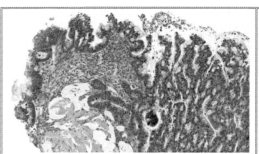
Pancreatobiliary type with high-grade dysplasia

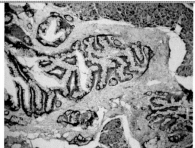
MUC-2 and MUC-5AC   Courtesy: Michele Angelo, MD (@BellaMicheleang)

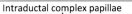
Intraductal complex papillae

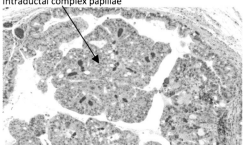
Eosinophilic cytoplasm & round nuclei

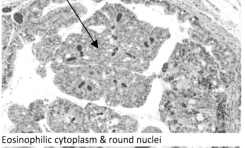
Courtesy: Dr. Olca Basturk, MD (@OlcaBasturk)

INTRADUCTAL ONCOCYTIC PAPILLARY NEOPLASM (IOPN)
MORPHOLOGY
- Gross: Cystic dilation of ducts with friable red-tan papillary or nodular projections
- Microscopy: Intraductal **complex arborizing** papillary growth pattern, lined by **2-5 layers of cuboidal cells**
- Cells have abundant eosinophilic cytoplasm and round, uniform nuclei with a prominent nucleoli
- Intraepithelial lumina impart a **cribriform** architecture
- IHC: **(+) MUC6, Hep Par1, MUC1**

OTHER HIGH YIELD POINTS
- Unlike IPMNs, IOPNs **lack KRAS, GNAS, and RNF4** mutations
- A subset of IOPNs harbors **DNAJB1-PRKACA** fusions, the same fusion as in fibrolamellar HCC
- Most exhibit high-grade dysplasia and invasive carcinoma (occurs in 30% of IOPNs)
- **Indolent** behavior, even with invasive carcinoma

Path Presenter

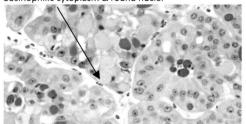
Back-to-back tubules   Growth as multiple nodules

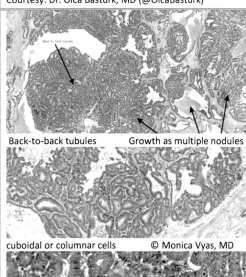
cuboidal or columnar cells   © Monica Vyas, MD

INTRADUCTAL TUBULOPAPILLARY NEOPLASM (ITPN)
MORPHOLOGY
- Gross: **Nodular solid** masses within dilated ducts; cystic change is less evident
- Microscopy: Intraductal epithelial neoplasm that features predominantly **back-to-back tubules**, resulting in a **cribriform** architecture, and lined by cuboidal or columnar cells
- Can have **focal papillary** growth, and there is no overt mucin production
- Often have **high-grade dysplasia, brisk mitotic** activity, and **necrosis**
- IHC: **(+) CK7, CK19, MUC1,** and variable MUC6; MUC2 and MUC5AC (a marker of all types of IPMNs) are negative

OTHER HIGH YIELD POINTS
- Unlike IPMNs, ITPNs **lack KRAS and GNAS** mutations
- May show **PIK3CA** mutation
- Invasive carcinomas are of **tubular** type and characterized by irregular infiltrating glands associated with a desmoplastic stromal reaction
- Overall **prognosis better than ductal adenocarcinoma**

Path Presenter

Low-grade PanIN

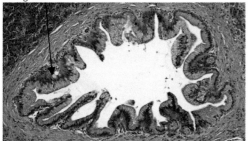

High-grade PanIN (loss of nuclear polarity)

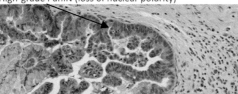

PANCREATIC INTRAEPITHELIAL NEOPLASIA (PanIN)

MORPHOLOGY

- Non-invasive, non-mass forming pancreatic ductal epithelial neoplasm, usually < 5 mm in diameter
- Microscopy: Low-grade and high-grade PanIN
- **Low-grade PanIN:** Flat or papillary mucin-producing epithelium, basally located or pseudostratified nuclei with mild to moderate cytologic atypia
- **High-grade PanIN** (carcinoma in situ): Severe cytologic atypia **with loss of nuclear polarity** and often **abnormal architecture** (papillary, micropapillary, or cribriform)

OTHER HIGH YIELD POINTS

- High-grade PanIN is the main **precursor** to ductal adenocarcinoma
- **KRAS** mutations (seen in >90% of PanIN) and **telomere shortening** are early molecular changes; *p16 (CDKN2A)* mutations are seen in **high-grade PanIN**

Path Presenter

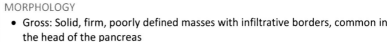

PANCREATIC DUCTAL ADENOCARCINOMA (PDAC)

MORPHOLOGY

- Gross: Solid, firm, poorly defined masses with infiltrative borders, common in the head of the pancreas
- Microscopy: Differentiation varies from well to moderately to poorly differentiated, showing haphazardly infiltrating duct-like glandular structures that elicit an **abundant desmoplastic** response
- Cells usually contain mucin, and clear cell change is common; variable nuclear pleomorphism (3-4 times the size of non-neoplastic nuclei) and there are several histologic subtypes
- **Adenosquamous carcinoma:** Glandular and squamous differentiation, the **squamous** component should account for ≥ **30%** of the tumor; worse prognosis than conventional PDAC
- **Colloid carcinoma**: ≥ **80%** of the neoplastic epithelium suspended in extracellular mucin, most arise in association with intestinal-type IPMN; better prognosis than conventional PDAC
- **Hepatoid carcinoma:** ≥ **50%** of tumor displays histologic and immunohistochemical evidence of hepatocellular differentiation
- **Medullary carcinoma**: Poorly differentiated, syncytial growth with abundant tumor-infiltrating lymphocytes, often microsatellite-instable; **better** prognosis than conventional PDAC
- **Invasive micropapillary carcinoma**: ≥ **50%** of tumors show small solid nests of cells suspended within stromal lacunae; aggressive behavior
- **Signet-ring cell (poorly cohesive) carcinoma:** At least **80%** of the tumor consists of individual poorly cohesive cells
- **Undifferentiated carcinoma with osteoclast-like giant cells**: contains three cell types- neoplastic mononuclear cells, non-neoplastic osteoclast-like multinucleated giant cells, and a mononuclear histiocytic component
- **Undifferentiated carcinoma**: Diffuse growth pattern without overt glandular differentiation. There are three morphologic patterns:
  - ➢ **Anaplastic** undifferentiated: At least 80% tumor is comprised of solid sheets of bizarre cells
  - ➢ **Sarcomatoid** undifferentiated: At least 80% of the tumor is comprised of spindle cells ± heterologous elements, loss of INI 1 is seen

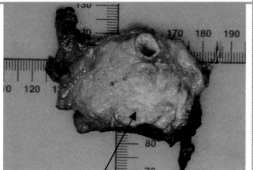

Infiltrating glands surrounded by desmoplastic stroma

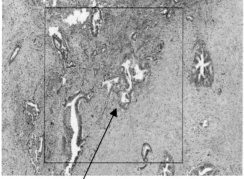

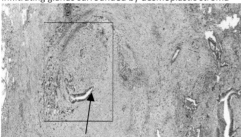

Perineural invasion

Solid ill-defined mass with a white cut surface

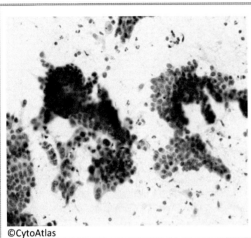

©CytoAtlas

> ➤ **Carcinosarcoma**: Sarcomatoid and epithelial elements each constitute at least 30% of the neoplasm
- **IHC: (+) CK7, CK8, CK18, CK19, and MUC1**
- **Loss of nuclear expression** of SMAD4/DPC4 and p16 in 50% of cases
- **Altered p53** expression (overexpression or null) in 75-80% of tumors

OTHER HIGH YIELD POINTS
- Most common mutations include **KRAS, TP53, CDKN2A, and SMAD4 (DPC4)**
- Precursor lesions: IPMN, MCN, and PanIN
- Perineural and lymphovascular invasion is common
- T stage is based on **tumor size** and is independent of any extrapancreatic tumor extension
- **Prognosis: poor**, depends on stage

Path Presenter

PANCREATIC NEUROENDOCRINE NEOPLASMS
MORPHOLOGY
- Includes neuroendocrine tumors (**PanNET**) and neuroendocrine carcinomas (**PanNEC**).
  - ➤ PanNET: **Well**-differentiated and graded as **G1, G2, and G3**
  - ➤ PanNEC: **Poorly** differentiated and **high-grade** neoplasms
- Gross: **Solid well-circumscribed** mass, but cystic changes can be prominent
- Microadenoma: PanNET <0.5 cm in size
- Microscopy: Well-differentiated NET- Various architectural patterns like trabeculae, gyri, solid nests, rosettes, or gland-like; composed of uniform cuboidal cells with round nuclei and coarsely stippled (**salt and pepper**) chromatin
- Poorly differentiated NEC: Sheet-like growth; 2 types- **small cell and large cell** NECs
- Small cell NEC: **scant** cytoplasm, finely granular chromatin, nuclear **molding**, **abundant mitosis**, and foci of punctate to geographic **necrosis.**
- Large cell NEC: moderate to **abundant** cytoplasm, large nuclei with **prominent nucleoli**, and increased mitotic activity
- IHC: **(+) Synaptophysin, Chromogranin, INSM1**

OTHER HIGH YIELD POINTS
- Well-differentiated NET: associated with **_MEN1, VHL, NF-1,_ and _DAXX/ATRX_** mutations
  - ➤ Malignant but slow-growing, indolent progression.
  - ➤ **Mitotic rate and/or Ki-67** labeling index are required for accurate grading of NET
- Functioning NETs include: Glucagonoma, Gastrinoma, Insulinoma, Somatostatinoma, VIPoma
- Poorly differentiated NEC: **_TP53_ and _RB1_** mutations are common; rapidly growing aggressive malignancies; mitotic rate typically **>20 per 2mm²,** and Ki-67 labeling index ranges from **50-95%**

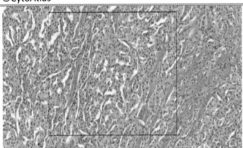

Well-differentiated NET, trabeculae of uniform cells
Credit: Elizabeth Montgomery, MD (@LizMontgomery)

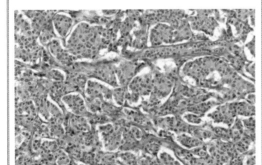

Well-differentiated NET   Synaptophysin
Credit: Upasana Joneja @Ujoneja

Path Presenter

NET Grade (G)	Mitotic rate (per 2mm²)	Ki-67 index (%)
G1	<2	<3
G2	2-20	3-20
G3	>20	>20

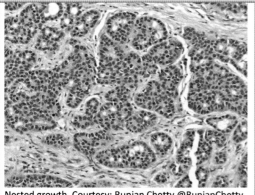

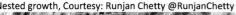

Nested growth, Courtesy: Runjan Chetty @RunjanChetty

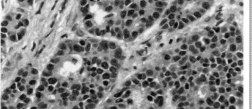

Path Presenter

ACINAR CELL CARCINOMA
MORPHOLOGY

- Gross: **Solid well-circumscribed** mass occasionally with necrosis or cystic change
- Microscopy: **Highly cellular**, lacks desmoplastic stromal response, with acinar, solid, trabecular, or nested growth patterns
- Cells have moderate amounts of **granular eosinophilic** cytoplasm (with or without **zymogen** granules), uniform nuclei with a single prominent nucleolus, and the **mitotic** rate is usually high
- It **can be mixed** with neuroendocrine or ductal carcinomas
- IHC: **(+) Trypsin, chymotrypsin, BCL10** (highly specific and sensitive), lipase or amylase, and cytokeratins (CK7, CK19)

OTHER HIGH YIELD POINTS

- Predominantly in **elderly men**
- Unlike PDAC, acinar cell carcinoma **lacks KRAS, CDKN2A, TP53, and SMAD4 mutations**
- Poor prognosis (better than PDAC, but less than Pancreatic NET)

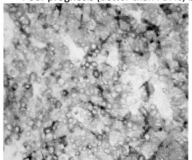 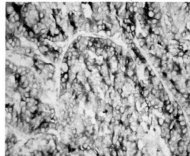

BCL10 and Trypsin. Courtesy: Anthony J Gill (@CaDxPath)

Pseudopapillary architecture

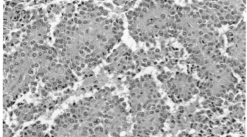

Hyaline globules

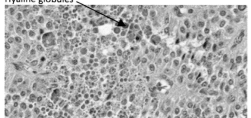

Credit: Elizabeth Montgomery, MD (@LizMontgomery)

Path Presenter

SOLID PSEUDOPAPILLARY NEOPLASM
MORPHOLOGY

- Gross: **Well-circumscribed solid** tumors with variable size, hemorrhagic necrosis, and pseudocystic changes in larger masses
- Microscopy: **Solid and pseudopapillary** structures admixed with hemorrhage and necrosis
- Solid tumor **resembles a neuroendocrine** tumor, composed of monomorphic, poorly cohesive cells
- Pseudopapillae are formed when cells detach from fibrovascular cores
- Tumor cells with eosinophilic or vacuolated cytoplasm often contain **PASD+ hyaline globules**, round to oval, often **grooved or indented** nuclei
- Cholesterol clefts, foamy histiocytes, and calcifications may occur in the stroma
- IHC: **Nuclear β-catenin+, loss of E-cadherin**, also (+) for cyclin D1, CD56, CD10, PR, CD99 (dot-like), sometimes express CK, CD117 or synaptophysin; however, **(-) for chromogranin and acinar markers (trypsin)**

OTHER HIGH YIELD POINTS

- Occur predominantly in **adolescent girls and young women** with a slight preference for the pancreatic **tail region**
- Somatic mutations in **CTNNB1 (encoding β-catenin)**
- **Excellent prognosis**: metastatic behavior cannot be predicted by perineural invasion, angioinvasion and deep infiltration into surrounding structures

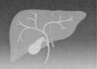
Highly cellular lobules separated by fibrous bands

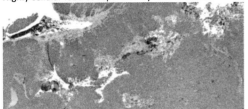

Squamoid nests

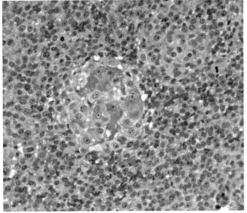

Courtesy: Miguel Reyes-Mugica (@mreyesm)

PANCREATOBLASTOMA
MORPHOLOGY
- Gross: **Solitary well-circumscribed solid lobulated mass**
- Microscopy: **Highly cellular lobules** with an acinar, solid, or trabecular pattern, separated by **fibrous bands**
- Most of the tumor looks like acinar cell carcinoma, a focal neuroendocrine component may be present, but **defining component** for establishing the diagnosis is **squamoid nests**
- Acinar differentiation shows cells polarized around small lumina with modest nuclear atypia and a single prominent nucleolus
- Squamoid nests are composed of epithelioid to spindle cells with eosinophilic/clear cytoplasm arranged in whorls; may show keratinization
- IHC: **Acinar** component stains **(+)** with trypsin, chymotrypsin, BCL10; **(+)** synaptophysin, chromogranin in **neuroendocrine** component and **squamoid nests** stain **(+)** with EMA and often nuclear β-catenin.

OTHER HIGH YIELD POINTS
- Most frequent pancreatic neoplasm in **childhood**
- Most are sporadic, but there is an association with **Beckwith-Wiedemann** and **Familial adenomatosis polyposis** syndrome
- Usually **indolent, curable** tumors with a more favourable outcome in children than adults; prognosis worse with metastatic and non-resectable tumors

Path Presenter

MiNEN (Mixed ductal-NET)

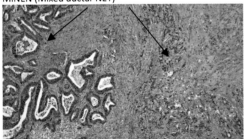

MIXED NEUROENDOCRINE NON-NEUROENDOCRINE NEOPLASM (MiNEN)
MORPHOLOGY
- Neoplasms composed of morphologically recognizable neuroendocrine and non-neuroendocrine components; **each comprises ≥ 30%** of tumor volume
- Gross: **Solid** tumors with focal necrosis
- Microscopy: Mixed ductal-NEC, mixed ductal-NET, mixed acinar-NEC, and mixed acinar-ductal-NEC are seen

OTHER HIGH YIELD POINTS
- A **monoclonal** origin for **both** components of the tumor
- Usually, metastasize to lymph nodes and the liver

Acinar atrophy and fibrosis

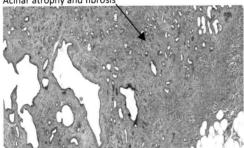

Foci of chronic inflammation

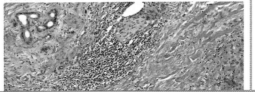

CHRONIC PANCREATITIS
MORPHOLOGY
- Gross: Diffuse **fibrosis** and induration, **cysts** of varying sizes, and calculi may be seen
- Microscopy: Varying degrees of **acinar atrophy**, **fibrosis**, and **ductal distortion** are the hallmark features
- Foci of **chronic inflammation** are seen but lesser than that in autoimmune pancreatitis
- **Pseudohypertrophic** appearance of islets due to loss of acinar tissue

OTHER HIGH YIELD POINTS
- The most common cause is **alcohol**
- **Groove (paraduodenal) pancreatitis** is a distinct form centered around the minor papilla and affects the duodenal wall and paraduodenal pancreatic tissue in the form of fibrosis and cystic changes
- Helpful features to distinguish from pancreatic ductal adenocarcinoma include
  ➤ **Retained lobular** architecture

> ➤ Absence of **cytologic** features of malignancy (nuclear size variation >4:1, nuclear membrane irregularities, pale vacuolated cytoplasm)
> ➤ Lack of single-cell infiltration, perineural invasion, and association of glands with arteries
> ➤ Retained SMAD4 and lack of aberrant p53 expression

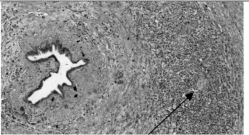
Storifirm fibrosis and Inflammation around the ducts

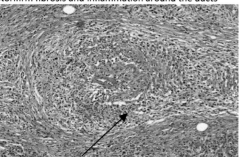
Fibrosis & obliterative phlebitis

AUTOIMMUNE PANCREATITIS (AIP)
MORPHOLOGY
- Gross: **firm pancreas**, occasionally mass forming and mimicking carcinoma
- Microscopy: two variants are there, type 1 and 2, both demonstrate **dense chronic inflammation centered around the ducts along with fibrosis**
- **Type 1(IgG4-related** pancreatitis or lymphoplasmacytic sclerosing pancreatitis): hallmark features of dense lymphoplasmacytic infiltrate, storiform fibrosis, and obliterative phlebitis
- Type 1 AIP can also have scattered eosinophilic infiltrates, lymphoid aggregates, and increased **IgG4+** plasma cells (>10/HPF in biopsies and >50/HPF in resection specimens, both with an **IgG4/IgG ratio of >40%)**
- **Type 2 AIP**: periductal lymphoplasmacytic infiltration, along with granulocytic epithelial lesions (**neutrophilic** infiltration of duct wall), lobular neutrophilic abscesses, fibrosis (not the typical storiform fibrosis as in type 1 AIP), and **absent or rare IgG4+** plasma cells

OTHER HIGH YIELD POINTS
- **Prognosis is good** in both types with steroid therapy

Lymphoepithelial cyst

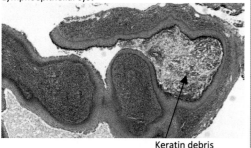
Keratin debris

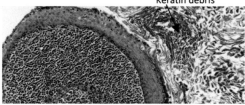
Lymphoepithelial cyst wall lined by squamous epithelium and surrounded by reactive lymphoid tissue

NON-NEOPLASTIC CYSTIC LESIONS OF PANCREAS
PSEUDOCYSTS
- Pancreatic or peripancreatic collection of enzyme-rich fluid, lacking lining epithelium and wall composed of fibrosis and granulation tissue
- Adjacent pancreas with features of resolving acute or chronic pancreatitis
- Cyst fluid demonstrates **high amylase** (>250 IU/mL) & **low CEA** (<200 IU/mL)

LYMPHOEPITHELIAL CYSTS
- Cyst lined by **squamous** epithelium and surrounded by **reactive lymphoid** tissue
- **Keratinaceous debris** may present within the cyst cavity

ACINAR CYSTIC TRANSFORMATION
- More common in the pancreatic **head,** unilocular or multilocular cysts filled with clear fluid.
- Lined by cells with pale or granular apical cytoplasm and basally oriented nuclei, the lining epithelium exhibit regions of either acinar or ductal differentiation

HEREDITARY PANCREATITIS
MORPHOLOGY
- **Early childhood** stages with **features similar to acute pancreatitis**, like necrosis and loss of acinar tissue
- **Late adult** stages with **fat replacement** of parenchyma, periductal and interlobular **fibrosis** as in chronic pancreatitis

OTHER HIGH YIELD POINTS
- Autosomal dominant disease; is caused by mutations in the **cationic trypsinogen gene (PRSS1)**; the two most common mutations are **R122H and N29I**
- **High risk** for developing pancreatic carcinoma
- Associated other gene mutations include *SPINK1, CFTR,* and *CTRC*

Chronic Cholecystitis

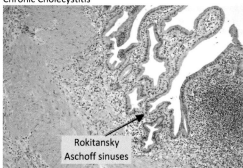

Rokitansky Aschoff sinuses

Acute cholecystitis

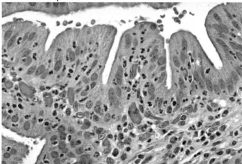

Porcelain Gall Bladder

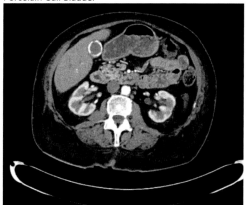

Emphysematous Cholecystitis

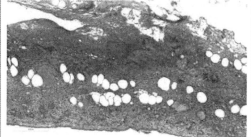

Path Presenter

GALLBLADDER AND EXTRAHEPATIC BILIARY TRACT
CHOLECYSTITIS
MORPHOLOGY

- Gross: Calculi may be seen in acute and chronic cholecystitis
- Features of acute cholecystitis: edema, congestion, and/or necrosis; chronic cholecystitis with **fibrosis** or **even grossly normal** appearing; **xanthogranulomatous** type may resemble carcinoma due to the presence of **firm yellow nodules or plaques**
- Microscopy: Variable picture depending on the clinical duration- acute neutrophilic inflammation with hemorrhage, necrosis, or gangrenous change in the acute phase; chronic phase- mononuclear inflammatory infiltrate, fibrosis, metaplastic changes, and **Rokitansky-Aschoff** sinuses (herniation of mucosa into or through muscularis)

OTHER HIGH YIELD POINTS

- Variants: **Xanthogranulomatous cholecystitis**- chronic inflammatory infiltrate composed of lipid-laden macrophages, lymphocytes, plasma cells, eosinophils, and neutrophils, admixed with fibrosis, cholesterol clefts, and giant cells, often produce mural or extramural nodule
- **Porcelain gallbladder**- diffuse dystrophic calcification with fibrosis; associated with a high risk of carcinoma
- **Emphysematous cholecystitis**- a variant of acute cholecystitis caused by gas-producing bacteria, particularly clostridial organisms

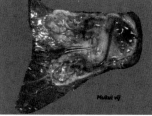

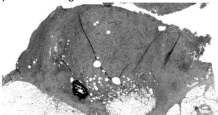

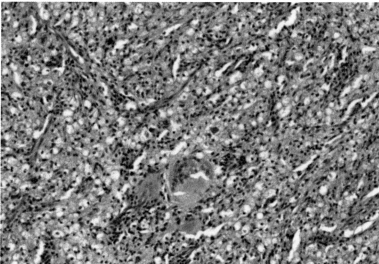

Xanthogranulomatous cholecystitis:
Characteristic yellowish wall thickening and ulceration Credit: Mukul Vij MD @vij_mukul
Microscopy: - lipid-laden macrophages with bile pigment, chronic inflammatory infiltrate, and giant cells, often producing mural or extramural nodule (low magnification image).

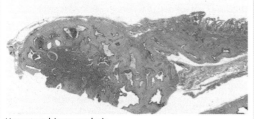
Cystically dilated glands

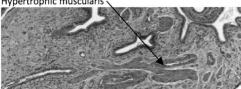
Hypertrophic muscularis

ADENOMYOMA/ADENOMYOMATOUS HYPERPLASIA
MORPHOLOGY
- Gross: Firm white nodular area usually in the **fundus** (adenomyoma- if solitary), but can also be a diffuse process
- Microscopy: **Cystically dilated benign biliary glands** along with **hypertrophic muscularis and fibrosis**

OTHER HIGH YIELD POINTS
- Other hyperplastic and metaplastic changes include hyperplastic polyps/mucosal hyperplasia (pedunculated or sessile), inflammatory polyps, pyloric metaplasia, intestinal metaplasia, and squamous metaplasia
- Among this pyloric gland metaplasia is a common finding associated with chronic injuries

Path Presenter

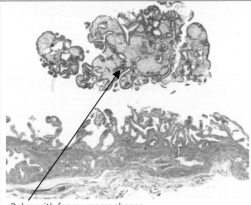

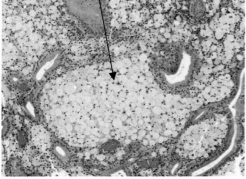
Polyp with foamy macrophages

CHOLESTEROL POLYP/CHOLESTEROLOSIS
MORPHOLOGY
- Gross: **Yellow flecks against a dark green background (strawberry gallbladder)** in cholesterolosis, and polypoid excrescences projecting into the lumen in cholesterol polyp
- Microscopy: Accumulation of **foamy macrophages** within lamina propria resulting in thickened folds or polyps and adjacent chronic inflammation if coexistent calculi present

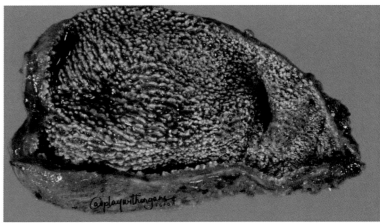

Path Presenter

Gross photograph: Strawberry gallbladder (©Cory Nash, MD)

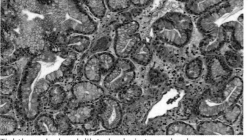
Tightly packed and dilated pyloric-type glands

PYLORIC GLAND ADENOMA (PGA)
MORPHOLOGY
- Gross: Sessile or pedunculated
- Microscopy: Non-invasive, benign glandular neoplasm composed of **mucinous glands with pyloric or Brunner gland-like features**
- Glands are tightly packed and maybe cystically dilated; cells feature abundant apical mucinous cytoplasm, peripheral nuclei, and minimal intervening stroma
- Paneth cells and neuroendocrine cells are often seen
- IHC: **(+) CK7, MUC6**

Path Presenter

OTHER HIGH YIELD POINTS

- **CTNNB1 mutations and nuclear β-catenin** immunohistochemical expression in 60% of PGAs
- If an invasive component is not present, it is usually cured by cholecystectomy, even when high-grade dysplasia is present.

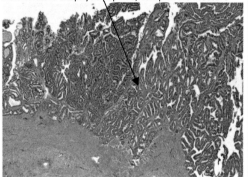

Non-invasive exophytic papillae, complex architecture

INTRACHOLECYSTIC PAPILLARY NEOPLASM (ICPN)

MORPHOLOGY

- Gross: **Granular, friable** excrescences or prominent **exophytic** growth, broad-based or with thin stalk which often detach into the lumen and mistaken as biliary sludge
- Microscopy: **Non-invasive back-to-back** epithelial units predominantly in **papillary or tubulopapillary** in the architecture
- Four morphological patterns, often with an intermixed pattern
- **Biliary-type:** most common, cuboidal cells with clear to eosinophilic cytoplasm, enlarged nuclei, and distinct nucleoli
- **Gastric-type:** elongated glands lined with tall columnar mucinous cells (resemble gastric foveolar epithelium) with abundant pale cytoplasm and peripheral nuclei
- **Intestinal-type:** resembles colonic adenomas, tall columnar cells with basophilic cytoplasm and pseudostratified cigar-shaped nuclei
- **Oncocytic-type:** least common, arborizing papillae lined by cells with abundant granular eosinophilic cytoplasm and nuclei with prominent nucleoli
- IHC: **Biliary type**: **(+)** CK7, MUC1; **Gastric-type**: diffuse **(+)** MUC5AC and some express MUC6; **Intestinal-type**: **(+)** CK20, CDX2, MUC2; **oncocytic-type**: **(+)** MUC1

OTHER HIGH YIELD POINTS

- **KRAS** mutation is common; TP53 and GNAS mutations are rare
- Invasive carcinoma is identified in half of the cases, particularly those with biliary morphology or high-grade dysplasia

Path Presenter

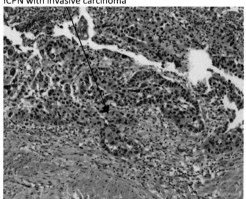

ICPN with invasive carcinoma

BILIARY INTRAEPITHELIAL NEOPLASIA (BilIN)

Features	Low-grade BilIN	High-grade BilIN
Microscopy	Flat or micropapillary Hyperchromatic nuclei High N: C ratio Nuclear stratification Preserved nuclear polarity	Flat or micropapillary Hyperchromatic, irregular nuclei High N: C ratio, pleomorphic, bizarre nuclei Complex nuclear stratification Loss of nuclear polarity
Biliary mucosal involvement	Relatively small foci	Relatively extensive
Peribiliary glands involvement	Infrequent	Frequent
IHC Ki-67 labeling index	Mildly to moderately increased	Markedly increased
S100	Mild to moderate	Diffuse and strong
p53	Wild-type	Frequently aberrant
p16	Relatively preserved	Decreased

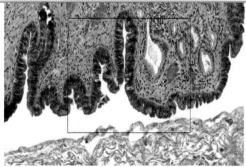

Low-grade BilIN

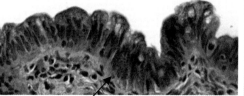

Nuclear stratification and preserved nuclear polarity

MORPHOLOGY

- Non-invasive flat or micropapillary dysplastic epithelial lesion confined to gallbladder lumen or biliary tree, grossly not visible. **Graded based on worst**

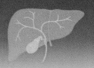

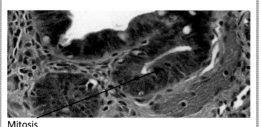

Mitosis

- **cytoarchitectural atypia** and is classified by current two-tiered grading system as low (includes previous BilIN-1 and 2) or high (previous BilIN-3)
- High-grade BilIN can extend to peribiliary glands and Rokitansky-Aschoff sinuses (feature should not be confused for invasion)

OTHER HIGH YIELD POINTS

- Cholelithiasis, FAP, Primary sclerosing cholangitis (PSC), choledochal cyst, and anomalous union of pancreatobiliary ducts are the **predisposing factors**
- **KRAS** mutations are seen in ~40% of cases (early molecular event), and TP53 mutations are late events in high-grade BilIN
- Low-grade BilIN is of no clinical significance
- Most cases of high-grade BilIN can be **cured by cholecystectomy**, usually multifocal disease due to a field effect and lead to recurrences and metastasis

Biliary-type adenocarcinoma:

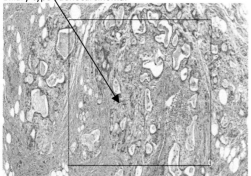

Cuboidal cells lined infiltrating tubules

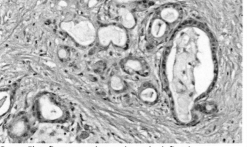

Gross: Flat, firm, granular, and poorly defined

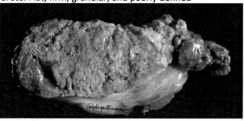

CARCINOMA OF GALLBLADDER

MORPHOLOGY

- Gross: Most carcinomas are located in the **fundus**, variable gross appearance- usually flat, firm, granular, and poorly defined
- Microscopy: Various histologic subtypes
- **Biliary-type adenocarcinoma**: Most common subtype, morphology, and behavior similar to pancreatic ductal adenocarcinoma, composed of infiltrating tubules lined with cuboidal cells embedded in a desmoplastic stroma.
- **Intestinal-type adenocarcinoma**: Resemble colonic adenocarcinoma, tubular configuration with columnar cells featuring elongated, pseudostratified nuclei, uncommon type so important to rule out a metastatic colonic adenocarcinoma
- **Mucinous adenocarcinoma**: >50% of the tumor contains extracellular mucin with single cells or strips of neoplastic cells floating in mucin and is more aggressive than ordinary gallbladder carcinomas
- **Clear cell carcinoma**: Sheets of clear cells in an alveolar arrangement separated by sinusoidal vessels mimic clear cell renal cell carcinoma
- **Poorly-cohesive carcinoma ± signet-ring cells**: Poorly cohesive individual cells or cords forming a diffuse infiltrative pattern and is more aggressive than ordinary gallbladder carcinomas
- **Adenosquamous carcinoma**: Squamous elements constitute ≥25% of the tumor admixed with an adenocarcinoma component
- **Squamous cell carcinoma**: Rare type with an aggressive behavior

OTHER HIGH YIELD POINTS

- Most common biliary tract carcinoma, more frequent in females
- **Risk factors**: Gall stones (most common), PSC, aflatoxin B1, infections (Salmonella typhi, Opisthorchis viverrini), pancreatobiliary maljunction, syndromic predisposition (FAP, Lynch)
- **TP53** mutations are seen in >50% of cases; other common mutations include **CDKN2A or CDKN2B, ARID1A, PIK3CA, and CTNNB1**
- The **tumor stage is the most important prognostic factor**, early gallbladder carcinomas (Tis/T1a/T1b) have a better prognosis compared to the advanced ones, and in T2 tumors: T2a (tumor invades peritoneal side connective tissue) has a better prognosis than T2b (tumor invades hepatic side)

Cystic dilatation of the biliary tree

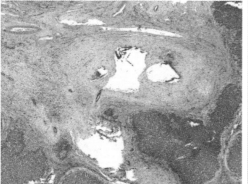

Cystic dilatation of the biliary tree

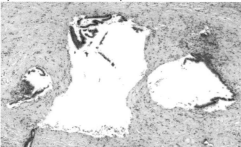

Todani classification: created using Biorender by Manju Ambelil, MD

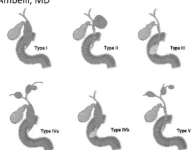

CHOLEDOCHAL CYSTS
MORPHOLOGY

- **Cystic dilatation of the biliary tree**; predominant in the **pediatric** population, and most patients have an anomalous pancreatobiliary junction which may result in reflux of pancreatic enzymes to the bile duct
- Gross: Fibrotic cyst wall with variable sizes, contains bile or stones and shows a distal narrowing
- Microscopy: **Cyst wall** composed of **dense fibrous** tissue featuring variable amounts of **smooth muscle and chronic inflammation**; a columnar epithelial lining may be focally seen and is most often is damaged and denuded

OTHER HIGH YIELD POINTS

- **Increased risk** of developing carcinoma, risk increases with age
- Other complications include pancreatitis, cholelithiasis, cholangitis, secondary biliary cirrhosis and spontaneous rupture
- Todani classification of choledochal cyst

Type	Findings
I	Segmental or Fusiform dilatation of common bile duct
II	Focal saccular dilatation or diverticulum of common bile duct
III	Cystic dilatation of common bile duct within the duodenal wall (choledochocele)
IVa	Combined intrahepatic and extrahepatic cystic dilatation of bile ducts
IVb	Multiple cystic dilatations of extrahepatic bile duct only
V	Multiple intrahepatic biliary cysts (Caroli disease)

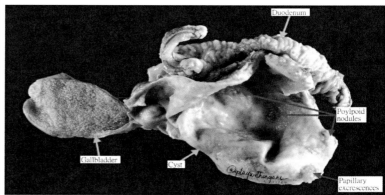

Image credits: Cory Nash

Papillary premalignant growth in dilated bile ducts

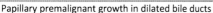

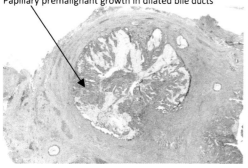

INTRADUCTAL PAPILLARY NEOPLASM OF THE BILE DUCTS (IPNB)
MORPHOLOGY

- Gross: **Polypoid or papillary** premalignant growth in dilated bile ducts which can lead to obstruction and duct dilatation
- Microscopy: Papillary structures with fine fibrovascular cores surfaced by cuboidal or columnar epithelial cells which show intestinal, biliary, gastric-type, or oncocytic differentiation like in ICPN, with variable cytologic atypia
- Two-tiered grading system: low and high-grade dysplasia
- Recently proposed classification divide IPNB into type 1 and type 2
  - ➤ **Type 1:** histologically similar to **IPMN** of the pancreas, with a regular papillary/villous growth pattern, mucin production, more frequent in **intrahepatic** bile ducts, and **less aggressive**

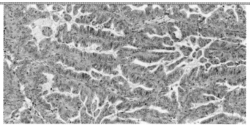
Intraductal papillary growth

Path Presenter

> **Type 2:** irregular papillae with **cribriform and solid** areas, rare mucin production, frequent in **extrahepatic** bile ducts and **more aggressive**

OTHER HIGH YIELD POINTS
- Risk factors include PSC, hepatolithiasis and liver fluke infection (clonorchiasis and opisthorchiasis)
- **KRAS, GNAS, and RNF4** mutations in those with **mucinous** morphology/**low-grade** dysplasia and **TP53 mutations in high-grade neoplasms**
- Prognosis depends on the presence of invasive carcinoma, but still, IPNB with invasive carcinoma have a **better prognosis than conventional cholangiocarcinoma**

CARCINOMA OF THE EXTRAHEPATIC BILE DUCTS

MORPHOLOGY
- Gross: **Sclerosing** (most common), nodular or papillary growths
- Microscopy: Most carcinomas are **pancreatobiliary-type** adenocarcinoma/cholangiocarcinoma, with widely spaced, irregular glands and small tumor clusters infiltrating through desmoplastic stroma and frequently with perineural and lymphovascular invasion
- Other histologic patterns of adenocarcinoma include intestinal-type, foveolar-type, mucinous, signet-ring cell, clear cell, hepatoid, and micropapillary-type
- Rare subtypes: squamous cell, adenosquamous, sarcomatoid, and undifferentiated carcinomas
- IHC: **(+) CK7, CK19, CEA, CA19-9**

OTHER HIGH YIELD POINTS
- Risk factors: PSC, cholelithiasis, choledochal cysts, and liver fluke infection (Clonorchis Sinensis and Opisthorchis viverrini)
- BilIN and IPNB are precursor lesions
- **Klatskin tumors: Perihilar** tumors occurring at the confluence of the right and left hepatic ducts
- **KRAS** mutations are early events, followed by **TP53** mutations (these can also be seen in intrahepatic cholangiocarcinoma)
- Extrahepatic cholangiocarcinoma specific alterations are PRKACA/PRKACB fusions, ELF3 and ARID1B mutations
- **Prognosis** depends on the stage at presentation and resectability

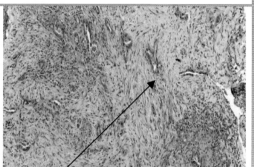
Irregular glands and tumor clusters in desmoplastic stroma

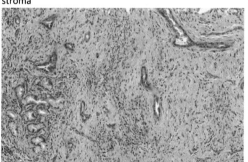

Path Presenter

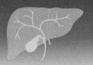
Diagnostic Algorithm for Pancreatic Tumors

Figure adapted from WHO

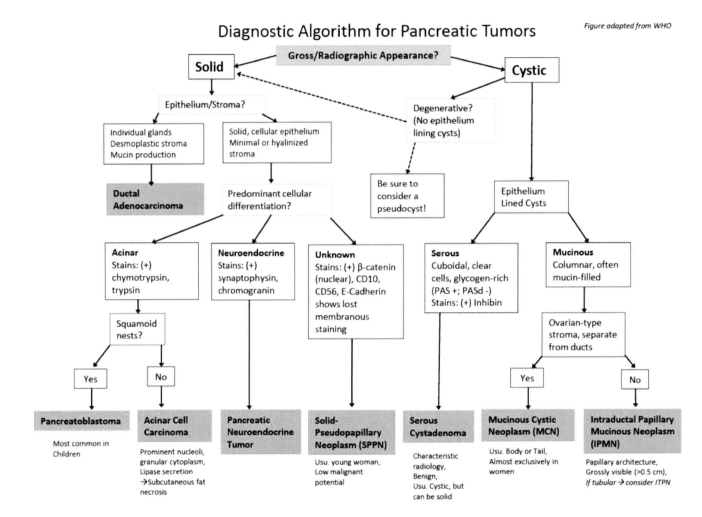

Ductal Adenocarcinoma	Chronic Pancreatitis
Haphazard, irregular architecture	Lobular, organized architecture
Incomplete luminal spaces with gland rupture	Complete luminal spaces
Cellular pleomorphism (4:1 variation in size)	Less pleomorphic
Perineural invasion	Absent
Vascular/perivascular invasion	Absent
Extrapancreatic invasion	Absent
Mitoses and nucleoli are often prominent	Often absent
Can extend outside of the pancreas into fat, etc.	Confined to pancreas

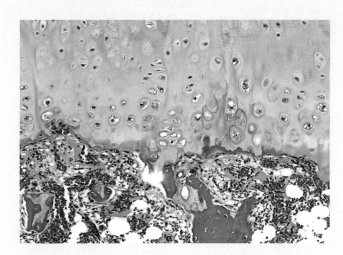

Osteochondroma (H&E stain). Courtesy: Akanksha
Gupta, MD

CHAPTER 8: BONE AND SOFT TISSUE
PATHOLOGY

Terrance Lynn, MD
Kenechukwu Ojukwu, MD
Manita Chaum, MD
Amandeep Kaur, MD
Snehal Sonawane, MD
Dinesh Pradhan, MD

Image courtesy: Cedars Sinai Medical Center, Department of
Pathology and Lab Medicine, Los Angeles, CA (images
contributed by Dr Bonnie Balzer, Vice Chair of Department)

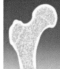
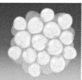

ADIPOCYTIC TUMORS

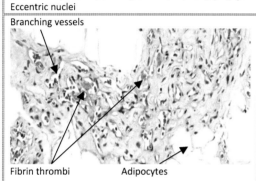

Mature adipocytes

Eccentric nuclei

LIPOMA
MORPHOLOGY
- **Mature adipocytes** with single large fat droplet and eccentric nuclei

OTHER HIGH YIELD POINTS
- Clinically presents as a **painless** mass and is superficial/subcutaneous
- Most common mesenchymal tumor in adults, M=F
- **Gross exam: well-circumscribed**, **homogenous cut surface**, <5 cm
- If retroperitoneal/large, **must** exclude well-differentiated liposarcoma
- **Recurrence uncommon**, slightly higher risk if incompletely resected
- **FISH:** Absence of MDM2 amplification
- **Molecular:** Rearrangements of *HMGA1, HMGA2*

Path Presenter

Courtesy of
John Cummings

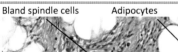
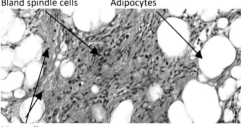

Branching vessels

Fibrin thrombi   Adipocytes

ANGIOLIPOMA
MORPHOLOGY
- Mature adipocytes, **branching vascular network, fibrin thrombi**

OTHER HIGH YIELD POINTS
- Clinically presents as a **painful** mass on the forearm
- Seen in 2-3rd decade with male predominance
- Gross: Circumscribed dense nodule, <2cm, and vascular
- **Molecular:** *PRKD2* mutations (>80%), activating *PIK3CA* seen also

Path Presenter

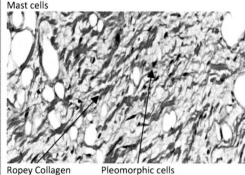

Bland spindle cells   Adipocytes

Mast cells

Ropey Collagen   Pleomorphic cells

Path Presenter

SPINDLE CELL & PLEOMORPHIC LIPOMA
MORPHOLOGY
- **Mature adipocytes** with bland **spindle cells** and **ropey collagen**
- Variable myxoid background and mast cells

OTHER HIGH YIELD POINTS
- **Uncommon** tumor with **cape-like distribution**: Neck, shoulder, back
- Mainly **middle age** to **elderly men**
- **Can have a spectrum of histology:** can be primarily fatty with minimal spindle cells, or can have minimal fat and composed of largely spindle cell component → mimics DFSP
- **Pleomorphic lipoma:** ropey collagen, pleomorphic spindle & **floret** cells, myxoid background
- **Floret cells:** giant cells with multiple nuclei arranged along the peripheral edge and central eosinophilic cytoplasm
- **IHC:** Spindle & floret cells → CD34 (+), loss of nuclear Rb1

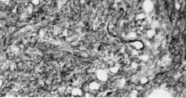
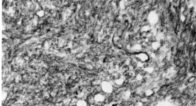
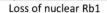

CD34+   Loss of nuclear Rb1

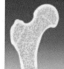
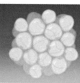

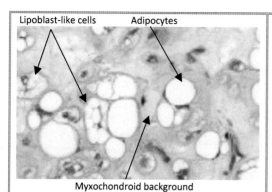

Lipoblast-like cells   Adipocytes

Myxochondroid background

CHONDROID LIPOMA
MORPHOLOGY

- Nests/cords of **"lipoblast-like"** or **chondrocyte-like** vacuolated cells
- **Chondromyxoid background**
- Prominent **vascular network** +/- hemorrhage
- **Absence of pleomorphism, atypia**, mitoses, necrosis

OTHER HIGH YIELD POINTS

- Predominantly in **females**, 3rd-4th decade
- Mostly seen in **limb girdles/proximal** extremities
- No metastasis, no recurrence
- **Molecular: t(11;16)(q13;p12-13) translocation** → fusion of **C11orf95** and **MRTFB** genes

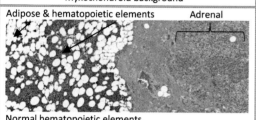

Adipose & hematopoietic elements   Adrenal

Normal hematopoietic elements

MYELOLIPOMA
MORPHOLOGY

- **Mature adipocytes** with **normal marrow elements**
- Often have adjacent adrenal parenchyma

OTHER HIGH YIELD POINTS

- Most common in the **adrenal medulla**
- Presents in 5-7th decade, **M=F, unilateral**, imaging is diagnostic
- Can become very large and weigh in kgs
- **Grossly**: Adipose tissue with hemorrhage (from marrow)
- No association with hematopoietic disorders
- **Pathogenesis:** unknown
- **Primary differential:** extramedullary hematopoiesis

Path Presenter

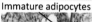

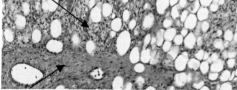

Immature adipocytes

Fibrous tissue   Myxoid   Spindle cells

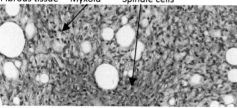

LIPOBLASTOMA
MORPHOLOGY

- **Immature adipocytes** separated by connective tissue that has a loose myxoid appearance
- Adipocytes are seen at various points of maturation (including **spindle cells**)
- **Plexiform vascular** pattern

OTHER HIGH YIELD POINTS

- Rare tumors seen in infants, **male predominance**
- Presents as a **painless** soft tissue mass
- Localized → Lipoblastoma; Diffuse→ Lipoblastomatosis
- Molecular: Chromosomal rearrangement of 8q11 →**HAS2-PLAG1** and **COL1A2-PLAG1; t(3;8)(p13;q21.1)** also seen

Path Presenter

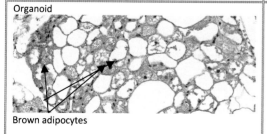

Organoid

Brown adipocytes

HIBERNOMA
MORPHOLOGY

- **Organoid arrangement** of **brown adipocytes** with **granular** and **vacuolated cytoplasm**
- Vacuoles in adipocytes are **small** and **uniform**
- Delicate **branching capillaries**

OTHER HIGH YIELD POINTS

- Rare tumor, seen in 3rd – 4th decade, no sex predilection
- Common locations: thigh, axilla, back

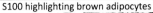
S100 highlighting brown adipocytes

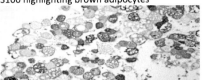

- Can **produce steroids**
- **IHC:** generally not needed, but (+) **UCP-1, S100**; (-) **CD34** (+ in spindle variant)
- **Molecular:** may have rearrangements in 11q13-21

Path Presenter

Lipoblast

Adipocytes   Atypical cells

Inflammatory cells

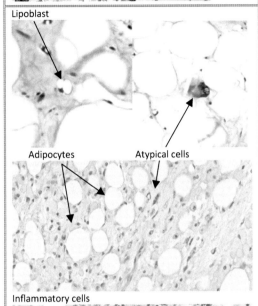

Path Presenter

ATYPICAL LIPOMATOUS TUMOR (WELL-DIFFERENTIATED LIPOSARCOMA)
MORPHOLOGY
- Variable amounts of **lipoblasts and mature adipocytes**
- **Atypical** cells **most commonly seen** near/in the **fibrous septae**

OTHER HIGH YIELD POINTS
- **Most common form** of liposarcoma
- Often are large, >10 cm
- No metastatic potential but recurs locally and can de-differentiate
- Subtypes:
  - **Lipoma-like:** Most common, frequently contain lipoblasts, grossly indistinguishable from lipoma
  - **Sclerosing type:** Second most common, usually paratesticular, or retroperitoneal, has collagenous fibrosis with scattered atypical multinucleated stromal cells
  - **Inflammatory:** Rare, chronic inflammatory cells (more commonly B>T) in a fibrocollagenous stroma, rare, atypical multinucleated cells
  - **Mixed:** Combination of the above
- **IHC:** (+) **S100, MDM2,** CDK4, p16; less common: (+) CD34, Desmin
- **FISH:** for **MDM2 and CDK4 amplification (can use real-time PCR)**

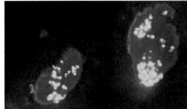
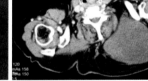

MDM2 amplification using FISH courtesy of: Amal Alodaini @DrAlodaini

Radiology of Liposarcoma courtesy of Dr. Panoraia Paraskeva

Delicate vessels   Spindle cells

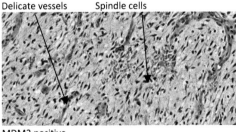

MDM2 positive

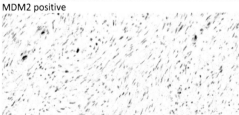

Credit: Raul Perret, MD, MSc @kells108

DEDIFFERENTIATED LIPOSARCOMA
MORPHOLOGY
- High grade component has entrapped lipoblasts and often looks sarcomatous (like fibrosarcoma) and has **multinucleated cells, pleomorphic cells, and/or spindled cells**
- Low grade component may resemble fibromatosis
- **Delicate branching vessels**

OTHER HIGH YIELD POINTS
- Better prognosis than other high-grade sarcomas
- Most common site is retroperitoneum, also in extremities and spermatic cord
- Metastasizes in 15-20% of cases, recurs in ~40-50%
- **IHC: (+)** MDM2, CDK4
- Molecular:
  - Amplification of **12q14**
  - FISH for **MDM2** and **CDK4** amplification (can use real-time PCR)

Path Presenter

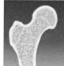

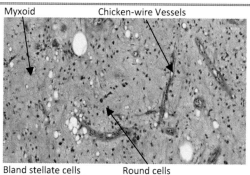

Myxoid — Chicken-wire Vessels

Bland stellate cells — Round cells

Breakpoint at 12q13.1

DDIT3 →

Chromosome 12

MYXOID LIPOSARCOMA
MORPHOLOGY
- Proliferation of bland monomorphic **stellate and fusiform cells**
- High-grade → cells are **rounded** and **more primitive**
- Abundant **myxoid matrix** and **chicken-wire vasculature**
- Lipoblasts with variable vacuolation

OTHER HIGH YIELD POINTS
- Usually in younger individuals, most common in thigh
- Higher grade → less myxoid component and more-round cell
- Metastasizes in 10-60% of cases (risk varies by grade), recurs in ~30%
- IHC: **(+)** for **DDIT3 and S100**; **(-)** for MDM2 and CDK4
- **Molecular/FISH:** *FUS-DDIT3* → **t(12;16)(q13;p11.2)**
  - ➤ **Uncommon:** EWSR1-DDIT3 → t(12;22)(q13;q12)

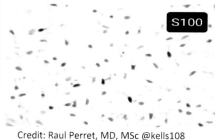

S100

Credit: Raul Perret, MD, MSc @kells108   Courtesy of Dr. Jordi M I Nogue

Path Presenter

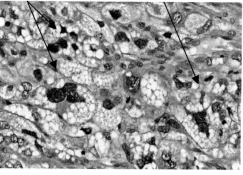

Pleomorphism — Bizarre cell

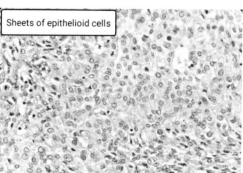

Sheets of epithelioid cells

PLEOMORPHIC LIPOSARCOMA
MORPHOLOGY
- **Pleomorphic cells (giant, bizarre)**, lipoblasts, many mitoses, necrosis

OTHER HIGH YIELD POINTS
- Least common liposarcoma
- **Grossly:** large, multi-nodular, and white-yellow, foci of necrosis
- **Molecular: (-)** MDM2 and CDK4
  - ➤ Complex karyotype but not specific

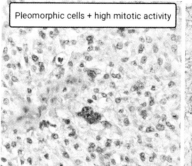

Pleomorphic cells + high mitotic activity

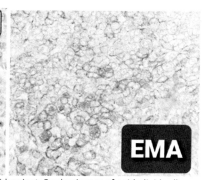

EMA

Pleomorphic liposarcoma : Epithelioid variant: Predominance of epithelioid cells
(may express EMA/CK) Credit: Raul Perret, MD, MSc @kells108

Path Presenter

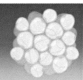

FIBROBLASTIC & MYOFIBROBLASTIC TUMORS

"Tissue culture" appearance

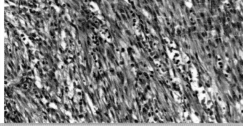

Spindle/Stellate cells | Extravasated RBC

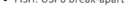

NODULAR FASCIITIS
MORPHOLOGY
- **Bland stellate/spindle cells** with a **"tissue culture"** pattern
- **Torn stroma** with "S" and "C" shapes
- **Extravasated red blood cells**
- Older lesions are collagenous/scarred

OTHER HIGH YIELD POINTS
- **Benign, self-limiting**, rapid growth, **mass-forming** subcutaneous lesion
- Most common in the **upper extremity** or **head** and **neck** of **kids**
- **Variants**: Ossifying fasciitis, intravascular fasciitis, cranial fasciitis
- IHC: (+) **SMA, MSA, Calponin**; (+) **Desmin**
- Molecular: **MYH9-USP6**; Other partners: *COL1A1, CTNNB1*, others
- FISH: USP6 break-apart probe

Path Presenter

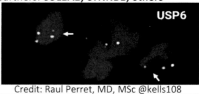

Credit: Raul Perret, MD, MSc @kells108

Ganglion-like cells

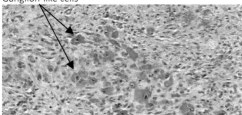

"Tissue culture" appearance

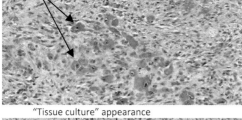

PROLIFERATIVE FASCIITIS/MYOSITIS
MORPHOLOGY
- **"Tissue culture"** pattern of prominent large, basophilic **ganglion-like cells** with one or more vesicular nuclei with conspicuous nucleoli
- **Extravasated red blood cells** and **arborizing vascular network**
- Variable mitotic activity but no atypical mitosis

OTHER HIGH YIELD POINTS
- **Most commonly seen** in **adults** (>50) on the **forearm**
- **Rapidly growing**, **poorly circumscribed** mass but **benign**
- If arising in muscle → Proliferative myositis
- **Childhood variant** → **more cellular, pleomorphic ganglion-like** cells with a "rhabdomyoblastic" look; can have necrosis and many mitoses and inflammation; pushing border (unlike adults → infiltrative)
- IHC: (+) SMA, MSA; Ganglion-like cells → (+) vimentin

S100 IHC

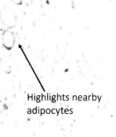

Highlights nearby adipocytes

Path Presenter

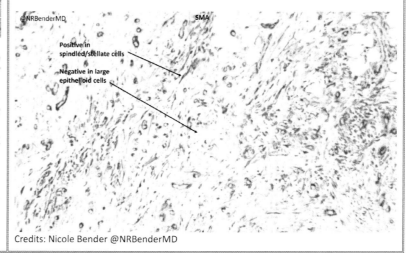

Credits: Nicole Bender @NRBenderMD

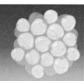

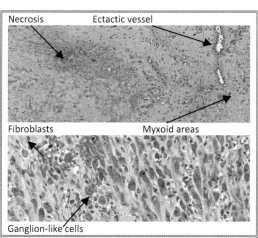

Necrosis   Ectactic vessel

Fibroblasts   Myxoid areas

Ganglion-like cells

ISCHEMIC FASCIITIS
MORPHOLOGY
- **Zonal fibrinoid necrosis** with **prominent myxoid areas**
- Ectatic, **thin-walled blood vessels** +/- atypical endothelial cells
- Fibroblasts with degenerative changes → mimic **ganglion-like cells**

OTHER HIGH YIELD POINTS
- Occurs in immobilized individuals in shoulder, coccyx, chest wall

Path Presenter

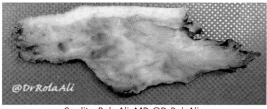

@DrRolaAli

Credits: Rola Ali, MD @DrRolaAli

Abnormal elastic fibers

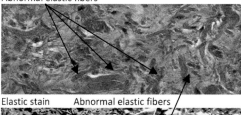

Elastic stain   Abnormal elastic fibers

Orcein stain

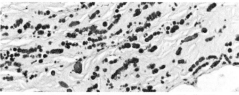

Image Credit: Raul Perret, MD, MSc @kells108

ELASTOFIBROMA
MORPHOLOGY
- **Thickened and fragmented elastic fibers, collagenous stroma** & variable fat

OTHER HIGH YIELD POINTS
- Association → **repetitive physical movements**
- Female predominance, **older age** (>50 years)
- Site → Scapula (inferior margin) on chest wall
- Clinically **slow growing painless** mass, Size → 3-10 cm
- **Gross**: Tan-**white to yellow firm mass** with poorly defined margins
- **Special stains: Elastin stain** → highlights abnormal elastic fibers
- Molecular: X-inactivation or gains of Xq; Rearrangements in 1p and 7q

Path Presenter

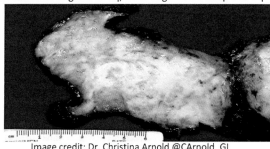

Image credit: Dr. Christina Arnold @CArnold GI

Paucicellular   Collagen bundles

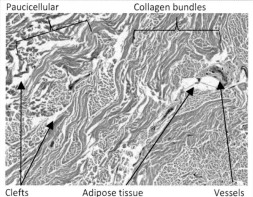

Clefts   Adipose tissue   Vessels

NUCHAL-TYPE FIBROMA
MORPHOLOGY
- Paucicellular **fibrocollagenous** proliferation composed of **patternless collagen** bundles separated by **clefts** (artifactual separation)
- Can have entrapped nerves, adnexal structures, vessels, or fat

OTHER HIGH YIELD POINTS
- Most commonly occurs on the posterior neck
- Strong male predominance, 3rd-5th decade of life
- Clinically: Solitary and painless mass
- IHC: **(+)** CD34 in spindle cells; **(-)** nuclear beta-catenin, SMA, desmin

Path Presenter

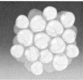

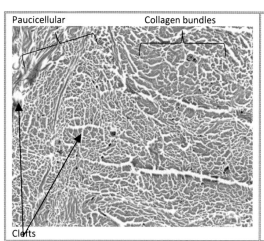

Paucicellular | Collagen bundles | Clefts

GARDNER-TYPE FIBROMA
MORPHOLOGY
- Patternless proliferation of **paucicellular collagen bundles** separated by **clefts** (artifactual separation)
- Infiltrative growth pattern +/-trapped fat, vessels, and nerves

OTHER HIGH YIELD POINTS
- **Rare benign tumor**, may occur **sporadically** or be **syndromic**
- **FAP Syndrome** → adenomatous polyps, osteomas, Epidermoid & Dermoid cysts, Gardner fibroma
- Often seen in the **first decade** of life, **slight male predominance**
- Occurs mostly in the **subcutis of the back** and **paraspinal**
- **IHC: (+)** nuclear **Beta-catenin**
- **Molecular:** Germline *APC* gene mutation in FAP

Path Presenter

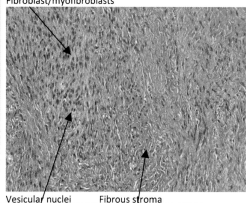

Fibroblast/myofibroblasts | Vesicular nuclei | Fibrous stroma

FIBROMA OF TENDON SHEATH
MORPHOLOGY
- Proliferation of **fibroblasts and myofibroblasts** with vesicular nuclei, single conspicuous nucleolus, and abundant granular eosinophilic to amphophilic cytoplasm
- "Slit-like" spaces seen at peripheral edge lined by flat endothelial cells
- Variable fibromyxoid stroma +/- cystic areas and storiform foci

OTHER HIGH YIELD POINTS
- Uncommon benign lesion, often middle-aged Males >> females
- Most common site is **upper extremities (~80% occur in hand**, mostly fingers)
- IHC: **Focally () for SMA** ; (-) Desmin
- **Molecular:** *USP6* gene rearrangements (similarly to nodular fasciitis)

Path Presenter

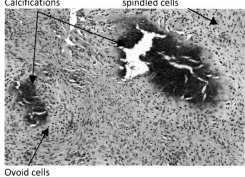

Calcifications | spindled cells | Ovoid cells

CALCIFYING APONEUROTIC FIBROMA
MORPHOLOGY
- Ovoid to spindled fibroblasts lacking nuclear atypia in a background of collagenous stroma with variable cellularity
- Scattered calcifications or cartilaginous foci with rimming by osteoclast-like giant cells
- Absence of mitoses

OTHER HIGH YIELD POINTS
- Rare, occurring mostly in male children on finger or palm
- Local recurrence ~50%

Path Presenter

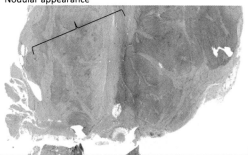

Nodular appearance

FIBROMATOSIS
MORPHOLOGY
- Infiltrative **proliferation of myofibroblasts** in **sweeping fascicles**
- Myofibroblasts have **regularly spaced nuclei** with **smooth** nuclear **contours**, small **conspicuous nucleolus**, and **lack atypia**; cytoplasm can be **stellate**
- **Collagen in the background** (can be keloidal-like) with **small vessels** and occasional lymphocytic infiltrate and scattered giant cells

OTHER HIGH YIELD POINTS
- **Variable presentation** in males and females based on subtypes, recurrence common

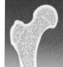
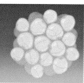
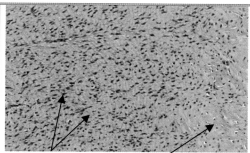

Myofibroblasts   Collagen

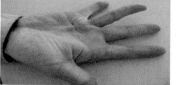

Path Presenter

Courtesy of Dr. Frank C. Muller

- ➢ **Palmar (Dupuytren Contracture):** volar surface nodular myofibroblastic proliferation, predominantly male adults >50 years old, no metastasis, rare in non-white individuals
- ➢ **Plantar:** plantar surface of foot nodular myofibroblastic proliferation, middle-aged individuals, slight male predominance, no metastasis
- ➢ **Penile (Peyronie Disease):** Fibrous proliferation/lesion which causes penile deformities and painful erections and often reports of erectile dysfunction; occurs in white adult males >50
- ➢ **Deep (Desmoid tumor):** myofibroblastic proliferation in deep soft tissue, can cause skeletal muscle atrophy
- Associated with **Familial Adenomatous Polyposis Syndrome** → dramatically increased risk (~1000x general population) → associated with cicatricial variant of fibromatosis
- **IHC:** (+) **Nuclear Beta Catenin,** SMA; variable CD117, calretinin expression; (-) for keratin, desmin
- **Molecular:** Testing for APC or CTNNB1 mutations
  - ➢ **Familial/FAP → APC**
  - ➢ **Sporadic → CTNNB1**

INFLAMMATORY MYOFIBROBLASTIC TUMOR
MORPHOLOGY

- Ovoid to **spindled/stellate myofibroblastic cells** in either a loose **myxoid background, sclerotic matrix, storiform pattern,** or **fascicles**
- **Myofibroblastic cells:** vesicular nuclei and 1-2 nucleoli, +/- smudgy chromatin, eosinophilic cytoplasm; smudgy chromatin → may have macronucleolus
- **Inflammatory cells present** and variable in number → lymphoplasmacytic predominance

OTHER HIGH YIELD POINTS

- Rare and **occurs in young and old; slight female** sex **predilection**
- Low rate of metastasis, recurrence seen in ~40% of cases
- IHC: **(+) ALK (cytoplasmic)** (~50% of cases), SMA; +/- desmin, Keratin; **(-)** S100P, CD117, EMA, myogenin
- **Molecular:** ALK rearrangement (2p23) and promiscuous
  - ➢ **Partners:** KLC1, THBS1, EML4, RANBP2, TPM4, ATIX, TPM3, IGFBP5
  - ➢ Epithelioid inflammatory myofibroblastic sarcoma
    - ▪ **ALK-RANBP2 →** most common
  - ➢ **ALK-1 expression →** seen in **younger patients**
  - ➢ **ALK negative →** consider testing for ROS1, PDGFRB, NTRK3, RET fusions
- Treatment: Complete resection +/- targeted therapy with TKI based on molecular findings

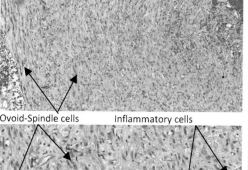

Ovoid-Spindle cells   Inflammatory cells

Myofibroblastic cell

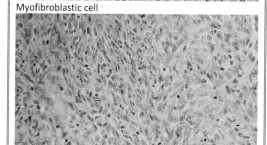

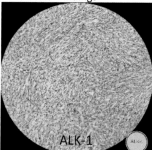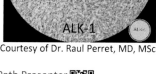

ALK-1

Courtesy of Dr. Raul Perret, MD, MSc

Path Presenter

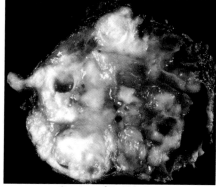

Courtesy of Dr. Yale Rosen

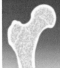
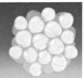

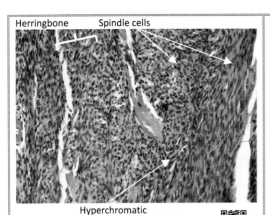

Herringbone   Spindle cells

Hyperchromatic

Path Presenter

FIBROSARCOMA (ADULT TYPE)
MORPHOLOGY
- **Uniform** and **hyperchromatic fibroblast**-like spindle cells with elongated nuclei and variable cytoplasm
- Spindle cells in a **herringbone pattern** and **intervening collagen fibers**
- **Mitoses** are present
OTHER HIGH YIELD POINTS
- **Malignancy** but **rare** and seen in **middle-aged** to **older adults**
- If subcutis → consider DFSP with fibrosarcomatous transformation
- **Metastatic sites**: **lung** (common), bone, liver
- **Low-grade** → better prognosis; general mortality ~50%
- **Pleomorphism** → think undifferentiated pleomorphic sarcoma (UPS)
- **IHC** (non-specific): (+) SMA; (-) S100, CD34, desmin, EMA, keratins
- No specific or diagnostic molecular abnormality

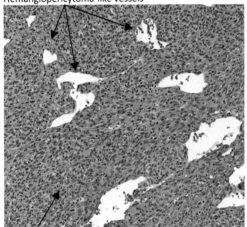

Hemangiopericytoma-like vessels

Spindle cells

INFANTILE FIBROSARCOMA (CONGENITAL FIBROSARCOMA)
MORPHOLOGY
- Infiltrative **monomorphic spindle cells** in sheets or **sweeping fascicles**
- May have a **primitive (round cell) component** and **brisk mitotic activity**
- Hemorrhage and necrotic foci common
- Hemangiopericytoma-like vessels or myxoid change, or necrosis
OTHER HIGH YIELD POINTS
- **Majority** of cases **occur within 1st year** of life, **slight male** predilection, **nearly 50%** of cases are **congenital**
- Clinically presents as a **rapidly growing solitary mass** +/- skin changes
- Often in distal extremities (most common), head and neck, or trunk
- **Favorable prognosis** (mortality rare) but **recurrence in 50%** of cases
- IHC: **(+) PanTRK positivity**
- **Molecular**: *ETV6-NTRK3* → t(12;15)(p13;q25)

Path Presenter

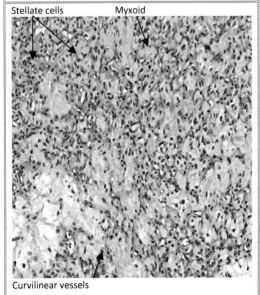

Stellate cells   Myxoid

Curvilinear vessels

MYXOFIBROSARCOMA
MORPHOLOGY
- Spectrum of morphology and cytologic features based on grade
- **Low grade** → predominant **myxoid component** with **scattered discohesive spindle to stellate cells** with enlarged **hyperchromatic nuclei**; **curvilinear vessels**, **rare mitosis**, no necrosis
- **Intermediate grade** → More **cellularity**, **increased pleomorphism**, more **mitotically active**, presence of **curvilinear vessels**, absence of **necrosis** and sheets of cells
- **High grade** → Predominantly **cellular component** with **fascicle formation** or solid sheets of cells with marked cytologic atypia (**multinucleation**, **bizarre forms**), many **mitotic figures** (and **atypical**), and **necrotic**
OTHER HIGH YIELD POINTS
- **Most common sarcoma** in the **elderly population** with slight M>F
- **Recurrence is common** and unrelated to the grade of the tumor
- **Metastasis**: low-grade → rare; intermediate and high grade → ~40%
- Prognosis dependent on size, grade, margins; overall ~60% 5-year survival
- **Epithelioid variant is aggressive** → majority have recurrence and half will have metastasis
- **IHC**: nonspecific and variable **(+)**CD34, MSA, and SMA; **(+)** CD34 in superficial

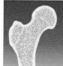

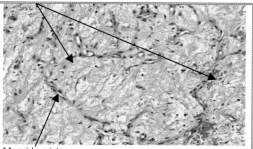

Myxoid matrix

- **Molecular**: Complex karyotypes but non-specific

<u>Path Presenter</u>

Image credit: Pedro Aleixo @pbaleixo

Spindle cells   vessels

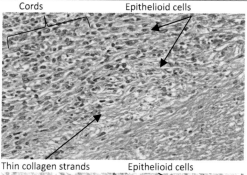

Perivascular sclerosis

LOW-GRADE FIBROMYXOID SARCOMA
MORPHOLOGY

- **Bland spindle cells** with **indistinct cytoplasm** in **small fascicles** and **whorled patterns** and **fibrocollagenous** and myxoid component
- **Myxoid foci** → arcades of vessels +/- perivascular sclerosis

OTHER HIGH YIELD POINTS

- **Malignant but** has **indolent** nature
- Wide variation in age and ~20% occur in pediatrics (<18 years old)
- IHC: **(+)MUC4**, (+/-) DOG1; (-) Claudin-1, EMA, CD34, p40, keratins, S100
- **Molecular:** Chromosomal translocations
  - ➤ *FUS-CREB3L2* fusion → t(7;16)(q33;p11) most common
  - ➤ *FUS-CREB3L1* fusion → t(11;16)(q11;p11)

<u>Path Presenter</u>

Cords   Epithelioid cells

Thin collagen strands   Epithelioid cells

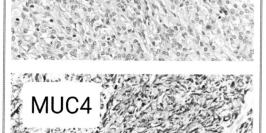

MUC4

SCLEROSING EPITHELIOID FIBROSARCOMA
MORPHOLOGY

- **Small** to **medium-sized epithelioid cells** with **variable** clear to eosinophilic **cytoplasm** and **bland ovoid nuclei**
- Epithelioid cells **arranged** in **chains**, **cords**, or **nests reminiscent of a pseudoalveolar** or **pseudoacinar** appearance
- **Dense hyalinized and sclerotic matrix** with thin collagen strands

OTHER HIGH YIELD POINTS

- Rare, **occurs in middle-aged** or **older individuals** in **lower limbs/girdles**
- **Prognosis** → poor, **metastasis to CNS**, bone, lung/pleura
- **IHC: (+)** MUC4; **(+/-)** EMA; **(-)** for keratins, SATB2, S100, SMA, CD34
- **Molecular** → *EWSR1-CREB3L1* fusions

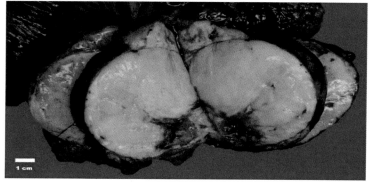

Credit: Raul Perret, MD, MSc @kells108

<u>Path Presenter</u>

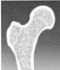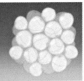
NERVE SHEATH TUMORS

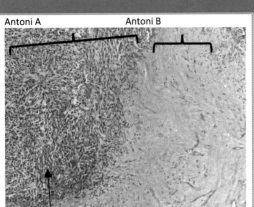

Antoni A · Antoni B

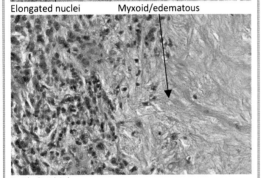

Elongated nuclei · Myxoid/edematous

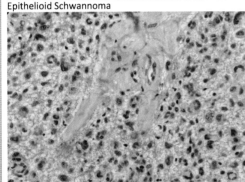

Epithelioid Schwannoma

SCHWANNOMA (NEURILEMMOMA)

MORPHOLOGY

- **Antoni A: spindle cells** arranged in **small fascicles** (loose or tight) with **whorling and nuclear palisading** → **Verocay body**
- **Antoni B:** Ovoid to spindle cells suspended in a **myxoid/edematous matrix**, often has **cystic changes** with inflammatory infiltrate
- **Spindle cells** (Schwann cells) have elongated or "carrot-like" nuclei +/- nuclear inclusions with no significant atypia and cytoplasm with indistinct borders; **Nuclear atypia → degeneration** (ancient change)
- Can have **metaplastic changes** → bone formation, calcifications
- Epineural capsule surrounds the entire lesion

OTHER HIGH YIELD POINTS

- **Benign, painless neoplasm** occurring in **head/neck**, and **extremities**
- Occurs in **all ages**, no sex predominance, **majority are sporadic**
- **Syndromic association → multiple meningiomas** (most common), **NF2**, **schwannomatosis**, NF1 (extremely rare)
- May be seen in other organs → GI, renal, or pancreaticobiliary
- Many **morphologic variants:**
  - ➤ Ancient, cellular, plexiform, epithelioid, pseudoglandular, neuroblastoma-like, reticular/microcystic-like
- **IHC: (+)** for S100, SOX10, H3K27me; **(-)** for EMA, CD34, GLUT1
  - ➤ **Epithelioid variant → loss of INI1** in ~50% of cases
  - ➤ **Retroperitoneal, posterior mediastinal, GI → GFAP and CKAE1/AE3 +**

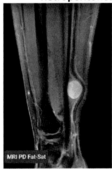
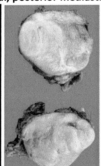
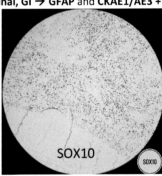

MRI PD Fat-Sat · SOX10

Credit: Raul Perret, MD, MSc @kells108

Path Presenter

NEUROFIBROMA

MORPHOLOGY

- Spindle cell tumors composed of **perineural-like cells, fibroblasts,** and **Schwann cells**
- **Cellularity** is **variable** and has **interspersed mast cells**

OTHER HIGH YIELD POINTS

- **Most common peripheral nerve sheath tumors**, majority (~90%) are sporadic
- Wide age range with no sex predominance, **slow-growing mass**
- **Factors predisposing** to **malignant** transformation
  - ➤ **NF1 patients**
  - ➤ **Plexiform and intraneural** → most common precursor to **MPNST**
- **IHC: (+)** for S100 and SOX10, CD34 (fibroblasts), EMA (perineural cells); intact H3K27me

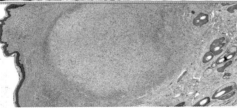

Spindle cells · Mast cell

Path Presenter

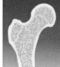
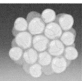

Spindle cells

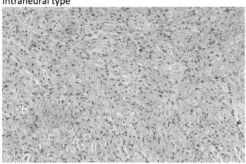

Intraneural type

Sclerosing subtype

Path Presenter

PERINEURIOMA
MORPHOLOGY
- Cytologically **bland spindle cells** with **variable nuclei** (round to wavy) **arranged** in **various patterns** (fascicular, lamellar, storiform, whorling)
- **Myxoid** to **collagenous stroma**
- **Unencapsulated**

OTHER HIGH YIELD POINTS
- Rare **benign neoplasm** arising from **perineural cells**
- Generally, **no sex predominance** and occurring in **adults**
  - ➢ **Sclerosing variant → male** predominance
- Clinically: **slow-growing, painless mass** seen in extremities or trunk
- **Morphologic variants**:
  - ➢ **Intraneural:** Bland perineural cells with characteristic "onion-skin" (concentric layers) around nerve axons → expanded nerve tissue
  - ➢ **Sclerosing:** Epithelioid to plump spindle cells arranged in a trabeculae, cords, or whorled pattern, hyalinized stroma with blood vessels with thin walls
  - ➢ **Reticular:** Thin fusiform spindle cells with lace-like anastomosis, pseudocystic spaces and conspicuous myxedematous stroma
  - ➢ **Plexiform:** Serpiginous pattern of perineurioma
- **IHC: (+)** for **GLUT1, claudin1, EMA**; variable CD34; **(-)** for MUC4, SMA, keratins, desmin, and S100
- **Molecular**:
  - ➢ **22q abnormalities (most common)**, Less commonly→ del 17q
  - ➢ **Sclerosing perineurioma → Deletions or rearrangements of 10q**
  - ➢ **Intraneural perineurioma → TRAF7 mutations**

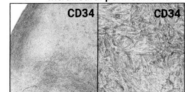
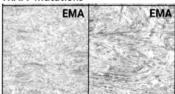

Credit: Raul Perret, MD, MSc @kells108

Polygonal cells   PEH

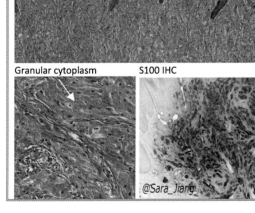

Granular cytoplasm   S100 IHC

@Sara_Jiang

GRANULAR CELL TUMOR
MORPHOLOGY
- **Polygonal cells** with **granular eosinophilic cytoplasm** arranged in **cords, nests, and sheets** in a **collagenous stroma**
- **Overlying epithelium → pseudoepitheliomatous hyperplasia**

OTHER HIGH YIELD POINTS
- **Benign** tumor cells of **Schwannian origin**
- **Most common: middle-aged females**, high incidence →**Black women**
- **Clinically:** slow-growing mass/plaque/nodule in head and neck
- If **malignant → ~50% metastasize** and 30% recur
- **Adverse prognosis:** metastasis, recurrence, size > 5cm, older age
- IHC: **(+)** for **S100, TFE3, SOX10,** CD68, inhibin, MITF, calretinin; **(-)** for ALK, GFAP, HMB45, NF, SMA, desmin, myogenin
- **EM: Rudimentary intercellular junctions, pleomorphic secondary lysosomes**

Path Presenter

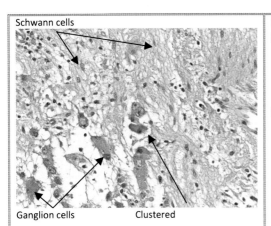

Schwann cells

Ganglion cells   Clustered

GANGLIONEUROMA
MORPHOLOGY
- Monotonous **spindled Schwann cells** with **elongated/wavy nuclei** arranged in **fascicles or no specific pattern**
- **Collagenous stroma**
- **Ganglion** cells arranged singly, in small nests or clusters

OTHER HIGH YIELD POINTS
- Rare, **benign tumor** from **neural crest**, sympathetic/peripheral nerves
- Usually seen in **young adults** with no sex predilection
- Most common locations: **posterior mediastinum**, **retroperitoneum**
- Large tumors can **secrete catecholamines** → **sweating** and **diarrhea**
- IHC: **(+) S100, NF** (Schwann, ganglion), **synaptophysin** (ganglion)

Path Presenter

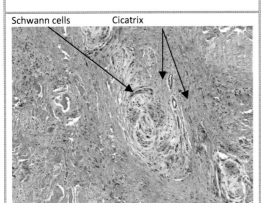

Schwann cells   Cicatrix

TRAUMATIC NEUROMA
MORPHOLOGY
- Hyperplastic **proliferation** of **cytologically bland spindled Schwann cells** with elongated nuclei and eosinophilic cytoplasm with indistinct borders
- **Unencapsulated nerve fibers** arranged in **irregular fascicles** in **cicatrix**

OTHER HIGH YIELD POINTS
- Occurs after **trauma** → amputation, injury, etc
- **Clinically** presents as a **painful mass**
- **IHC**: Not generally needed for diagnosis

Path Presenter

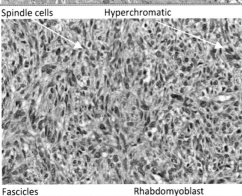

Spindle cells   Hyperchromatic

Fascicles   Rhabdomyoblast

MALIGNANT PERIPHERAL NERVE SHEATH TUMOR (MPNST)
MORPHOLOGY
- **Proliferation** of variably cellular **hyperchromatic uniform spindled cells** with pale cytoplasm arranged in fascicles, whorls, herringbone
- Background stroma: **collagenous to myxoid** and is **vascular**
- May have a primitive component

OTHER HIGH YIELD POINTS
- **Patients with NF1:** present **younger age** with **male** predominance
- Heterologous differentiation may be present
- Majority arise from **major nerves** → **Sciatic (most common)**
- **Poor prognosis: metastasis in ~60%** and recurrence in almost 50%
- **Adverse factors** → central location, >5 cm, recurrence, high-grade
- IHC: **Diffuse loss of nuclear H3K27me; (+)** for **SOX10, S100**; (+/-) CD34, GFAP; negative for SMA, desmin, MART-1, and keratins
- **Molecular:** Numeric chromosomal abnormalities

Malignant Peripheral Nerve Sheath Tumor with Rhabdomyoblastic Differentiation (Malignant Triton Tumor)
- **Associated with NF1**
- **Rhabdomyoblasts** (mature with abundant eosinophilic cytoplasm) scattered throughout MPNST
- May show epithelial, chondroid or osteoid differentiation
- **IHC: (+) for Desmin, Myogenin, and MyoD1**
- **Poor prognosis**

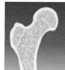

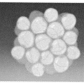

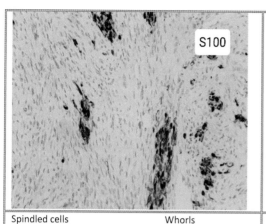

S100

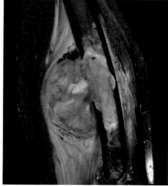

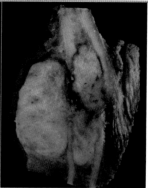

Credit: Raul Perret, MD, MSc @kells108

Path Presenter

Spindled cells — Whorls

Fibrous septae — Verocay-like bodies

NERVE SHEATH MYXOMA
MORPHOLOGY

- **Lobular proliferation** of **epithelioid to spindled cells** and suspended in a **myxoid matrix**
- Often have **interconnecting networks, syncytial nests, verocay-like bodies**, and **ring-like structures**
- Lobules are separated by dense **fibrocollagenous septae**
- Cells **lack atypia** and without **mitosis**

OTHER HIGH YIELD POINTS

- **Extremely rare tumor**, mostly seen in adults **in 3rd decade**
- Most common location is **hands/fingers** or **pretibial skin**
- Presents as a **painless, slow-growing** mass
- Recurrence rate in half of cases
- IHC: **(+)** for **S100** (image below), **GFAP** (in most)

Cytoplasmic processes

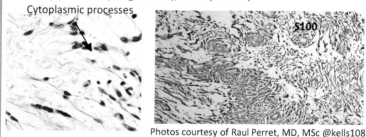

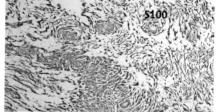

S100

Photos courtesy of Raul Perret, MD, MSc @kells108

Spindle cells — Clefting

Plump bland spindle cells — Palisade

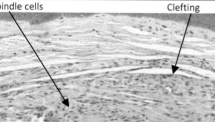

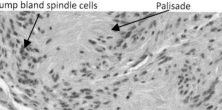

SOLITARY CIRCUMSCRIBED NEUROMA (PALISADED ENCAPSULATED NEUROMA)
MORPHOLOGY

- **Plump bland spindle** cells arranged in **interlacing fascicles** with a **collagenous** stromal background and **"clefting"**
- Palisading may be subtle or obvious
- Degenerative changes → often seen hyperchromasia

OTHER HIGH YIELD POINTS

- **Benign** tumors arising in **middle age to older adults** with no sex predilection and found on the **head and neck**
- Most common cutaneous sites → **lips, nose, forehead**
- Most common non-cutaneous site → **oral mucosa**
- IHC: **(+)** for **S100 protein**, SOX10 (Schwann cells), NF (axons)
- **No association** to **NF1** or **MEN2B syndromes**

Path Presenter

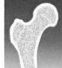

PERIVASCULAR TUMORS

GLOMUS TUMOR
MORPHOLOGY
- Proliferation of **small nests** of **glomus cells** which have **round nuclei** with single **small nucleolus** and **amphophilic to eosinophilic cytoplasm**
- Cells organized around **vascularized hyalinized** to **myxoid stroma**
- Absence of necrosis

OTHER HIGH YIELD POINTS
- **Mostly young adults**; female predominance in **subungual tumors**
- **Clinically**: small red-blue painful nodule on **stimulation & cold temperatures**
- **IHC**: **(+)** for **SMA, caldesmon**, and variable TLE1
- **Molecular**: NOTCH gene rearrangements

Path Presenter

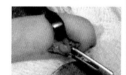

Courtesy of Dr. S. Koch

MYOPERICYTOMA
MORPHOLOGY
- **Uniform plump** ovoid to **spindle cells** with **cytologically bland nuclei** and have **concentric growth** pattern **around thin-walled blood vessels**
- May have **degenerative changes** → myxoid stroma, atypical nuclei, hemorrhage, hyalinization, infarction, **metaplastic bone formation**
- Mitotic activity is rare

OTHER HIGH YIELD POINTS
- Usually seen in **middle-aged adults** with **male** predominance
- Clinically presents as a **single, painless, slow-growing** mass on the distal **lower extremities** in deep soft tissue
- Unlikely to have a local recurrence
- **IHC**: **(+)** for h-caldesmon; **(-)** for CD31/CD34, keratins
- **Molecular**: Alteration in **PDGFRB**

Path Presenter

Courtesy of Dr. W. Paulus

PERIVASCULAR EPITHELIOID CELL TUMOR (PEComa)
MORPHOLOGY
- **Epithelioid** to **spindled cells** with round to oval nuclei and lightly **eosinophilic cytoplasm** and arranged in **nests, sheets,** or **trabeculae** and **radiate outward from vessels**
- Few multinucleated giant cells may be seen
- Can have melanin pigment

OTHER HIGH YIELD POINTS
- Rare tumors occurring **mostly in middle-aged females**
- **Can arise anywhere** but uncommon in bone, skin, and extremities
- Clinically presents as a **painless mass** +/- site-specific symptoms
- **Morphologic variants**
  - ➢ **Fibroma-like** PEComa → **associated with TS**
  - ➢ **Sclerosing PEComa** → **not** associated with **TS**
- Features with risk of malignant behavior (**Folpe** criteria)
  - ➢ **High risk:** >5 cm, cellular, high nuclear grade, mitoses, necrosis, vascular invasion, infiltrative growth pattern
  - ➢ **Likely benign:** <5cm in size and <2 high-risk features

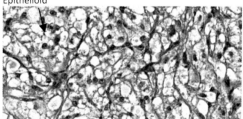

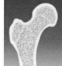
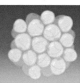
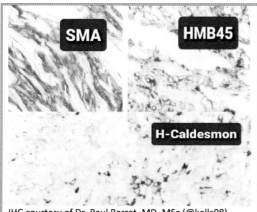

- **Uncertain malignant potential**: size 5 cm or greater, no other high-risk features, or multinucleated giant cells/or pleomorphism only
- **Malignant:** Two or more high-risk features
- **IHC: Myomelanocytic phenotype→ (+)** for **HMB-45**, MiTF, MART-1 **SMA**, desmin, caldesmon
  - **HMB-45** and **SMA most sensitive** markers
- **Pathogenesis:** TSC2 deletion → mTOR pathway activation
- **Molecular:**
  - **TSC2 deletion-related →** mTOR pathway activation
  - **Non-TSC2 related → TFE3 mutations or SFPQ-TFE3 fusion**

Path Presenter

IHC courtesy of Dr. Raul Perret, MD, MSc (@kells08)

SMOOTH MUSCLE TUMORS

Nodular appearance   White whorled cut surface

LEIOMYOMA
MORPHOLOGY
- **Uniform spindle cells** in **short fascicles** or **aggregates**
- Spindle cells have **"cigar-shaped" nuclei** and **eosinophilic cytoplasm**
- **No pleomorphism**, significant mitotic activity or necrosis

OTHER HIGH YIELD POINTS
- **Older patients**, no sex predominance (except pelvic tumors, F>>M)
- Mitotic rate and relation to sex and location
- Gross examination: Tan-white, whorled cut surface
- **Deep tissues:**
  - <1mitosis / 50HPF → Benign leiomyoma
  - 1 to 5 /50HPF → Smooth muscle tumor of uncertain malignant potential (STUMP)
- **Retroperitoneal/Pelvic in women**
  - <5mitosis / 50HPF → Benign leiomyoma
  - 5 to 10 /50HPV → STUMP
- **Retroperitoneal/Pelvic in men**
  - <1mitosis / 50HPF → Benign leiomyoma
  - 1 to 5 /50HPV → STUMP
- **IHC: (+)** for MSA, SMA, desmin, h-caldesmon
  - Female pelvic/retroperitoneal tumors positive for WT-1, ER, and PR
- **Molecular:** Genetic heterogeneity
  - **EWSR1-PBX3 or KAT6B-KANSL1 fusions → retroperitoneum**
  - PLAG1 or HMGA2 gene aberrations

Path Presenter

Courtesy of Dr. Ed Uthman (@euthman)

Spindle cells   "Cigar-shape" nuclei

Leiomyosarcoma   Necrosis

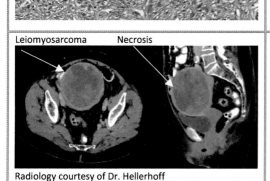

LEIOMYOSARCOMA
MORPHOLOGY
- **Spindle cells** with **intersecting fascicles** with **infiltrative borders**
- Spindle cells have **"cigar-shaped" nuclei, atypia, mitoses** and **necrosis**

OTHER HIGH YIELD POINTS
- **Malignant tumor**, older adults, no sex predilection (**pelvic → F>>M**)
- **Sites**: retroperitoneum, inferior vena cava, lower extremities, viscera
- **Poor prognosis** and **majority have metastasis**
  - **Most common** site is the lung
  - **Hematogenous route of metastasis**

Radiology courtesy of Dr. Hellerhoff

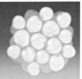
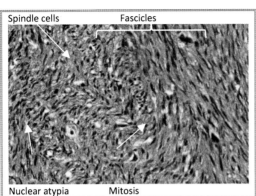

Spindle cells | Fascicles

Nuclear atypia | Mitosis

- **Morphologic variants:**
  - ➤ **Pleomorphic**: marked pleomorphic tumor cells resembling undifferentiated pleomorphic sarcoma
  - ➤ **Myxoid**: low grade, abundant myxoid stroma
  - ➤ **Epithelioid**: small cells with scant eosinophilic cytoplasm or large eosinophilic cells with macronucleoli arranged in nests and sheets
- **IHC**: **(+)** for **SMA**; **(+/-)** caldesmon and desmin; **(-)** p63, CD34, HMB-45, MART-1, CD117, ALK1, S100
- **Molecular**: **Complex karyotypes**

Path Presenter

Round | Spindled

Syncytialized | Vessel

Credit: Raul Perret, MD, MSc (@kells108)

Path Presenter

EBV-ASSOCIATED SMOOTH MUSCLE TUMOR
MORPHOLOGY
- Tumor cells are variable in morphology
  - ➤ **Round (primitive) to spindled** and may be **syncytial**
- Tumor cells form **storiform fascicles** or **faint fascicles**
- **Rarely pleomorphic** and **necrosis** typically **absent**
- **Mitotic activity is high** but **lacks atypical forms**
- **Prominent vascularity** is seen

OTHER HIGH YIELD POINTS
- **Very rare indolent tumor** but commonly seen in **immunosuppressed patients**, with **majority** having **had a renal transplant**
- Average age is **50 years old** and **no sex predilection**
- Most common in **larynx** in the **true vocal cords**
- **IHC**: **(+)** for **SMHC, MSA, SMA, p53**, and **h-caldesmon**; **(-)** for p63, S100, SOX-10, HMB-45, TLE1, EMA, CD99, and panCK
- **In situ hybridization**: **EBER strongly positive** and diffuse in nucleus

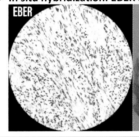
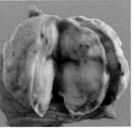

SKELETAL MUSCLE TUMORS

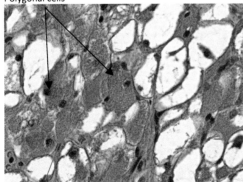

Polygonal cells

Cross striations

RHABDOMYOMA
MORPHOLOGY
- Large **polygonal tumor cells** with **central or eccentric nuclei**, **finely granular** eosinophilic **cytoplasm**, arranged in **small nests** and **sheets**
- Cytoplasm often has **cross striations** and +/- inclusions
- **Delicate capillary** network
- Absence of necrosis and mitosis

OTHER HIGH YIELD POINTS
- Predominantly occur in the **head** and **neck** of **middle-aged men**
- Clinically presents as a **painless, slow-growing** mass
- May be **multifocal**, seen in **~20%** of cases
- About **60% of cases do not have** a **recurrence**
- Other Rhabdomyoma types:

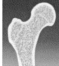
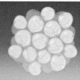

"Spider web" cell

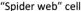

- ➤ **Cardiac type:** hearts of infants and children, associated with TSC, has "spider web cells"
- ➤ **Fetal type:** head and neck and occur at any age
- IHC: **(+)** for **MYOD1**, **desmin**, myogenin; **(-)** for CD163, PAX-8, TFE3, keratin, CD68, and synaptophysin
Path Presenter

Ovoid   Hyperchromatic

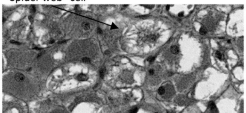

Botryoid type

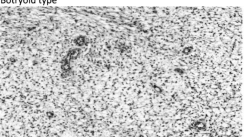

Anaplastic

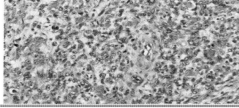

EMBRYONAL RHABDOMYOSARCOMA
MORPHOLOGY
- Tumor cells with **variable morphology** (spindle, stellate, ovoid) with **hyperchromasia**
- **Variable cellularity** and described as **"marbled"** appearance → **alternating cellular** and **hypocellular** foci
- Tumor cells may show **rhabdomyoblastic differentiation**→ **eccentric nuclei** and prominent **eosinophilic cytoplasm** +/- **striations**
- Other tumor cells can be described as **"tadpole cells"** or **"strap cells"**
- **Mitoses frequently seen** and necrosis is variable
OTHER HIGH YIELD POINTS
- **Most common sarcoma in children** in first decade, **slight male predominance**
- Often occur in the **head and neck** region or **genitourinary system**
- **Morphologic variants:**
  - ➤ **Botryoid type:** **densely cellular layer** below cambium layer (epithelial surface) and separated by **hypocellular zone**; presents as a **grape-like mass** from the **vagina** or **nasal cavity**
  - ➤ **Anaplastic type:** pleomorphic nuclei with atypical mitotic figures
- **Prognosis greatly affected** by stage, age, location, and histologic grade
- IHC: **(+) MYOD1 and Myogenin (nuclear)**, **desmin**; **(+/-)** keratin, SMA
- **Molecular:**
  - ➤ **Complex karyotypes** → gains of chromosomes in 2, 8, 12, 14
  - ➤ Characteristic **loss of heterozygosity** of **11p15.5**
  - ➤ **Absence of PAX7-FOXO1 and PAX3-FOXO1 fusions**
Path Presenter

Septa   Pseudoalveolar

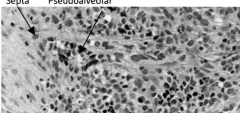

Atypical mitoses

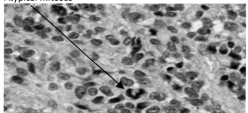

ALVEOLAR RHABDOMYOSARCOMA
MORPHOLOGY
- Sheets of **primitive monomorphic round cells** ("round blue cell") with **hyperchromatic nuclei** and a few with **small nucleoli** and **scant cytoplasm**
- Dense **variably-thick fibrous septa** separate nests and sheets of round cells imparting a **"pseudoalveolar"** pattern
- **Necrosis is seen**, especially within central parts of nests/sheets of cells
- **Mitotic activity** is **conspicuous**
- Multinucleated cells, peripherally located nuclei → **"wreath-like"** cells
OTHER HIGH YIELD POINTS
- **Second most common type** of rhabdomyosarcoma and **seen in adolescents** and **young adults** (M=F)
- Seen in **deep tissue of the extremities** but can be seen in the **head and neck, paraspinal, retroperitoneum,** and **perineal areas**
- **Clinically:** **rapidly-growing mass** and symptoms depend on location
- Morphologic variant → **Solid-type** which **lacks pseudoalveolar pattern**

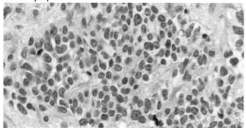
Scant cytoplasm

Path Presenter

- **Prognosis**: worse compared to embryonal type rhabdomyosarcoma
- Clinically **high stage at presentation**
- **IHC: (+) for MyoD1, Myogenin, MSA, desmin, ALK**; variable keratin (patchy), synaptophysin, CD56, CD99 expression
- **Molecular**: Two main recurrent chromosomal translocations
  - ➤ **Most common: PAX3-FOXO1 → t(2;13)(q35:q14)**
  - ➤ **PAX7-FOXO1 → t(1;13)(q36:q14)**
  - ➤ Alternative fusions seen in ~20% and negative by RT-PCR → consider INO80D, NCOA1 as possible partners; some cases may be truly lacking a fusion
  - ➤ **Fusion negative is more common** in **mixed embryonal/alveolar** or **solid** growth **patterns**

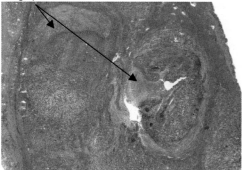
Geographic necrosis

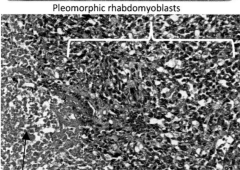
Pleomorphic rhabdomyoblasts

Necrosis

PLEOMORPHIC RHABDOMYOSARCOMA
MORPHOLOGY
- Tumor composed of **significantly pleomorphic rhabdomyoblasts**, which have a variety of morphology
- **Unlikely to see cross-striations** in any cell
- **Three morphologic patterns**:
  - ➤ **Round cell pattern**: pleomorphic rhabdomyoblasts in clusters and medium-round cells in the background
  - ➤ **Classic pattern**: pleomorphic rhabdomyoblasts in sheets
  - ➤ **Spindle cell pattern**: pleomorphic spindle cells in storiform arrangement, rarely fascicular pattern, few pleomorphic rhabdomyoblasts seen throughout
- **Mitoses are conspicuous** and have **atypical forms**
- **Necrosis** is typically seen **in a geographic pattern**
OTHER HIGH YIELD POINTS
- Mostly seen in **middle-aged adults**
- **Clinically: lower extremity** deep **soft tissue mass** → particularly **thigh**
- **Very aggressive high-grade sarcoma** with early metastasis
- **Prognosis is poor** and **mortality high** (~70%)
- **IHC: (+) for MyoD1** (strong), desmin, actin; **variable** keratins; **(-)** for S100, CD45, melanocytic markers
- Molecular findings are non-specific, most have complex karyotypes

Path Presenter

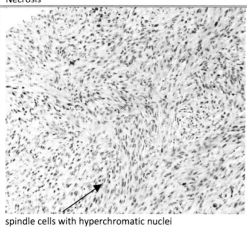
spindle cells with hyperchromatic nuclei

SPINDLE CELL RHABDOMYOSARCOMA
MORPHOLOGY
- **Uniform spindle cells** with **hyperchromatic nuclei** that are **ovoid or wavy** and have **variable nucleoli** and **scant eosinophilic to amphophilic cytoplasm**
- **Spindle cells** usually in **fascicular pattern** but can have foci of herringbone or storiform patterns
- Uncommon to have necrosis
OTHER HIGH YIELD POINTS
- Seen in both **children (first decade)** and **adults** (3rd decade)
- Location is variable based on age
  - ➤ **Children: paratesticular; Adults**: 50% in **head and neck**
- Clinically presents as a **painless mass** that is deep
- Prognosis is dependent on the age group
  - ➤ **Children: good if at low stage**, 95% survival at 5 years
  - ➤ **Adults: Metastasis, recurrence in 50%; Metastasis: lungs, lymph node**

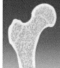
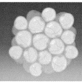

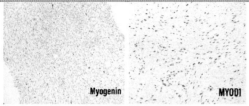

Credit: Raul Perret, MD, MSc @kells108

- **IHC**: **(+)** for **MyoD1** and **Myogenin** (both nuclear), **Desmin** (diffuse cytoplasmic), **Actin**; **(-)** for keratins, caldesmon, S100, CD34, TLE1, and beta-catenin
- **Molecular**: No genetic findings as seen in alveolar or embryonal RMS
  - ➤ **Spindle cell type**: recurrent **MYOD1** mutations
  - ➤ **Infantile/congenital spindle cell RMS**: few reports of NCOA2 and VGLL2 rearrangements

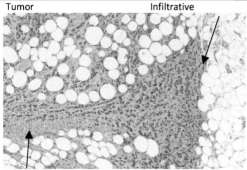

Tumor | Infiltrative

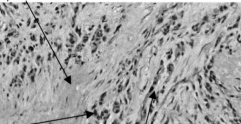

Hyalinized stroma

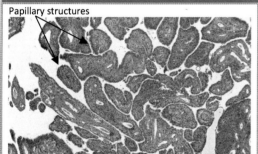

Round cells | Ovoid cells

SCLEROSING RHABDOMYOSARCOMA
MORPHOLOGY

- Tumor cells are **variable in morphology, primitive**, and range from **round-ovoid to spindled cells** with **eosinophilic to clear cytoplasm** in a nested or cord pattern
- **Hyalinized collagenous stroma** → mimics vascular spaces or osteoid
- **Mitoses are common**, peripheral edge of tumor shows infiltration

OTHER HIGH YIELD POINTS

- Rare and **variable age at presentation, strong male predominance**
- Clinically presents as a **deep, painless mass** in the **extremities**
- **Prognosis**: **poor and 50% will have metastasis** and recurrence
  - ➤ **MYOD1 mutation** → **worst prognosis**
- **IHC**: **(+)** for MyoD1 (diffuse), Myogenin (focal), and **Desmin** (perinuclear dot-like); **(+/-)** SMA; **(-)** for keratins, SATB2, S100, CD31, and CD34
- **Molecular**: Lacks genetic findings seen in embryonal and alveolar type
  - ➤ Recurrent MYOD1 mutations and/or PIK3CA mutations
  - ➤ MYOD1 suggestive of common pathogenesis for Sclerosing and spindle cell RMS

Path Presenter

FIBROHISTIOCYTIC TUMORS

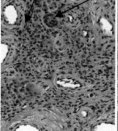

Papillary structures

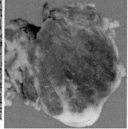

Epithelioid cells | Giant cells

Image Credit: Raul Perret, MD, MSc @kells108

TENOSYNOVIAL GIANT CELL TUMOR (DIFFUSE TYPE)
MORPHOLOGY

- **Large epithelioid cells** with nuclei that are **round to ovoid** and **eccentrically** located with **conspicuous nucleoli** and **ample eosinophilic**
- **Osteoclast-like giant cells**, macrophages, hemosiderin present
- **Mitotic** figures **frequently seen**
- Lesion is **well-circumscribed**

OTHER HIGH YIELD POINTS

- **Rare benign tumor** with **wide age of occurrence, slight female predominance**
- Most common in **intraarticular spaces** → majority in the **knee** (~80%), and hip (10-15%); can be **extraarticular as well** → **knee still most common**
- Clinically **presents as a painful mass** that has been **present for years**, and **limits the range of motion** of affected joint; body fluid (synovial) often shows hemorrhagic effusion with inflammatory cells
- **Prognosis**: Recurrence/relapse is high (~50%)
  - ➤ **Very rare transformation to malignancy** → seen in **radiation exposure**
  - ➤ Rare metastasis
- **IHC**: **(-)** for H3.3 G34W
- **Molecular**: **COL6A3-CSF1** fusions commonly seen

 Path Presenter

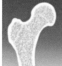

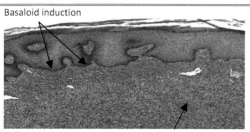

Basaloid induction

Collagen trapping   Spindle cells

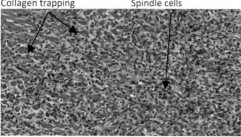

FIBROUS HISTIOCYTOMA (DERMATOFIBROMA)
MORPHOLOGY
- **Plump cytologically bland, ovoid to spindled cells** with **vesicular chromatin** and **delicate nucleoli** and **eosinophilic cytoplasm** with indistinct borders, arranged in **storiform or short fascicles**
- **Collagen trapping** at edges
- Overlying epidermis may show **basaloid induction**
- Vessels often have a "**staghorn**" appearance
- Lesion is **well-circumscribed** with **thin pseudocapsule**

OTHER HIGH YIELD POINTS
- **Rare neoplasm**, wide age of presentation, **slight male sex predilection**
- **Painless, slow-growing mass** in the **extremity** subcutaneous tissue
- **Recurrence** after surgery is **frequent, metastasis is very rare**
- **Variants**: Deep benign, plexiform, aneurysmal, epithelioid, cellular
- **IHC: (+) for CD34 and Factor XIIIA; (-)** STAT6, EMA, desmin

Path Presenter

TUMORS OF UNCERTAIN DIFFERENTIATION

Spindle cells   Myxoid matrix   Vasculature

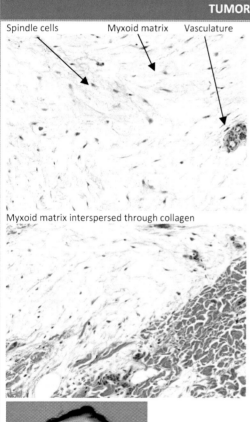

Myxoid matrix interspersed through collagen

Path Presenter

MYXOMA
MORPHOLOGY
- **Bland, uniform spindled** to **stellate cells** with oval nuclei and **fibrillary** or **tapered cytoplasm** suspended in a **myxoid matrix**
- **Sparse vasculature** and spindle cells lack condensation around vessels
- **No necrosis, no mitosis**
- Often has cystic change and myxoid matrix can intersperse through collagen

OTHER HIGH YIELD POINTS
- Can arise in various locations in the body
- **Intramuscular:** female predominance, most common in thigh
- **Juxta-articular:** male predominance, majority occur in knee
- **Cardiac:**
  - ➤ **Sporadic type** (majority of cases) → females
  - ➤ **Familial type** → males
- May be associated with **genetic syndromes** → **Mazabraud syndrome**
  - ➤ **Mazabraud: Intramuscular myxoma** and **fibrous dysplasia**
- **IHC:** most important → **(-) for MUC4**; variable CD34 and SMA
- **Molecular:** Activating mutation of *GNAS* at codon 201
  - ➤ Seen in **sporadic, cellular, non-cellular,** and Mazabraud syndrome
  - ➤ **Juxta-articular does not have GNAS mutations**
  - ➤ **Familial cardiac myxomas** → heterozygous **PRKAR1A (17q24) mutation**
  - ➤ **Sporadic cardiac myxomas** → **no GNAS, no PRKAR1A** mutations

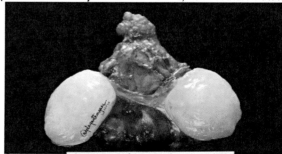

Gross photograph courtesy of Cory Nash, MS, PA (@iplawithorgans)

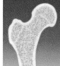

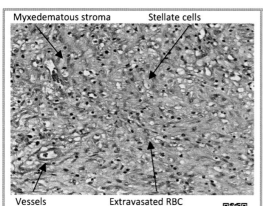

Myxedematous stroma — Stellate cells

Vessels — Extravasated RBC

Path Presenter

DEEP AGGRESSIVE ANGIOMYXOMA
MORPHOLOGY
- **Spindled to stellate cells** with **no significant atypia** that are suspended in **abundant myxoedematous** stroma
- **Vascularity has variation** (thin-wall capillaries → thick-walled vessels)
- **Collagen fibers scattered** throughout **myxedematous stroma**
- Often **low cellularity** and has an **infiltrative growth** pattern
- **Extravasated red cells** and **scattered mast** cells common

OTHER HIGH YIELD POINTS
- **Benign tumors** occurring mainly in **women** in a wide age range
- Clinically presents as a **slow-growing mass** in the **pelvicoperineum**
- Recurrence is seen in ~40% of cases
- **IHC: (+)** for ER, PR, and desmin
- **Molecular:** Rearrangements in **HMGA2 (12q13-15)** → t(8;12) or t(11;12)

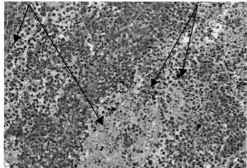

Rhabdoid cells

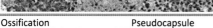

Necrosis — Hemosiderin

EXTRARENAL RHABDOID TUMOR
MORPHOLOGY
- **Polygonal rhabdoid cells** with **eccentric vesicular nuclei, conspicuous nucleoli, +/- intranuclear** inclusions, and **glassy eosinophilic cytoplasm**
- **Rhabdoid cells** are arranged in **trabeculae** or **solid sheets**
- **Necrosis** and **hemosiderin** are seen in the background
- Infiltrative peripheral borders

OTHER HIGH YIELD POINTS
- Rare, **highly malignant neoplasms** seen in **infants** and **young children**
- Mainly in **axial locations** → neck, spine, **retroperitoneum**, thigh
- **Clinically:** **rapidly enlarging mass** that ulcerates overlying skin
- **Prognosis: very poor, ~10% survival** → often recurrence/metastasis
- **Treatment:** Total neoadjuvant then surgical resection
- **IHC: (+) CD99** (~50%), **synaptophysin** (~50%), vimentin, keratins (CK8, CK18), and SALL4; **(-) for INI1** (non-specific)
- **Molecular:**
  - ➤ **Homozygous deletions** or **monosomy of chromosome 22q11.2** → **SMARCB1/INI1** tumor suppressor gene
  - ➤ Translocations involving 1p, 6p, 11p, or 18q

Path Presenter

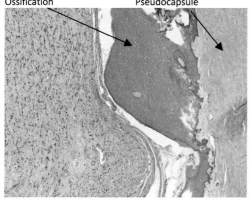

Ossification — Pseudocapsule

OSSIFYING FIBROMYXOID TUMOR
MORPHOLOGY
- **Uniform** oval to round tumor cells, **bland nuclei** and **pale eosinophilic cytoplasm**; arranged in nodules with **fibrous pseudocapsule**
- **Stroma is variable** → fibromyxoid, myxoid, or hyalinized
- **Ossification present**, no necrosis or vascular invasion

OTHER HIGH YIELD POINTS
- **Rare tumor** occurring in **middle-aged** with a **2:1 male predominance**
- Morphologic variants
  - ➤ **Atypical OFMT:** increased mitotic activity (>2/ 50 HPF) or high cellularity and low mitotic rate (<2 mitoses /50HPF)
  - ➤ **Malignant OFMT:** high nuclear grade, >2 mitoses/50HPF, extracellular matrix absence and overlapping nuclei in a single 4x field; typically has necrosis
- **IHC: (+) S100**; +/- neuroendocrine markers; loss of nuclear INI1

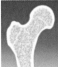

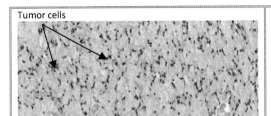

Tumor cells

- Molecular: Rearrangements of *PHF1* (6p21) seen in majority of cases
  - ➢ **Most common fusion: EP400-PHF1**
  - ➢ **Alternative fusions:** EPC-PHF1, ZCH7B-BOR, CREBBO-BCORL1, KDM2A-WWTR1, or MEAF6-PHF1
  - ➢ **PHF1** seen in **benign, atypical,** and **malignant OFMT**

Path Presenter

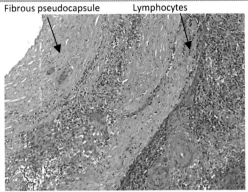

Fibrous pseudocapsule   Lymphocytes

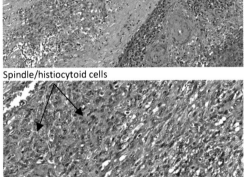

Spindle/histiocytoid cells

Path Presenter

ANGIOMATOID FIBROUS HISTIOCYTOMA

MORPHOLOGY

- Spindled to **histiocytoid appearing bland cells** arranged in **short fascicles, loose swirls,** or **storiform** pattern
- **Lymphocytic rim "cuffing"** surrounding the entire fibrous pseudocapsule of the lesion. Stroma is variable → fibrosclerotic to myxoid. Variably sized pseudoangiomatous spaces

OTHER HIGH YIELD POINTS

- Rare, **seen in children and young adults, slight female predominance**
- **Clinically:** a painless, **slow-growing** mass in superficial extremities
- Recurrence rate is variable, metastasis is rare
- **IHC: (+) for ALK,** desmin; **(-)** for MyoD1, myogenin, CD31, S100
- **Molecular:** Chromosomal translocations
  - ➢ **Most common (90%): EWSR1-CREB1 → t(2;22)(q33:q12)**
  - ➢ **Extrasomatic cases: EWSR1-ATF1 → t(12;22)(q13:q12)**
  - ➢ **Uncommon: FUS-ATF1 → t(12;16)(q13:q12)**

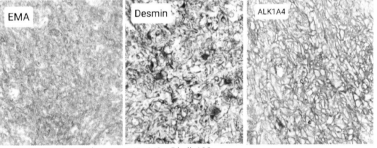

EMA   Desmin   ALK1A4

Image Credit: Raul Perret, MD, MSc @kells108

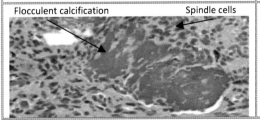

Spindle cells   Epithelial cells   Lymphocytes

ECTOPIC HAMARTOMATOUS THYMOMA

MORPHOLOGY

- **Haphazard proliferation** of **epithelial** cells, **spindle cells,** and **adipocytes**
- Bland spindle cells seen in sheets, storiform, lattice, or short fascicles
- Epithelial cells are **predominantly squamous**
- **Low mitotic activity;** lymphocytic infiltrate present but subtle

OTHER HIGH YIELD POINTS

Path Presenter

- **Extremely rare,** seen in male adults
- Unrelated to the thymus (despite name)

Flocculent calcification   Spindle cells

PHOSPHATURIC MESENCHYMAL TUMOR

MORPHOLOGY

- **Bland spindled and stellate cells** in a background of **chondromyxoid** or **hyalinized matrix material,** scattered **flocculent calcifications**
- Stromal capillary vasculature; osteoclast-like multinucleated cells

OTHER HIGH YIELD POINTS

- **Very rare, middle-aged adults** with pain/stress fractures in thigh, foot

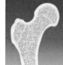
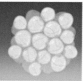
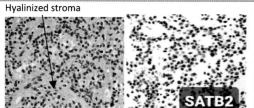

Hyalinized stroma

SATB2

Image Credit: Raul Perret, MD, MSc @kells108

- **Mechanism of development**:
  - ➤ **Produces FGF23** → **inhibits** proximal renal tubule **re-uptake of phosphorus** → **osteomalacia**
- **Laboratory** abnormalities **common** → **hypophosphatemia** and **hyperphosphaturia** but **calcium is normal**
- **IHC**: **(+)** for **FGF23, SATB2, ERG**, and **CD56**; **(-)** for STAT6, DOG-1, and CD34
- Molecular: **FN1-FGFR1 fusion** seen in ~50% of cases

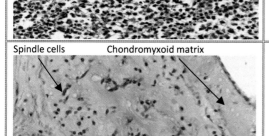

Dense collagen   Delicate collagen

Ovoid cells   Pigment

CLEAR CELL SARCOMA OF SOFT TISSUE
MORPHOLOGY
- **Monotonous ovoid to spindle cells** with nuclei that have **conspicuous nucleoli**, and **clear cytoplasm** and arranged in **fascicles** and **nests**
- Cells may also have **melanin pigment** (often focal)
- **Collagen separates nests** and is either sclerotic/dense or delicate
- Scattered **multinucleated giant cells** with **peripherally located nuclei** characteristic → **"wreath cells"**
OTHER HIGH YIELD POINTS
- **Rare malignancy** seen in predominantly **white young adults**
- Clinically: **mass arising in the extremities** → **feet** most common
- **Prognosis is poor**, 20-year survival is <10%
- **Important prognostic factors**: recurrence, size (>5 cm), necrosis
- Often has **late metastasis** or recurrence up to **20 years later**
- **IHC**: **(+)** for **all melanocytic markers**
- **Molecular**: Most have translocations
  - ➤ **Most common: EWSR1-ATF1** → **t(12;22)**
  - ➤ Uncommon: EWSR1-CREB1 → t(2;22)

Path Presenter

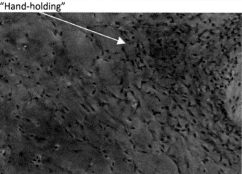

Spindle cells   Chondromyxoid matrix

"Hand-holding"

Path Presenter

EXTRASKELETAL MYXOID CHONDROSARCOMA
MORPHOLOGY
- **Monotonous proliferation** of round to **spindle-shaped cells** with minimal **eosinophilic cytoplasm**; arranged in **cords, clusters**, and **nests** with a "hand holding" type of look
- Background has **abundant chondromyxoid matrix**
- **Necrosis, hemorrhage**, and hemosiderin are common
OTHER HIGH YIELD POINTS
- **Rare sarcoma**, seen in **middle-aged men** as a **lower extremity mass** with larger tumors decreasing range of motion
- **Most common site** of **metastasis** is the lungs
- **IHC**: **(+)** for S100 and EMA but non-specific
- **Molecular**: Various fusions with NR4A3 are reported
  - **Most common: EWSR1-NR4A3** → t(9;22)(q22;q12.2)
  - Others: t(9;17)(q22;q11.2)

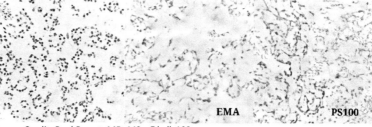

EMA   PS100

Image Credit: Raul Perret, MD, MSc @kells108

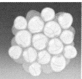
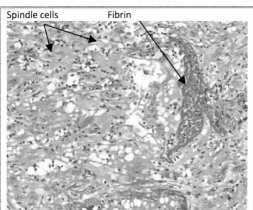

Spindle cells   Fibrin

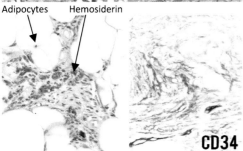

Adipocytes   Hemosiderin

CD34

Image Credit: Raul Perret, MD, MSc @kells108

PLEOMORPHIC HYALINIZING ANGIECTATIC TUMOR/HEMOSIDEROTIC FIBROLIPOMATOUS TUMOR

MORPHOLOGY
- **Spindle cells** with **nuclear hyperchromasia** and **conspicuous nuclear pleomorphism** adjacent to **variably sized blood vessels** lined by **fibrin**
- Adipocytes with admixed hemosiderin-laden spindle cells

OTHER HIGH YIELD POINTS
- Rare, **middle-aged slight female predominance**; **foot/ankle mass**
- High local **recurrence rate** (up to 50%), no metastasis
- **Molecular**: TGFBR3 or **MGEA5** rearrangements, CD34+/-

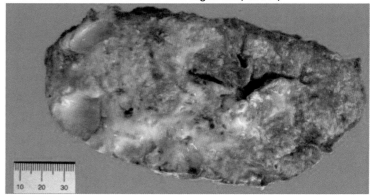

Path Presenter   Image Credit: Raul Perret, MD, MSc @kells108

Glandular structures

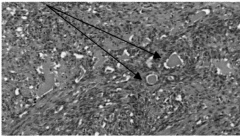

Spindle cells

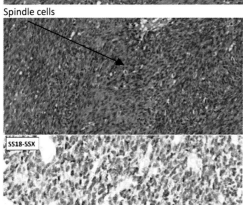

SS18-SSX

Courtesy of Raul Perret, MD, MSc @kells108

SYNOVIAL SARCOMA

MORPHOLOGY
- **Spindle cells** with **ovoid nuclei** and **minimal cytoplasm** arranged in **cellular sheets** or **fascicles**
- **Variable collagenous stroma** and may be **wiry** and **have calcifications**
- Can have an **epithelioid component** with round to ovoid nuclei, conspicuous nucleoli, and eosinophilic cytoplasm arranged in nests or glandular structures
- Prominent vessels seen and are "**staghorn**" in appearance

OTHER HIGH YIELD POINTS
- Typically seen in **young adults <50 years** old
- Most arise in **extremities near joints** → particularly the **knee**
- Deep situated, slow-growing mass and 50% are painless
- Histologic variants:
  - ➤ **Monophasic:** spindle component only
  - ➤ **Biphasic:** spindle and epithelioid component
- **Metastasis** in about 50% of cases
- **Unfavorable prognostic** factors:
  - ➤ **Large** tumor **size**
  - ➤ **Age >40**
  - ➤ **Poorly differentiated** in 20% or more of tumor
  - ➤ **High-stage** at diagnosis
- **IHC**: (+) for **SSX**, **SS18**, **TLE1**, CD56, CD99, keratin, EMA; (-) for NKX2.2, PAX3, CD34, myogenin
- **Molecular**: Characteristic translocation
  - ➤ **Most common: SSX1-SS18 fusion** → t(x;18)(p11;q11)

Path Presenter

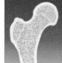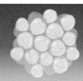
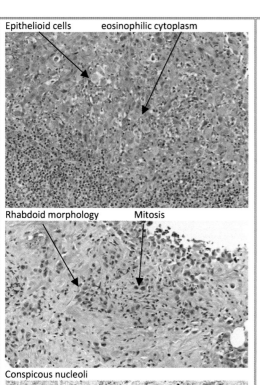

Epithelioid cells   eosinophilic cytoplasm

Rhabdoid morphology   Mitosis

Conspicous nucleoli

EPITHELIOID SARCOMA
MORPHOLOGY
- **Classic type:** Cellular nodules of epithelioid to spindled cells with vesicular nuclei, **conspicuous nucleoli**, and **eosinophilic cytoplasm**; can look granulomatous
- Often have central degeneration and necrosis
- **Proximal type:** sheet-like growth of large pleomorphic rhabdoid-appearing cells with similar nuclear features to spindled cells
- Mitosis is very common

OTHER HIGH YIELD POINTS
- Rare, aggressive sarcoma, seen in young adult males or older males
- Two main types:
  - ➢ **Conventional/Classic** → seen in **young** adult **males**
  - ➢ **Proximal** → seen in **middle-aged** or **older male** adults
- **Majority** of cases recur, and half metastasize to lymph nodes and lungs
- Proximal type has a worse prognosis → 5-year survival is 30%
- Adverse prognostic factors:
  - ➢ **Location** (proximal or deep sites), **male sex**, and size **>5cm**
- **IHC:** Loss of INI1; **(+)** for EMA, keratins, CD34, ERG, GLUT1; **(-)** for FLI-1 and PROX1
- **Molecular:** Deletion of 22q11 → SMARCB1 (INI1)

Path Presenter

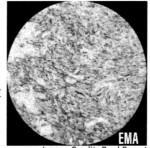
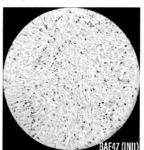

EMA   BAF47 (INI1)

Image Credit: Raul Perret, MD, MSc @kells108

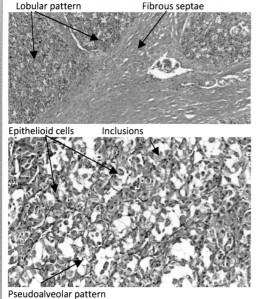

Lobular pattern   Fibrous septae

Epithelioid cells   Inclusions

Pseudoalveolar pattern

ALVEOLAR SOFT PART SARCOMA
MORPHOLOGY
- Large, **uniform epithelioid cells** with **round nuclei** and **conspicuous nucleoli**, and **abundant** granular **eosinophilic cytoplasm**
- **Compartmentalization** → **lobules**, nests with **fibrocollagenous septa**
- Rod to rhomboid-shaped intracytoplasmic inclusions
- **Pseudoalveolar pattern** → **tumoral nests** with an **empty central portion** due to **absence of cohesion** and degeneration
- **Necrosis** is **uncommon** and mitotic activity is low

OTHER HIGH YIELD POINTS
- **Rare** and predominantly seen in **infants** and **young adults** with a **female predominance**; **slow-growing mass** in **anterior thigh/buttocks**
- **Metastasis present in 50%** of patients at diagnosis
- **Poor prognosis** → present with metastasis to lung and brain
- Most important **favorable factors:**
  - ➢ **Small size (<5 cm), young age** at diagnosis **(<10), no metastasis**
- **IHC: (+)** for TFE3; variable S100 and desmin
- **Special stains:** PAS highlights intracytoplasmic inclusions
- **Molecular: der(17)t(X;17)(p11.2;q25)** → ASPSCR1 (ASPL)-TFE3 fusion

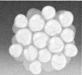

Irregular nuclei   Discohesive

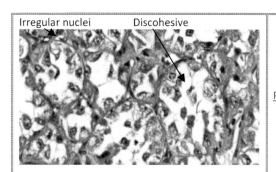

Path Presenter

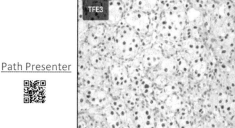
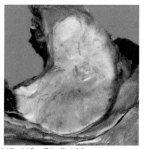

Image Credit: Raul Perret, MD, MSc @kells108

Round cells

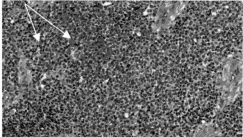

Lobular pattern

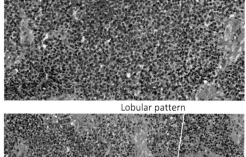

Variable fibrosis

EWING SARCOMA
MORPHOLOGY

- **Uniform round blue** cells with **finely granular chromatin** and **occasional nucleoli**, and **vacuolated cytoplasm**
- **Sheet-like or lobular growth** pattern; **rosettes** may be seen
- **Inconspicuous mitosis**
- **Necrosis** and **apoptosis** are typical and scattered about

OTHER HIGH YIELD POINTS

- **Young adults**, painful mass, **fever**, **weight loss**, **pathologic fracture**
- **Most** common **affected** bones are the **femur**, **tibia**, and **humerus**
- **Radiographic**: "moth-eaten" appearance of bone
- **Metastasis** occurs early → typically to the lungs
- **Favorable prognosis**: age (**<10**), **location** (non-pelvic bone), <8 cm size
- **IHC**: **(+)** for **CD99**, vimentin, and **FLI1**
- Molecular: Several translocations
  - ➢ **Most common (95%):** EWSR1-FLI1 → t(11;22)(q24;q12)
  - ➢ Type 1 fusion **better prognosis**: EWSR1 exons 1-7 fuse to FLI1 exons 6-9
  - ➢ **Less common:** EWSR1-ERG → t(21;22)(q22;q12)
  - ➢ Alternatives, less than 5% of cases:
    - EWSR1-E1AF → t(17;22)(q12;q12)
    - EWSR1-PATZ1 → t(1;22)(p36;q12)
    - EWSR1-ETV1 → t(7;22)(p22;q12)
    - EWSR1-FEV → t(2;22)(q33;q12)

Muscle infiltration   "Round blue cells" on Cytologic Prep

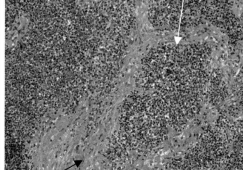

CD99

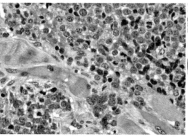

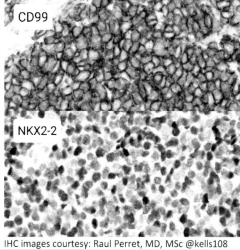

NKX2-2

Images courtesy: Raul Perret, MD, MSc @kells108

Path Presenter

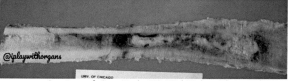

Courtesy of: Cory Nash, MS, PA (@iplaywithorgans)

IHC images courtesy: Raul Perret, MD, MSc @kells108

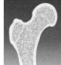

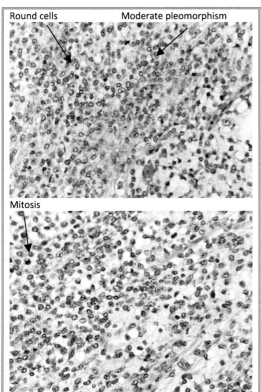

Round cells — Moderate pleomorphism

Mitosis

UNDIFFERENTIATED ROUND CELL SARCOMA WITH CIC-DUX4 TRANSLOCATION
MORPHOLOGY
- **Proliferation of small round** cells with **moderate nuclear pleomorphism, coarse chromatin, conspicuous nucleoli**, and indistinct cytoplasm
- Lobular architecture and has **geographic necrosis**
- Most have a **myxoid matrix**, and **numerous mitoses** are seen

OTHER HIGH YIELD POINTS
- **Very rare; seen in children** and **young adults; extremity** or **trunk mass**
- Majority have metastasis at diagnosis → lung; most dead at 2 years
- IHC: **(+)** for **WT1, ETV4, CD99**
- **Molecular:**
  - ➤ **CIC-DUX4 translocation → t(4;19)(q35;q13.1)**
  - ➤ **Alternative:** t(10;19)(q26.3;q13)
  - ➤ **Trisomy 8 frequently** seen
  - ➤ **Post treatment → complex karyotype**

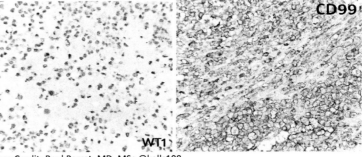

Image Credit: Raul Perret, MD, MSc @kells108

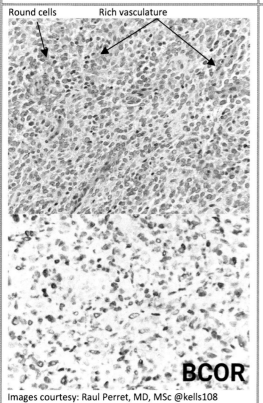

Round cells — Rich vasculature

BCOR

BCOR-CCNB3 Fusion-Positive Sarcoma
MORPHOLOGY
- **Small round** to **plump spindled cells** with **monomorphic round nuclei, fine chromatin** and **scant** eosinophilic **cytoplasm**
- **Solid arrangement** of tumor cells with rich vascular stroma
- **Necrosis** is **variable**

OTHER HIGH YIELD POINTS
- **Very rare**, mostly **adolescents** & **young adults**, majority **males**
- Clinically presents as **swelling** and **pain** in the affected bone
- **Uncommon to have metastasis** at the time of diagnosis
- **Survival is better than CIC-rearranged** and similar to Ewing sarcoma
- **5-year survival ~75%** and similar disease-free survival
- IHC: **(+)** for **BCOR**, CCNB3, CD99, SATB2, TLE1; variable NKX2.2, PAX-8; negative for WT1, ETV4
- **Molecular: Inversion of X chromosome → BCOR-CCNB3** fusion
  - ➤ **Less common:** BCOR-MAML3; BCOR internal tandem duplication

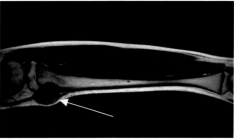

Images courtesy: Raul Perret, MD, MSc @kells108

Images courtesy: Raul Perret, MD, MSc @kells108

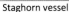

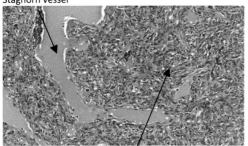

Staghorn vessel

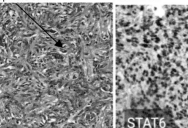

Spindle cells   Patternless

STAT6

Image Credit: Raul Perret, MD, MSc @kells108

SOLITARY FIBROUS TUMOR

MORPHOLOGY
- Ovoid to spindled fibroblastic cells with vesicular nuclei and scant cytoplasm
- Tumor cells are in a "patternless" pattern
- Cellularity is variable
- Prominent vessels with thin walls and branching → "Staghorn" appearance
- Mast cells commonly present

OTHER HIGH YIELD POINTS
- Usually seen in adults with no sex predilection with few exceptions
  - **Lipomatous variant**: slight **male** predominance
  - **Superficial variant**: strong **female** predominance
- Often occurs **thoracic cavity**, **extremities**, viscera, head and neck
- **Risk stratification** based on tumor size, age, mitotic activity, and necrosis
  - **Atypical features:** >4 mitoses /10HPF, cellular, pleomorphism, necrosis, infiltrative margins
  - **Malignant features:** abrupt transition to high-grade sarcoma, heterologous elements
  - **Heterologous elements:** rhabdomyosarcomatous or osteosarcomatous
- **IHC: (+)** for **STAT6**, CD34
- **Molecular: NAB2-STAT6** gene fusion

Path Presenter

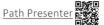

Spindle cells

Severe pleomorphism

INTIMAL SARCOMA

MORPHOLOGY
- **Poorly differentiated spindle cells**, **moderate** to **severe pleomorphism**
- Tumor cells **arising in the wall of large** blood **vessels**
- Often has **seeding tumor emboli**
- May have **myxoid** (common) or fascicular patterned areas

OTHER HIGH YIELD POINTS
- **Rare** and **occurs** in **older adults**
- Usually in the **pulmonary trunk** or **artery** with **direct extension into** the **pulmonary valve** and **right ventricle**
- Has **distant metastasis**: liver, peritoneum, bone, and mesenteric lymph nodes
- Most common to be **discovered at autopsy**
- **Mortality is >80%** at one year
- **IHC: (+)** for **MDM2** (nuclear); **(-)** for **endothelial markers**
- **Molecular:** Chromosomal gains or amplifications (MDM2, EGFR, PDGFRA)

Path Presenter

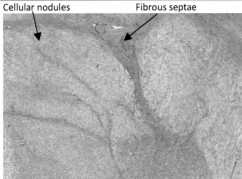

Cellular nodules   Fibrous septae

UNDIFFERENTIATED SARCOMAS

MORPHOLOGY
- **Highly cellular tumor** composed of **atypical spindled** or **polygonal cells** with **marked nuclear pleomorphism**, **multinucleation** or **bizarre nuclei**, and amphophilic to **eosinophilic cytoplasm**
- **Variable stroma**, most often **collagenous** or focally myxoid & sclerotic
- **Abundant mitosis** (and atypical) and **necrosis**

OTHER HIGH YIELD POINTS
- Most common in **older to elderly males** (Males >> females)
- **Subfascial mass** of **lower extremity** → most common is **thigh**
- May be associated with the **history of radiation** to the area
- **Morphologic variants** are **named** based **on morphology**
  - Undifferentiated spindle cell sarcoma

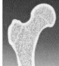

Nuclear pleomorphism

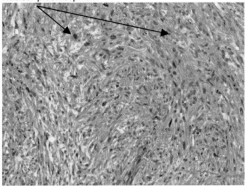

- ➢ Undifferentiated round cell sarcoma
- ➢ Undifferentiated epithelioid sarcoma
- ➢ Undifferentiated pleomorphic sarcoma (Malignant fibrous histiocytoma)
- **Local recurrence** is seen **in ~30-40%**
- **Distant metastasis:**~50% of cases → **most common** is **lung**
- **Poor outcome**, survival at 5 years is ~50%,
- **IHC: (-)** for keratins, CD31, CD34, S100, CD163, CD68, CD45, CD30, SMA, desmin, myogenin, MyoD1, ERG, p63
- **Molecular**: nonspecific complex karyotypes

Path Presenter

VASCULAR LESIONS

Small vessel component

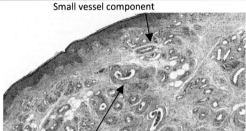

Large tortuous arteries

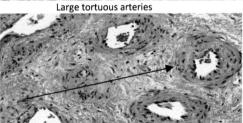

Thick-walled

VASCULAR MALFORMATIONS
MORPHOLOGY
- Large **tortuous arteries** with **fragmented elastic lamina**, associated with **thick-walled veins** and variable small vessel component

OTHER HIGH YIELD POINTS
- **Venous malformations** (venous hemangiomas) are poorly circumscribed collection of abnormal veins
  - ➢ Vary in size/proportion
  - ➢ Often abnormally thick or thin walls
  - ➢ Includes cavernous hemangiomas (collection of large, dilated veins with thin walls)
- **Cutaneous capillovenous malformation**
  - ➢ Often diagnosed clinically (e.g. Telangiectasia)
  - ➢ Associated with a variety of conditions (e.g. Osler-Weber-Rendu)
- **Intramuscular hemangioma** shows small vessels (often parallel) in muscle

Path Presenter

Anastamotic channels

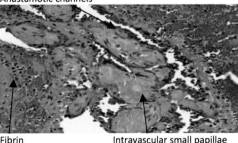

Fibrin   Intravascular small papillae

Image courtesy of Dr. Michael Bonert

PAPILLARY ENDOTHELIAL HYPERPLASIA (*aka Masson Tumor*)
MORPHOLOGY
- **Intravascular** exuberant **proliferation** of **endothelial cells** with **fibrin**
- **Small papillae** covered by a single layer of endothelium with a **collagenized fibrin core**
- Papillae can fuse, forming **anastomotic channels**
- **No atypia or mitoses**

OTHER HIGH YIELD POINTS
- **Can mimic angiosarcoma** and can be distinguished by exclusively intravascular growth and **lack of mitosis/atypia**

Path Presenter

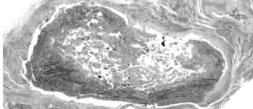

Image courtesy of Dr. Michael Bonert

Plump endothelial cells

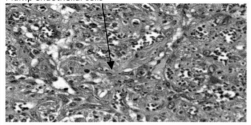

Warthin-Starry stain   Organism

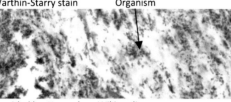

Provided by: Kauczuk on Wikimedia

BACILLARY ANGIOMATOSIS
MORPHOLOGY
- Lobules of capillary-sized vessels with plump endothelium with clear to eosinophilic cytoplasm
- Associated with **neutrophilic infiltrate**
OTHER HIGH YIELD POINTS
- Pseudo-neoplastic vascular proliferation caused by **Bartonella**
- Can be **Bartonella Henselae** or **Bartonella Quintana**
  - ➢ Gram-negative **intracellular** bacilli
  - ➢ Can see concomitant Cat-Scratch Disease
  - ➢ **B. Henselae** transmitted by **cat**
  - ➢ **B. Quintana** transmitted by **flea or louse bites**
- **Special stains: Warthin-starry** stain highlights the organisms, but can be difficult to read due to stain precipitation
- Treatment includes antibiotics

Path Presenter

Small or large caliber thin-walled blood vessels

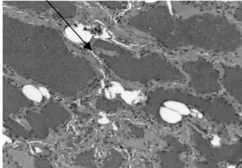

HEMANGIOMA
MORPHOLOGY
- Tumor composed of **small or large caliber thin-walled** blood **vessels**
- Single layer of non-atypical endothelial cells
OTHER HIGH YIELD POINTS
- **Benign neoplasm**
- Categorized by vessels size/appearance
  - ➢ **Lobular Capillary Hemangioma** ("Pyogenic granuloma")
  - ➢ **Infantile (Juvenile) Hemangioma**
  - ➢ **Rarer subtypes:** Hobnail hemangioma, Anastomosing hemangioma, Spindle cell hemangioma

Path Presenter

Large epithelioid cells with dense eosinophilic cytoplasm

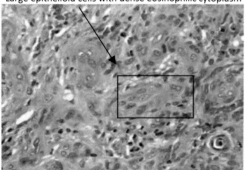

EPITHELIOID HEMANGIOMA
MORPHOLOGY
- Large **epithelioid endothelial cells** with densely eosinophilic cytoplasm, distinct **vasoformation**, **lobular architecture** and can have solid areas
- Mitoses are infrequent and not atypical
- Often rich inflammatory infiltrate comprising of **eosinophils**
OTHER HIGH YIELD POINTS
- **Benign** neoplasm seen in wide age range   Path Presenter
- Presents as a **slow-growing** dermal nodule
- IHC: **(+) for vascular markers** (ERG), keratins, EMA; **(-)** for **HHV8**
- Molecular: **Rearrangements of FOS** or **FOSB** (seen in **atypical** cases)

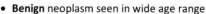

Dilated lymphatics with fluid

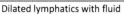

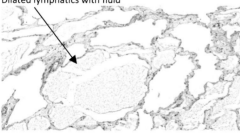

LYMPHANGIOMA
MORPHOLOGY
- Thin-walled, variable **dilated** lymphatics, lined by **flattened endothelium**
- Frequently surrounded by lymphoid aggregates
- Contain grossly "milky" lymphatic fluid
OTHER HIGH YIELD POINTS
- Associated with **Turner syndrome (XO)**
- Endothelium expresses **D2-40, PROX1** (specific for lymphatics) and **CD31**   Path Presenter

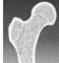

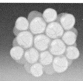

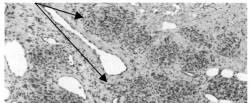
Cannon-ball infiltration

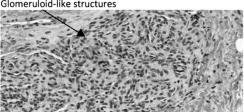
Glomeruloid-like structures

KAPOSIFORM HEMANGIOENDOTHELIOMA
MORPHOLOGY
- Infiltrate the soft tissue in **"cannon-ball fashion"**
- Different areas have features of both capillary hemangioma and Kaposi sarcoma (spindle cells)
- Tightly coiled **glomeruloid-like** structures which **may have thrombi**
- **Minimal atypia** is seen in the lesion

OTHER HIGH YIELD POINTS
- Locally aggressive vascular tumor seen in children (50% of cases in 1st year)
  - ➤ Nearly 50% occur within first year of life
- Presents as a **painful mass** or **violaceous plaques**
- Often associated with **Kasabach-Merritt phenomenon**
  - ➤ Consumptive **coagulopathy & thrombocytopenia**
- IHC: **(+) for ERG**, CD34, CD31, PROX1, D2-40; **(-)** for **HHV8, GLUT1**

Path Presenter

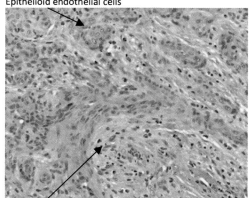
Epithelioid endothelial cells

Myxohyaline stroma

EPITHELIOID HEMANGIOENDOTHELIOMA
MORPHOLOGY
- Cords and nests of epithelioid endothelial cells within **myxohyaline stroma**
- Larger cells with **abundant eosinophilic cytoplasm**, some have **intracytoplasmic lumina with RBCs** ("Blister cells")

OTHER HIGH YIELD POINTS
- Malignant (but less aggressive than angiosarcoma), common in liver
- In soft tissue, often angiocentric, expands wall and obliterates lumen
- **High-risk features:** >3cm or >3 mitoses per 50 hpf
- IHC: **(+)** for vascular markers, keratins, EMA, **CAMTA1, TFE3 (minority)**
- **Molecular:**
  - ➤ **WWTR1-CAMTA1** fusion → **t(1;3)(q36;q25)** (majority of cases)
  - ➤ **YAP1-TFE3 fusion** (minority of cases)

Path Presenter

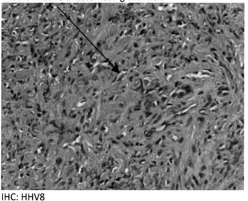
Vasoformative anastomosing channels

IHC: HHV8

KAPOSI SARCOMA
MORPHOLOGY
- Proliferation of bland spindle cells with slit-like vascular spaces containing erythrocytes
- Often associated with inflammatory infiltrate and hyaline globules
- **Patch stage:** Infiltrative vascular channels that dissect collagen fibers
- **Plaque stage:** Spindle cells infiltrate and destroy eccrine glands
- **Tumor stage:** Nodules of intersecting fascicles with "sieve-like" spaces

OTHER HIGH YIELD POINTS
- Locally aggressive, often multiple cutaneous lesions
- **Classic/endemic associated:**
  - ➤ **NOT associated with HIV,** and is **indolent**
  - ➤ Seen in equatorial Africa in children and adults
  - ➤ Association with **podoconiosis** (foot lymphedema from soil exposure)
- **AIDS Associated:**
  - ➤ **Most aggressive** and **presents at patch stage**
  - ➤ Usually is seen on the face, genitals, or extremities
  - ➤ **Co-infection** with **HIV1** and **HHV8**
  - ➤ May **regress** or **flare** with HAART

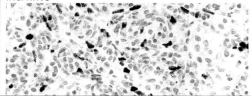

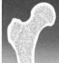

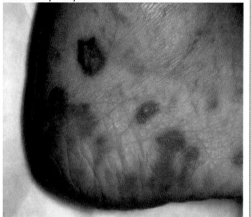
Provided by: Amylacea on Wikimedia

Heel with KS (Endemic): Provided by CDC on Wikimedia

Path Presenter

- **Iatrogenic:**
  - ➤ Immunosuppressed individuals and has variable behavior
- **Viral etiology:** caused by Human Herpes Virus 8 (HHV8)
- IHC: **(+)** for **HHV8 (LANA1)**, ERG, CD31, CD34, D2-40, FLI1

Patch/Plaque Stage of Kaposi Sarcoma   **Tumor stage of Kaposi Sarcoma**

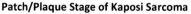
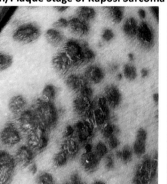
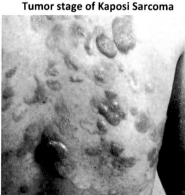

Photographs courtesy of the NIH on WIkimedia

Plump spindle cells with eosinophilic cytoplasm

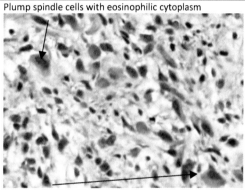

Rhabdomyoblast-like cells

PSEUDOMYOGENIC HEMANGIOENDOTHELIOMA
MORPHOLOGY
- **Infiltrative sheets** and **fascicles** of plump **spindle cells** with vesicular nuclei
- Abundant **brightly eosinophilic cytoplasm** (rhabdomyoblast-like)
- Mitoses and intralesional hemorrhage are not readily seen
- May have a brisk infiltrate of neutrophils

OTHER HIGH YIELD POINTS
- Most common in young adults and has a male predilection
- Mostly arise in the lower extremities
- IHC: **(+)** for **CKAE1/AE3**, **ERG**, **FOSB**, **INI1** (intact), variable CD31
- **Molecular: SERPINE1-FOSB fusion** → t(7;19)(q22;q13)

Path Presenter

Anastomosing growth   Hobnail

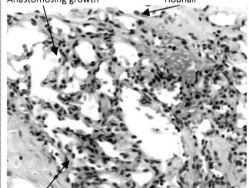

Lacks true cytologic atypia

ATYPICAL VASCULAR LESION
MORPHOLOGY
- **Irregularly shaped thin-walled vessels** with branching and anastomosing growth pattern
- Lined by a **single layer** of **endothelial cells** which may be **hyperchromatic** or demonstrate **hobnailing**
- **No true cytologic atypia or endothelial cell multilayering**

OTHER HIGH YIELD POINTS
- Benign, often small or multiple and typically seen in middle-aged individuals
- Frequently seen in **irradiated skin** (often breast) and may precede radiation-induced angiosarcoma (occurs ~10 years later)
- **No MYC overexpression or MYC amplification**

Path Presenter

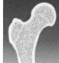

Vasoformative architecture

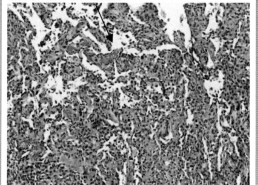

Prominent nuclear atypia

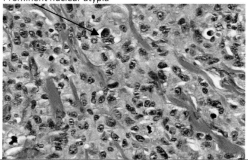

ANGIOSARCOMA
MORPHOLOGY
- Endothelial differentiation and can be epithelioid or spindled
- **Vasoformative architecture** and/or expression of endothelial markers
- Often epithelioid in bone with frequent solid growth
- Numerous **extravasated RBCs** and **variable inflammation**, and **necrosis**
- **Prominent nuclear atypia** and **readily observed mitoses**

OTHER HIGH YIELD POINTS
- **High-grade malignancy** which is seen typically in **elderly**
- Presents as a **red-purple "bruises", plaques,** or **nodules**
- **Post-radiation angiosarcoma** of the **breast**, occurs **~5 years post-radiation**
  ➢ Can occur in post-surgical lymphedema (**Stewart-Treves Syndrome**)
- Treatment is aggressive resection with wide margins and chemotherapy
- Poor prognosis with a 30% survival rate at 5 years
- IHC: (+) **vascular markers** and **frequent keratins**   Spider-leg chromatin
- Molecular: High-level amplification of MYC

IHC: MYC

Path Presenter

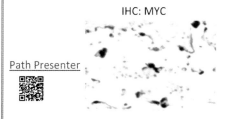

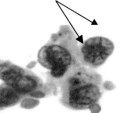

Image by: Dr. Terrance Lynn,

CARTILAGE/CHONDROBLASTIC TUMORS

Cartilage cap

OSTEOCHONDROMA
MORPHOLOGY
- **Cartilage cap** with growth plate-like architecture
- **Underlying** stalk with **medullary and cortical bone**
- No significant nuclear atypia or mitotic activity

OTHER HIGH YIELD POINTS
- **Most common bone tumor** and **occurs** largely in **first 2 decades**
- Usually in **metaphysis of distal femur**, **proximal tibia**, or **proximal humerus**
  ➢ Due to enchondral ossification (bones pre-formed by cartilage)
- **Hereditary osteochondromatosis:**
  ➢ Autosomal dominant inheritance
  ➢ Germline mutation in EXT1 (8q24.1), EXT2 (11p11-12), EXT3 (19p)

Cortical Bone

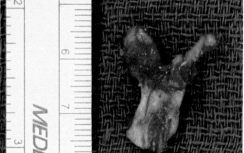

Tibial Osteochondroma by: Paigeblue08

Clinical Images of MO

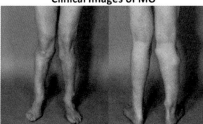

Images provided by: Dr. Judith VMG Bovee

Path Presenter

Multiple Osteochondromas

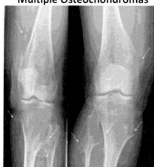

Provided by: Michielvds on Wikimedia

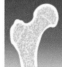

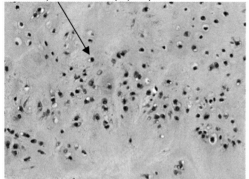

Chondrocytes with bland lymphocyte-like nuclei

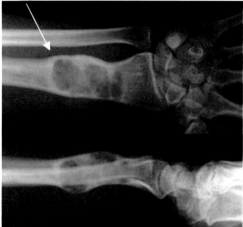

Radiograph of patient with Ollier Disease

Radiograph courtesy of: Dr. Hellerhoff

ENCHONDROMA
MORPHOLOGY
- Hypocellular, abundant hyaline cartilaginous matrix
- **Chondrocytes** in sharp-edged lacunae with **bland lymphocyte-like nuclei**
- No significant cytologic atypia, mitoses, cortical invasion, or soft tissue extension
- In small bones of hand, can have increased cellularity, myxoid cartilage, mild atypia and binucleation

OTHER HIGH YIELD POINTS
- Benign, relatively common
- Hyaline cartilage neoplasm arising within the medullary cavity
- Most frequently in short tubular bones of the hands, often in the metaphysis
- Often treated with curettage, if symptomatic
- Molecular: Frequent IDH1 and IDH2 mutations,
  - ➢ Germline IDH1/ IDH2 mutations → Multiple enchondromas
    - ▪ Consider **Ollier disease** and **Mafucci Syndrome**

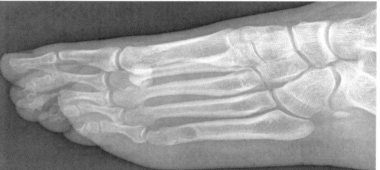

Radiograph courtesy of: Dr. Hellerhoff

Path Presenter

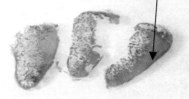

Cartilaginous cap

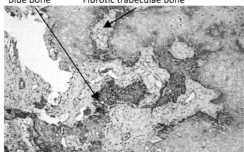

"Blue bone"   Fibrotic trabeculae bone

Images courtesy of Dr. Syed T. Hoda; Twitter: @01sth02

BIZZARRE PAROSTEAL OSTEOCHONDROMATOUS PROLIFERATION (BPOP)
(*also known as "Nora's Lesion"*)
MORPHOLOGY
- **Benign surface lesion** composed of spindle cells, cartilage, and bone
- Not contiguous with medullary cavity
- Surrounded by **cartilaginous cap** with central trabecular bone (via endochondral ossification) and hypervascular bland spindle cells.
- Between the cartilage and bone is characteristic "**Blue bone**" with basophilia
- The **chondrocytes** can show **moderate atypia**
- **Mitoses may be numerous** but are **not atypical**

OTHER HIGH YIELD POINTS
- **Rare** and the **exact incidence** is **unknown**
- **Most common** in **small bones** of the **hand** and **feet**, often phalanges
- Presents as a **mass** which **may be painful** or **cause bleeding** if the mass distorts the nail architecture
- Unclear if it is a reactive process or neoplasm but can be locally aggressive
- **Recurrence is common** in nearly half of all cases
- **Radiography**: Pedunculated and **well-delineated mass** that is **radiolucent early on** and then **becomes** more **radiodense**

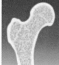
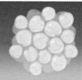
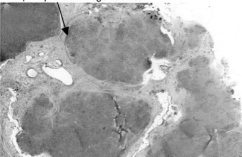

Multiple hyaline cartilage nodules

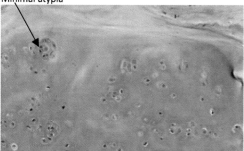

Minimal atypia

SYNOVIAL CHONDROMATOSIS

MORPHOLOGY

- **Multiple hyaline cartilage nodules** within synovium or loose joint space, chondrocytes cluster together in groups
- **Minimal atypia** is seen in the chondrocytes
- If significant atypia seen including loss of chondrocyte clustering, bone invasion, increased mitoses – increased concern for malignant status

OTHER HIGH YIELD POINTS

- Rare and peak age is **5th decade** with a **2:1 male to female** predominance
- Locally aggressive and can be multifocal
- Involves **large joints (knee is most common)** but can involve any joint
- **Molecular: FN1-ACVR2A** fusions

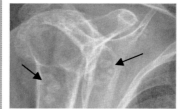

Radiograph By: Hellerhoff Wikimedia

Path Presenter

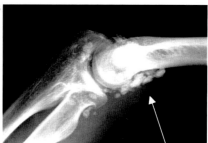

Radiograph courtesy: Nat Folk on Wikimedia

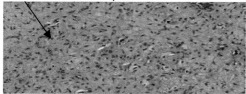

Stellate cells in chondromyxoid matrix

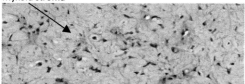

Myxoid stroma

CHONDROMYXOID FIBROMA

MORPHOLOGY

- Benign **lobulated lesion** with sharp margins
- Chondroid and **stellate cells** embedded in a chondromyxoid matrix
- Peripheral spindled cells and admixed giant cells

OTHER HIGH YIELD POINTS

- Benign lesion and typically seen in young adults
- Occurs in many sites, but often long bones near the knee
- Most arise within the medullary space and are frequently eccentric
- Treatment is variable based on location (curettage, en bloc resection)
- Radiograph: Multiloculated radiolucent lesion with a sharp sclerotic rim
- IHC: **(+)** S100 diffusely (like all cartilage)
- **Molecular: GRM1** fusions/upregulation

Path Presenter

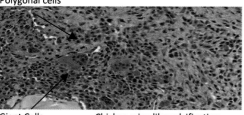

Polygonal cells

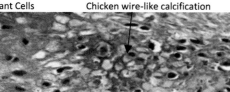

Giant Cells   Chicken wire-like calcification

CHONDROBLASTOMA

MORPHOLOGY

- Sheets of ovoid to **polygonal cells** with a single grooved nucleus and eosinophilic cytoplasm and interspersed multinucleated giant cells
- Characteristic "lace-like" or "chicken wire-like" calcification
- Islands of **eosinophilic chondroid** matrix
- Can have **cystic degeneration**, **nuclear atypia**, and **mitoses**

OTHER HIGH YIELD POINTS

- **Benign tumor** and is seen in first and second decade, more common in **males**
- Involves the **epiphysis of long bones, most common** in femur
- **Radiograph:** Radiolucent lesion with well-defined sclerotic margin
- IHC: **(+)** for **H3F3 K36M, S100, SOX9, DOG1**
- Molecular: **H3.3 K36M** substitution (similar histone to GCT of bone)

Path Presenter

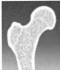

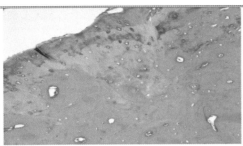

Image courtesy of Dr. Bonnie Balzer

SUBUNGUAL EXOSTOSIS
MORPHOLOGY
- **Benign osteocartilaginous surface lesion** in the distal phalangeal bone underneath the nail bed, most often big toe
- Sometimes cartilage is mildly atypical with mitoses
- No continuity with medullary cavity (as is seen in osteochondromas)

OTHER HIGH YIELD POINTS
- Often young adults
- **Cytogenetics:** Recurrent breakpoint resulting in increased IRS4 expression

Path Presenter

Abundant cartilaginous matrix (hyaline/myxoid)

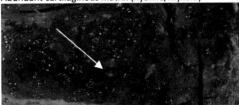

Bone entrapment

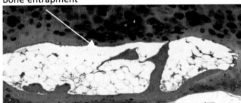

Increased cellularity, bland

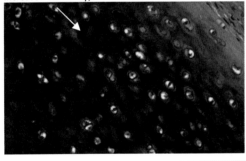

CONVENTIONAL CHONDROSARCOMA
MORPHOLOGY
- **Abundant** cartilaginous matrix (**hyaline/myxoid**)
- Lobular growth, **entrapment** of pre-existing **bone**
- **Increased cellularity**, but **bland** condensed nuclei, variable binucleation
- No significant nuclear atypia or mitotic activity
  - ➤ **Grade 1: Hypocellular**, nuclei are **lymphocyte-like**
  - ➤ **Grade 2:** More **cellular**, nuclei are **large** with **irregular contours** and have **coarse chromatin**, mitoses infrequent
  - ➤ **Grade 3: Hypercellular**, **severe pleomorphism** and mitoses; cells are often more spindled

OTHER HIGH YIELD POINTS
- Macroscopic Features
  - ➤ **Central:** arising in the **medulla** of the bone
  - ➤ **Central primary: no** pre-existing **precursor**
  - ➤ **Central secondary: arising** from an **enchondroma**
  - ➤ **Secondary peripheral: arising in** pre-existing **cartilaginous cap** of an **osteochondroma** (cap > 2cm)
- Appendicular skeleton (easier to resect) → atypical cartilaginous tumor
- Axial skeleton (harder to resect) = chondrosarcoma, grade 1
- **Molecular:** ~50% have **IDH1 or 2 mutations** (likely progressed from **enchondroma**)
  - ➤ **Higher-grade** tumors have **TP53, RB1, CDKN2A mutations**

Path Presenter

Abrupt transition from cartilage to non-cartilage

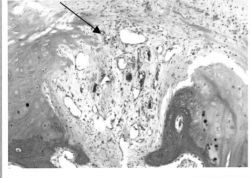

DEDIFFERENTIATED CHONDROSARCOMA
MORPHOLOGY
- Conventional chondrosarcoma with an **abrupt transition** to high-grade non-cartilaginous sarcoma

OTHER HIGH YIELD POINTS
- Seen in middle aged to elderly adults and develops in pelvis, or femur
- Very poor prognosis
- **Cytogenetics:** complex karyotypes
- **Molecular:** Frequent **IDH1/2** and **TP53** mutations

Path Presenter

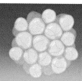

Islands of organized hyaline cartilage

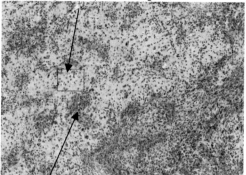

Undifferentiated component

MESENCHYMAL CHONDROSARCOMA
MORPHOLOGY
- Biphasic tumor with:
  - ➤ Islands of **organized hyaline cartilage**
  - ➤ **Undifferentiated component** with high nuclear to cytoplasm ratios
  - ➤ Frequent **staghorn vessels**
OTHER HIGH YIELD POINTS
- Aggressive and seen in young adults and adolescents
- Most often arises in craniofacial area (predilection for jaw)
- IHC: **(+)** for **S100**, CD99, **SOX9**, NKX2.2 (~70%), and vimentin
- **Molecular: HEY1-NCOA2** fusions (90%), IRF2BP2-CDX1 fusion
Path Presenter

Clear cells (glycogen)   Low-grade component

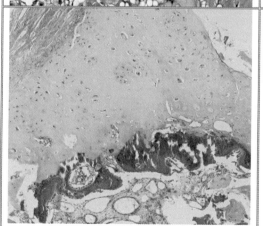

CLEAR CELL CHONDROSARCOMA
MORPHOLOGY
- **Clear cells** centrally placed nuclei, abundant **glycogen-rich** cytoplasm, and **well-defined** cytoplasmic **borders**
- Woven bone and osteoclast-like giant cells
- Minimal atypia and low mitotic activity
- Half of cases have conventional **low-grade chondrosarcoma component**
OTHER HIGH YIELD POINTS
- Low-grade malignancy that is seen in adults in 4th decade
- Usually affects the epiphysis or apophysis of long tubular bones
- IHC: strongly **(+) S100** in clear cells

Path Presenter

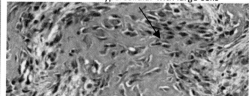
Image courtesy of Dr. Bonnie Balzer

PERIOSTEAL CHONDROSARCOMA
MORPHOLOGY
- **Cartilaginous tumor** on the surface of a bone with close association to periosteum with either:
  - ➤ Invasion of the underlying bone, or size >5.0 cm
OTHER HIGH YIELD POINTS
- **Located on the surface** of **long tubular bones**, usually the **distal femur**
- **Low metastatic rate**, grading not predictive
- **Molecular:** comparatively low IDH1/2 mutation rate
- **Differential diagnosis: Periosteal Chondroma**
  - ➤ Well-marginated, lobulated cartilaginous tumor arising on the bone surface, with elevation of the periosteum and erosion, but no invasion of the underlying bone cortex
  - ➤ Low to moderate cellularity, and relatively uniform chondrocytes
  - ➤ Usually <5 cm, benign, and treated with curettage
  - ➤ Frequently also has IDH1 mutations

BONE LESIONS

Woven Bone   Hypercellular with large cells

NORMAL BONE
MORPHOLOGY
- **Two main types of bone organization** (highlighted by polarization)
  - ➤ **Immature** → haphazard arrangement
  - ➤ **Mature** → parallel arrangement
- **Woven bone (Immature):**
  - ➤ Collagen fibers are **haphazardly arranged**

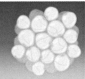

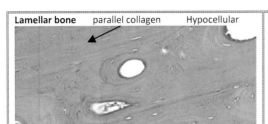

Lamellar bone   parallel collagen   Hypocellular

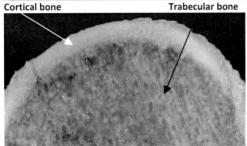

Cortical bone   Trabecular bone

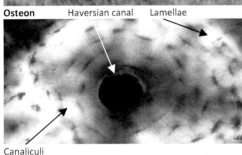

Osteon   Haversian canal   Lamellae

Canaliculi

- Formed during ossification and rapid bone growth/repair
  - Example: fracture callus
- Relatively hypercellular with large cells
- **Lamellar bone (Mature):**
  - Collagen fibers are organized in **parallel arrays**
  - Formed through **gradual remodeling** of woven bone
  - In adults, almost all bone are lamellar
  - **Hypocellular** with **small cells**
- Two main types of mature lamellar bone architecture:
  - **Cortical (Compact) Bone:** Dense lamellar bone with Haversian canals surrounded by concentric lamellar units
  - **Trabecular (Cancellous) Bone:** Connecting plates of lamellar bone

OTHER HIGH YIELD POINTS
- **Tumor Bone:** Typically, woven bone; either mineralized or unmineralized
- Deciding if it is bone/osteoid (unmineralized bone) versus collagen versus extracellular material
  - "Cement lines" (reversal lines)→ Thin, dark, linear lines are seen in osteoid, but not other substances (specific, but not sensitive)
  - SATB2 → expression supports osteoblastic differentiation

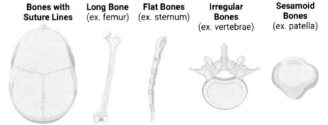

| Bones with Suture Lines | Long Bone (ex. femur) | Flat Bones (ex. sternum) | Irregular Bones (ex. vertebrae) | Sesamoid Bones (ex. patella) |

BONE AND JOINT INFECTIONS

ACUTE OSTEOMYELITIS
MORPHOLOGY

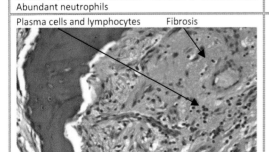

Empty lacunae   "Moth Eaten"

Abundant neutrophils

- **Necrotic bone** with **empty** osteocyte **lacunae**
- May see brisk osteoclast activity
- Bone often appears "**moth eaten**" (irregular erosions) with lots of "**rat bites**"

OTHER HIGH YIELD POINTS
- Often caused by **bacteria** (usually Staphylococcus)
- Can get from **hematogenous spread** ("**primary**," often in kids in **metaphysis** of **long bones** or adults in spine)
- Can also be from **direct inoculation**, often from trauma or ulceration ("**secondary**," often **adults**)    Path Presenter

CHRONIC OSTEOMYELITIS
MORPHOLOGY

Plasma cells and lymphocytes   Fibrosis

Image courtesy of Dr. Bonnie Balzer

- **Chronic inflammation with bone destruction**
- Marrow replaced by **fibrosis**, plasma cells and lymphocytes
- Often bone remodeling with osteoclasts and osteoblasts
- Similar irregular **rat/moth-eaten appearance**

OTHER HIGH YIELD POINTS
- **Necrotizing granulomas** → consider **Tuberculosis** ("**Pott's disease**" in spine)
- Can have sinus tract to surface lined by squamous epithelium → can turn into squamous cell carcinoma   Path Presenter

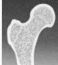

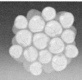

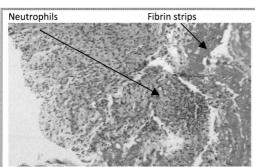

Neutrophils   Fibrin strips

Image courtesy of Dr. Bonnie Balzer

SEPTIC ARTHRITIS
MORPHOLOGY
- **Neutrophilic inflammation** of synovium with accumulation of **purulent debris** in joint space
- **Necrosis** and **fibrin strips**

OTHER HIGH YIELD POINTS
- Often clinical/lab diagnosis
- Caused by **bacteria**, often **Staphylococcus** (**S. epidermidis** with **prostheses**)
- Leads to **rapid cartilage destruction** → acute medical emergency that needs rapid treatment

Path Presenter

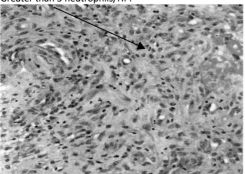

Greater than 5 neutrophils/HPF

Image courtesy of Dr. Bonnie Balzer

PERIPROSTHETIC JOINT INFECTION
MORPHOLOGY
- If there is a concern for infection, will often send joint capsule for frozen section neutrophil count
  - **Cutoff >5 neutrophils/HPF in 5 separate HPFs**, exclude surface fibrin
- Be SURE that it is PMNs → lymphocytes can be twisty and mimic PMNs

OTHER HIGH YIELD POINTS
- Can cause **prosthetic loosening**, requiring **revision arthroplasty**
- **Treatment** → **prosthesis removal** and subsequent reimplantation after eradication of the infection (may take weeks)
- Also evaluated clinically based on physical exam, culture, ESR, CRP, and synovial fluid studies

Path Presenter

DEGENERATIVE/REPARATIVE CHANGES

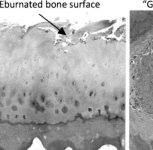

Eburnated bone surface   "Geode" Bone cyst

Courtesy of Dr. Michael Bonert & Dr. Bonnie Balzer

DEGENERATIVE JOINT DISEASE
MORPHOLOGY
- Non-inflammatory **loss of joint cartilage, subchondral bone sclerosis,** periarticular **bone cysts** (Geodes), **osteophyte formation**, and **synoviocyte hypertrophy/hyperplasia**

OTHER HIGH YIELD POINTS
- Also known as "DJD" or Osteoarthritis ("OA")
- Typically seen in **older individuals**
- Common result of a variety of factors including trauma, "**wear and tear,**" **metabolic diseases, avascular bone necrosis,** and **altered loading/anatomy**
- If treated surgically → joint arthroplasty

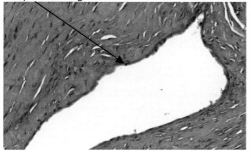

No epithelial lining

GANGLION CYST
MORPHOLOGY
- Cysts composed of fibrous tissue **without a lining**
- Contain **myxoid/mucous material**
- Can be **unilocular** or **multilocular**

OTHER HIGH YIELD POINTS
- Most common in young adults
- Usually occurs most often on **wrists** and **hand/feet**

Path Presenter

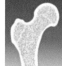

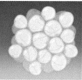

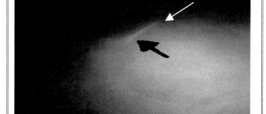

Granulation   Osteoblastic rimming

Woven bone   Depressed skull fracture

Radiograph provided by: A. E. Francis at the NIH

FRACTURE CALLUS
MORPHOLOGY
- Reparative changes seen at a site of prior bone fracture
- Stages to fracture repair:
  - ➤ **Stage 1: Hemorrhage** and **hematoma**
  - ➤ **Stage 2: Fibrocartilagenous matrix** forming a "soft callus"
  - ➤ **Stage 3:** Creation of a woven bony matrix by **osteoblastic rimming**
  - ➤ **Stage 4: Bone resorption** by multinucleated osteoclasts
- **Should NOT see atypical mitoses**, significant cytologic pleomorphism
OTHER HIGH YIELD POINTS
- In children, these findings should **raise suspicious for child abuse**
  - ➤ **Multiple fractures** at **different stages** of healing
  - ➤ **Pre-ambulatory children** and infants with **femur fractures**
  - ➤ **Fractures** to **ribs, skull,** or **scapula**
  - ➤ "**Bucket handle**" fractures or "**nightstick**" midshaft **fracture**

New Rib Fractures   Old Fractures

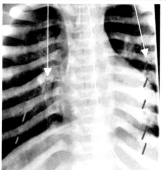

Spiral fracture of Tibia

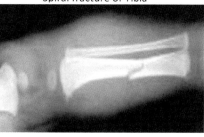

Path Presenter

Radiographs provided by: A. E. Francis at the NIH

"Crescent sign" of articular cartilage separation

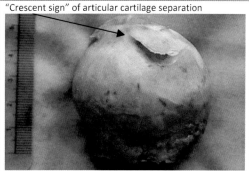

Courtesy of Dr. Steven Fruitsmaak, MD, PhD
Cartilage loosening

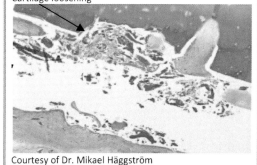

Courtesy of Dr. Mikael Häggström

AVASCULAR NECROSIS (ASEPTIC NECROSIS)
MORPHOLOGY
- Geographic area of **subchondral bone and marrow necrosis** with partially **separated articular cartilage** surface ("**crescent sign**")
- **Empty** osteocyte **lacunae**
- **Necrosis** throughout
OTHER HIGH YIELD POINTS
- **Risk factors:** Sickle cell disease, trauma, **steroids**, alcohol, **chemotherapy, collagen vascular disease**, pregnancy, **coagulopathy, cancer**, etc.

Necrosis of the osteocytes

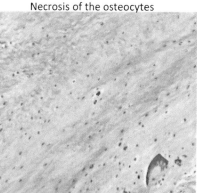

Courtesy of Dr. Mikael Häggström

Avascular Necrosis Femoral Head

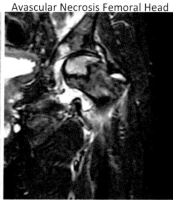

Courtesy of Dr. Jordi March I Nogue, MD

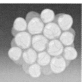

Pigmented debris in histiocytes

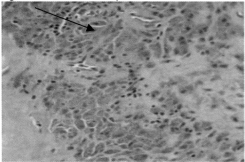

Image courtesy of Dr. Bonnie Balzer

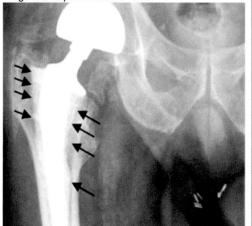

Photo courtesy of Zhenxin Shen et al.

ASEPTIC JOINT LOOSENING
MORPHOLOGY
- **Foreign material wear particles**
  - ➤ Fragments of **prosthetic material** that have broken off including **metal**, **polyethylene glycol**, **cement**, **ceramic**
- **Ingested by macrophages** → causes **inflammation** around joint → **osteolysis** and **joint loosening** around prosthesis
- Abundant **foamy histiocytes**, foreign body **giant cells**, and **inorganic particles**
- Particles from metal articular surfaces are small and appear black
- **Accumulate in macrophages** and fibrous tissue→ **"Metallosis"**

OTHER HIGH YIELD POINTS
- Metal can even make its way to regional lymph nodes
- **Aseptic Lymphocytic Vasculitis-associated Lesion (ALVAL)**
  - ➤ Seen with metal-on-metal articulation occur
  - ➤ Despite name, no true vasculitis is present
  - ➤ Three defining features:
    - ▪ **Prominent lymphoid aggregates**, often near venules
    - ▪ **Absence** of **obvious metal debris**
    - ▪ **Necrosis** of synovium

Metallic debris   Metallic debris

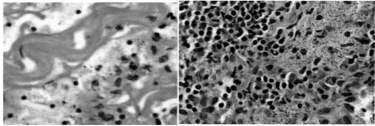

Courtesy of Dr. Frank Ingram

Cartilage   Laminated fibrin

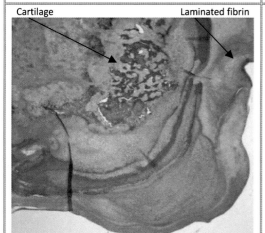

Courtesy of Dr. Bonnie Balzer, MD

LOOSE BODIES
MORPHOLOGY
- Fibrinous Loose bodies (**"Rice Bodies"**)
  - ➤ Consist of **laminated fibrin**
  - ➤ Grossly resemble **rice grains**
- **Osteochondral** or **Cartilaginous Loose bodies**
  - ➤ Detached fragments of **articular cartilage** with or without bone
  - ➤ Result from trauma and often **solitary**

OTHER HIGH YIELD POINTS
- Loose **fragments** of **tissue** found **free within** the **joint space**
- Can result from trauma, degenerative joint disease, or neoplasm
- Most common in knee → cause locking and pain
- Related entity: **Synovial Chondromatosis**
  - ➤ **Multiple hyaline cartilage** nodules in a synovium or loose in joint space
  - ➤ Chondrocytes cluster together in groups
  - ➤ **Molecular**: FN1-ACVR2A fusions

Path Presenter

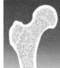

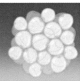

AUTOIMMUNE DISEASES

Proliferative synovium   Plasma cells

Lymphocytes

RHEUMATOID ARTHRITIS
MORPHOLOGY
Related entities
- **Chronic Synovitis:** Expands synovium with chronic inflammation (lymphocytes and plasma cells), often with lymphoid aggregates
  - ➢ Often reactive/hyperplastic synovium with surface fibrin/fibrinoid necrosis and granulation tissue
- **Pannus:** Synovium that erodes cartilage and other joint structures → characteristic marginal erosions of bone on X-ray
- **Rheumatoid nodule:** Necrotizing granulomas with central necrobiosis

OTHER HIGH YIELD POINTS
- **Most common primary** inflammatory **arthropathy**
- Chronic, idiopathic **erosive symmetric polyarthropathy**
- **Impacts all joints**, but worst impacted are small joints of hands
- Many extra-articular manifestations (e.g., Lung disease)
- Serology: **Positive Rheumatoid Factor (RF)**

CRYSTALLINE DISEASES

Fluffy pink deposits

Gout affecting first MTP joint

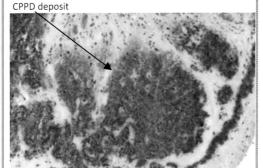

Gross examination of gout

GOUT
MORPHOLOGY
- **Fluffy pink deposits** with associated granulomatous inflammation
- Can have **scattered giant cells** surrounding deposits
- Joint fluid often **neutrophil-rich**
- Uric acid dissolves in water during staining process (not seen on H&E slides)
- Fresh touch preparations or unstained slides → **"needle-shaped" yellow, negatively birefringent crystals**

OTHER HIGH YIELD POINTS
- Usually seen in males
- Most common joint: **1st MTP**
- Presents as a very painful nodule

Path Presenter

Negatively Birefringent

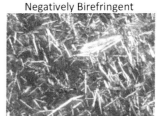

Courtesy of: Dr. Jeff Cloutier

CPPD deposit

Images courtesy of Dr. H. Yang (Twitter: @HENRYY_MD)

PSEUDOGOUT
MORPHOLOGY
- **Calcium Pyrophosphate Dihydrate (CPPD)** deposits in **cartilage** and in the soft tissue of the **joint**
- **Rhomboidal** purple-blue **positively birefringent crystals**
- **Well-demarcated basophilic material** with virtually **no inflammatory response**

OTHER HIGH YIELD POINTS
- Often associated with degenerative joint disease
- Often incidental finding in arthroplasty
- Crystals found inside leukocytes

Positively Birefringent

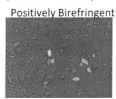

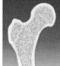 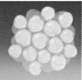

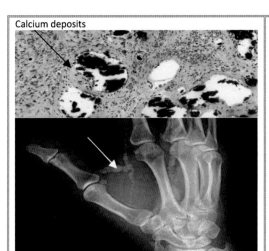

Calcium deposits

Radiograph courtesy of: Jto410 (Radiologist)

TUMORAL CALCINOSIS
MORPHOLOGY
- **Calcium hydroxyapatite deposits in** the **soft tissue**
- Lobules of **apatite-type calcifications** surrounded by **chronic inflammation** with a prominent **foreign body giant** cell reaction

OTHER HIGH YIELD POINTS
- Common locations: **hands, shoulder, sites of pressure**
- **Idiopathic/Sporadic** tumoral calcinosis (**most common**)
  - ➤ Seen in **ages < 20** and is usually painless
- Secondary tumoral calcinosis is trauma or due to a systemic disorder
  - ➤ **Renal failure** and on **dialysis** → electrolyte abnormalities
- **Familial tumoral calcinosis:** genetic-related
  - ➤ **Autosomal recessive,** more **common** in **African Americans**
  - ➤ **Hyperphosphatemia type:** Mutations in FGF23, KL, or GALNT3 genes
  - ➤ **Normophosphatemia type:** Mutations in SAMD9 gene

Path Presenter

SUMMARY OF CRYSTALLINE DISEASES

	Gout	Pseudogout	Tumoral calcinosis
Age	Middle age	Older	Young
Site	1st MTP	Knee	Shoulder, Hips
Crystal Shape	Needle	Rhomboid	Irregular gritty plates
Type	Uric acid	Calcium pyrophosphate	Calcium hydroxyapatite
Polarizable	Yes **Negative Birefringent**	Yes, **Positive birefringent**	**No**
Seen on H&E	**No**	Yes	Yes
Inflammatory reaction	Yes	**No**	Yes
Image			

METABOLIC/ENDOCRINE/IDIOPATHIC BONE LESIONS

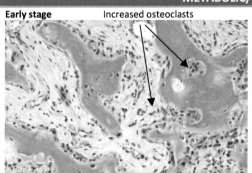

Early stage   Increased osteoclasts

PAGET DISEASE
MORPHOLOGY
- Localized **disorder of bone remodeling** characterized by focal areas of **increased turnover** with excess bone synthesis and resorption
- Unusually **large osteoclasts** with increased nuclei and prominent nucleoli
- Prominent **osteoblastic rimming**
- Paratrabecular **marrow fibrosis**
- Unusually thick and thin bone trabeculae
- Numerous irregular **reversal cement lines** and **bone scalloping**
- Mosaic pattern
- **Histology** is **variable** based on stage of disease

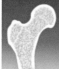
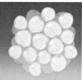

Courtesy of Dr. Raul Perret, MD (Twitter: @kells108)

Late stage   Fibrosis   Irregular cement lines

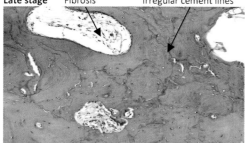

Thickened calvarium

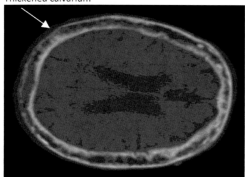

Courtesy of Dr. Laughlin Dawes

- ➢ **Early stage:** **more resorptive** and has **numerous osteoclasts, increased vascularity** and **resorptive** surfaces
- ➢ **Mid stage: more synthesis** due to **increased osteoblastic activity** and osteoclastic resorption (which slows)
- ➢ **End stage:** Extensively **sclerotic** bone

OTHER HIGH YIELD POINTS

- Etiology is unknown, does occur in clusters of families
- Often localized to a single bone (monostotic) in **elderly men**
- **Most common** sites are **pelvis**, femur, spine, and skull
- Monitoring of disease can be done using **Alkaline phosphatase**
- Grossly, bones can be **pumice (look like a sponge)** and have **thickened cortex**
- **Radiography:** can show "Blade of grass" sign or typical "cotton wool" or "ground glass" appearance due to osseous matrix synthesis
- **Familial cases** usually have **chromosomal abnormalities** and **autosomal dominant inheritance**
- **Confers** an **Increased risk** of **osteosarcoma**

Deformed bone   Pumice appearance of bone

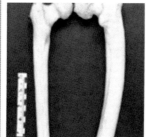
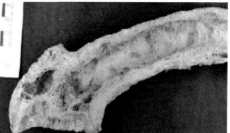

Photographs courtesy of Elena Nebot Valenzuela & peter Pietschmann

BROWN TUMOR OF HYPERPARATHYROIDISM

MORPHOLOGY

- Hemorrhage and extravasated **erythrocytes**
- **Hemosiderin-laden macrophages** and other inflammatory cells
- **Plump fibroblasts** and scattered **osteoclast-like giant cells**
- **Woven bone** with adjacent **fibrous tissue**

OTHER HIGH YIELD POINTS

- Usually seen in the **3rd to 4th decade** and **more common in females**
- Forms a **mass lesion** that **may be painful**
- May be **solitary** or involve **multiple bones**
- Frequently **arises in pelvis, clavicles & ribs, or extremities**
- **Radiology:** expansile **lytic lesion** which may have **trabeculations and may** have **well-defined margins**
- **Cause of lesion:** Hyperparathyroidism
  - ➢ **PTH** binds to surface **receptors** on **osteoblasts** → **RANKL** upregulated and **binds to RANK receptor** on **osteoclastic precursors** → **osteoclast development** and subsequent **resorption**
- Gross examination: Red-brown lobulated, hemorrhagic mass which expands (and thins) the bone cortex
  - ➢ May develop large, **blood-filled cysts** → **osteitis fibrosa cystica**
- **Biochemical test:** PTH and **serum calcium** will be **elevated**
- **Treatment:** parathyroidectomy → tumor will regress and new bone will form

Hemorrhage   Giant cells   Fibrous tissue   Remodeling

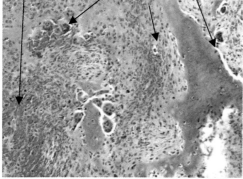

Courtesy of Dr. Michael Bonert, MD

Brown tumor on Radiograph

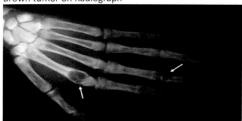

Radiograph courtesy of Dr. Frank Gaillard

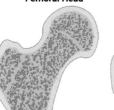

Normal Femoral Head | **Osteoporosis Femoral Head**

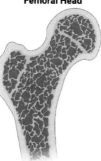

No osteoporosis | Osteoporosis

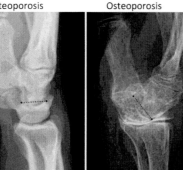

Courtesy of Dr. Nevit Dilmen and Dr. Mikael Häggström

OSTEOPOROSIS

MORPHOLOGY

- Cortical thinning and decreased bone volume
- Trabeculae are thin; lose their interconnections between each other, and have smooth contours (Trabeculae will be <10% of marrow area)
- May become fatty within the marrow space due to age related changes
- **Decrease in mass** of mineralized bone

OTHER HIGH YIELD POINTS

- **Primary osteoporosis:**
  - ➤ Frequent in **postmenopausal women**
  - ➤ **Mechanism: Decreased estrogen** acting on osteoclast receptors → **decreased FASL induction**→ osteoclasts have **longer lifespan** due to decreased apoptosis
  - ➤ **Decreased bone density** usually takes ~10 years to notice
  - ➤ **Risk factors:** low body weight, low BMI, low body fat (site of estrogen synthesis in post-menopausal), **smoking**, alcohol use
- **Secondary Osteoporosis:**
  - ➤ Usually caused by **systemic disorders** such as **malabsorption, hypothyroidism, hyperparathyroidism, hematologic** disorders, **corticosteroids, anti-hormonal medications**
- **Increased risk of fracture** over time**,** often **little force required** to cause
- **Gross examination**: Decreased bone mass → fragile
- **Radiology: DEXA Scan** → T-score below 2.5 standard deviations below normal aged-matched individuals

Path Presenter

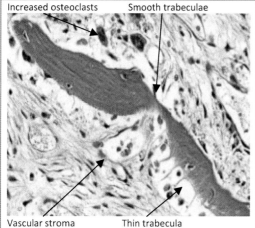

Increased osteoclasts | Smooth trabeculae

Vascular stroma | Thin trabecula

RENAL OSTEODYSTROPHY

MORPHOLOGY

- **Trabeculae are smooth** and is generally **unmineralized**
- Marrow space will demonstrate a **vascular stromal fibrosis**
- Thinning of the cortical bone as osteoclast activity increases

OTHER HIGH YIELD POINTS

- Usually seen in individuals with renal failure and on dialysis
- With renal failure → **decreased phosphate excretion**, which will result in **decreased serum calcium** levels → **increased PTH** → kidney unresponsive → **hydroxylation** of 25-0H vitamin D3 is **impaired** → **osteoclastic activity increases**
- **Radiology: increased radiolucency, DEXA** will show **similar** findings **to osteoporosis**
- **Treatment:** Phosphate binders; overtreatment → adynamic renal osteodystrophy → no osteoid formation and nearly no cellular activity

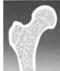

TUMORS OF THE BONE

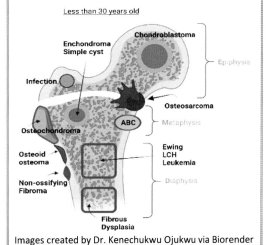

EPIDEMIOLOGY AND ANATOMIC SITES

- Overall, primary clinically significant bone tumors are rare
- Benign, incidental tumors (like non-ossifying fibroma) are relatively common, but are often clinically insignificant
- Primary bone sarcomas have a **bimodal** distribution:
  - ➢ **First peak in second decade (teens with actively growing skeleton):**
    - Osteosarcoma, Ewing sarcoma
  - ➢ **Second peak after age 60:**
    - Chondrosarcoma, Osteosarcoma
- Most common location is **near the knee**, which is the site of the fastest growing growth plate (although variable by tumor)
- Bone tumors are **most often de novo**
- **Risk-factors** that **predispose** an individual to **osteosarcoma**
  - ➢ Radiation, Paget's Disease of Bone, chronic osteomyelitis, bone infarctions, and prosthetic joints
- **Symptoms**: Often pain, which is classically worse at night, and a mass; Can have pathologic fractures, swelling, tenderness
- **Classic specific locations:**
  - ➢ **Anterior Cortex of Tibia:** Adamantinoma and osteofibrous dysplasia
  - ➢ **Posterior Cortex of Distal Femur:** Parosteal osteosarcoma
  - ➢ **Clivus, Vertebral bodies, Sacrum**: Chordoma
  - ➢ **Posterior Elements of Spine:** Osteoblastoma

Skeleton	Less than 30 years old	More than 30 years old
Axial (skull, vertebrae, pelvis)	Osteoblastoma, Langerhans cell histiocytosis, Aneurysmal bone cyst (ABC), Hemangioma	Metastases, Plasmacytoma, Hemangioma, Chordoma
Appendicular (arms and legs)	**Most tumors,** Osteosarcoma, Ewing sarcoma	**Most tumors,** Chondrosarcoma, Osteosarcoma
Acral (hands and feet)	Enchondroma	Enchondroma

Images created by Dr. Kenechukwu Ojukwu via Biorender

OSTEOGENIC TUMORS

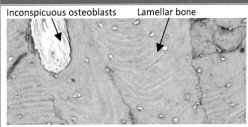

Inconspicuous osteoblasts   Lamellar bone

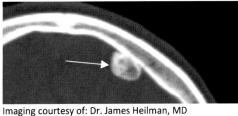

Radiodense

Imaging courtesy of: Dr. James Heilman, MD

OSTEOMA

MORPHOLOGY

- Composed of **lamellar/cortical-type bone with haversian-like systems**
- Inconspicuous osteoblasts
- May have a fibrous component → mimics a fibroosseous lesion

OTHER HIGH YIELD POINTS

- Benign tumor that is usually seen in middle-aged adults
- Usually occur on **face** or **jaw** bones → sites of membranous ossification
  - ➢ Most common is in **frontal & ethmoid sinuses**
  - ➢ Develops in medullary cavity→ called a "Bone Island"
- **Radiology:** Usually an incidental finding and is **uniformly radiodense**
- **Gross examination: Tan-white**, firm and usually <2 cm in size
- **Multiple osteomas** → consider **Gardner's syndrome** (subset of FAP)
- Generally, require no treatment unless symptomatic

Path Presenter

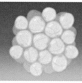

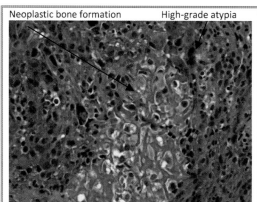

Neoplastic bone formation — High-grade atypia

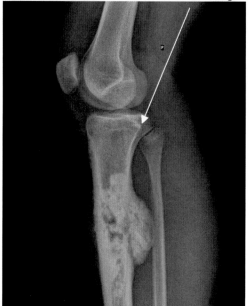

Tibia with Osteosarcoma — Codman Triangle

Radiograph courtesy ofL Dr. Yousef Samir

CONVENTIONAL OSTEOSARCOMA

MORPHOLOGY

- **High-grade** sarcoma in which tumor cells produce bone
- Requires **neoplastic bone** formation (any amount is sufficient for diagnosis)
- Woven bone will have disorganized trabeculae
- Has an infiltrative growth pattern
- **High-grade cytologic atypia** and "normalize" if surrounded by bone matrix
- Mitotic activity is brisk and has atypical forms
- Can have **various components**:
  - ➤ Cartilaginous (chondroblastic osteosarcoma)
  - ➤ Spindled cells (fibroblastic osteosarcoma)
  - ➤ Others: Giant cell-rich, telangiectatic, osteoblastoma-like

OTHER HIGH YIELD POINTS

- Usually seen in **ages 10-20** and **males** are **slightly more common**
- Most common to arise in long tubular bones
  - ➤ **Femur** > proximal tibia > proximal humerus
- Presents as a **painful, enlarging mass** and overlying skin may be erythematous
- Metastasis is **hematogenous** and most frequently to the **lung**
- IHC: (+) for **SATB2, CD99, S100** (cartilaginous areas); **variable** keratins
- **Molecular:** Typically arise de novo, but will have mutations in **RB1** and **TP53**
  - ➤ Chromosomal instability and abnormalities on karyotype
  - ➤ **MDM2 amplification** → arises from **low-grade central osteosarcoma**
  - ➤ Germline mutation in **RB1** → **Hereditary retinoblastoma**
  - ➤ Germline mutation in **TP53** → **Li-Fraumeni syndrome**
  - ➤ **Rothmund-Thomson Syndrome** → baseline skeletal abnormalities

Path Presenter

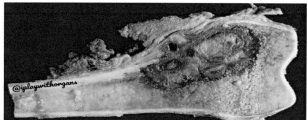

Courtesy of Cory Nash, MS, PA(ASCP) (Twitter: @iplaywithorgans)

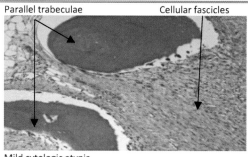

Parallel trabeculae — Cellular fascicles

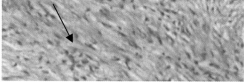

Mild cytologic atypia

Images courtesy of Dr. Bonnie Balzer

LOW-GRADE CENTRAL OSTEOSARCOMA

MORPHOLOGY

- Moderately **cellular fascicles** of **spindled cells** with only **mild nuclear atypia**
- Admixed (usually woven) **neoplastic bone**, which is composed of **long** and **thick bony trabeculae**, often **in parallel arrangement**

OTHER HIGH YIELD POINTS

- **Very uncommon**, low-grade malignancy (<1% of all osteosarcomas)
- Average age of diagnosis is in **3rd decade**, no sex predilection
- Arises in the **intramedullary cavity** of **long bones** at the **metaphyseal-diaphyseal area** → usually **femur** and **tibia, rare** in **flat bones**
- **Radiology:** Dense, **cloud-like** and mineralized lesion, few may be radiolucent
- **Gross examination:** tan-white, gritty, and has cortical destruction
- **Good prognosis** if widely resected but **can dedifferentiate** into conventional osteosarcoma
- IHC: (+) for **MDM2** and **CDK4**
- **Molecular:** MDM2 amplifications

Path Presenter

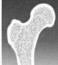
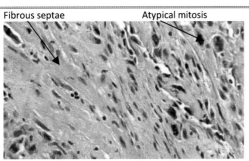

Fibrous septae · Atypical mitosis

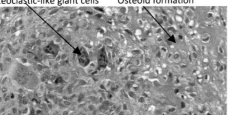

Osteoclastic-like giant cells · Osteoid formation

TELANGIECTATIC OSTEOSARCOMA
MORPHOLOGY
- **Blood-filled** or **empty cystic spaces** separated by variable **fibrous septae**
- **Pleomorphic malignant cells** with significant **nuclear atypia, hyperchromasia, atypical mitotic figures**, and variable cytoplasm
- Scattered **osteoclast-like giant cells**
- **Focal osteoid formation** and infiltrative border

OTHER HIGH YIELD POINTS
- **No prognostic significance** to this subtype of osteosarcoma
- Most common to **arise** in **long tubular bones**
  - ➢ **Femur** > **proximal tibia** > proximal humerus
- **Radiology**: Can **present exactly like** an **aneurysmal bone cyst (ABC)**
- Closely **resembles aneurysmal bone cyst** (ABC)
- **Molecular**: Identical to conventional

Path Presenter

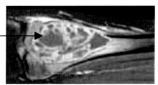

Tibia with cystic, blood-filled spaces

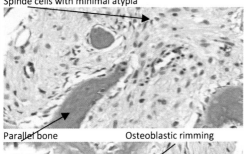

Spinde cells with minimal atypia

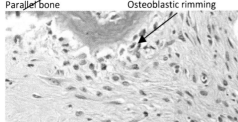

Parallel bone · Osteoblastic rimming

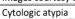
Images courtesy of Dr. Bonnie Balzer

PAROSTEAL OSTEOSARCOMA
MORPHOLOGY
- **Spindle cells** with **minimal atypia** and **mitotic** activity
- **Woven bone trabeculae** are long, well-formed, **arranged in parallel**, and have **cement lines** that are **well-visualized**
- Bone may have **osteoblastic rimming**
- **Can dedifferentiate** and have high-grade nuclei with coarse chromatin

OTHER HIGH YIELD POINTS
- **Most common surface**-located **osteosarcoma**
- Majority are in **young adult** to **middle-aged** with slight **female** predominance
- Presents as a **slowly enlarging, exophytic lobular mass** on **bone surface**
- Usually on **tubular bone surface** and majority **involve metaphysis**
- **Radiology**: Uniformly **radiodense, lobulated contour, surface based**
- **Molecular**: MDM2 amplifications (from **supernumerary ring chromosomes**)
- **Excellent prognosis** and has a **>90% survival** at **5 years**

Path Presenter

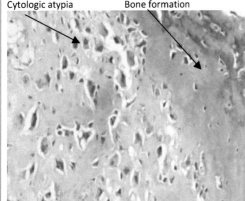

Cytologic atypia · Bone formation

Image courtesy of Dr. Bonnie Balzer

PERIOSTEAL OSTESARCOMA
MORPHOLOGY
- Predominantly a **myxo-hyaline chondroblastic** proliferation
- **Malignant cells** have **moderate to severe** cytologic **atypia** composed of **hyperchromatic nuclei, irregular nuclear contours,** variable cytoplasm
- Intervening **bands** of **primitive sarcoma show bone formation**

OTHER HIGH YIELD POINTS
- **Uncommon** variant, intermediate-grade osteosarcoma
- Usually seen in **young adults** (2-3rd decade) on **surfaces of long bones**
  - ➢ **Diaphysis** of **long bones**, especially **femur** and **tibia**
- Presents as a **slow growing, palpable mass** that is **non-mobile**
- **Radiology**: Fusiform mass with "sun-burst" or "hair on end" appearance
- Better prognosis than conventional osteosarcoma (~85%, 5-year)

Path Presenter

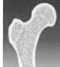
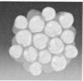
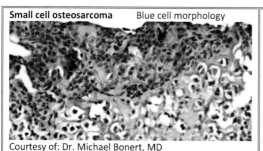

Small cell osteosarcoma   Blue cell morphology

Courtesy of: Dr. Michael Bonert, MD

OTHER OSTEOSARCOMA VARIANTS
MORPHOLOGY
- **Small cell osteosarcoma**: a subtype of conventional osteosarcoma with **small round blue cell** morphology with focal neoplastic bone formation
  - ➢ Tumor cells have **scant cytoplasm** and **fine to coarse chromatin**
  - ➢ Similar distribution to conventional osteosarcoma
- **High-grade surface Osteosarcoma**: histologically high-grade osteosarcoma, but arising on the surface of the bone, without substantial intraosseous involvement

HEMATOPOIETIC NEOPLASMS

Histiocytes   Fibrosis   Lymphocytes

ERDHEIM-CHESTER DISEASE
MORPHOLOGY
- Clonal systemic **histiocytosis** with **inflammation** and **fibrosis**
- Infiltration by **foamy, lipid-laden histiocytes**
- Variable amounts of mixed inflammatory cells including: **Touton giant cells**, small lymphocytes, neutrophils, and eosinophils
- Fibrosis is usually present and can be extensive

OTHER HIGH YIELD POINTS
- Extremely **rare disease** and arises in **middle-aged to elderly adults**
- Usually involves long bones, but is a multisystem disease
- **IHC: Foamy histiocytes** stain **(+)** with **CD68, CD163** and **(-)** for **CD1a**
- **Molecular**: BRAFV600E mutations (others: MAPK, ARAF, KRAS, NRAS)

OSTEOCLASTIC GIANT CELL RICH TUMORS

Spindle cells   Giant cells

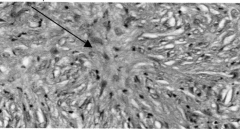

Storiform pattern

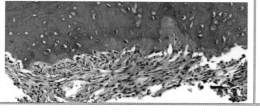

Reactive bone

NON-OSSIFYING FIBROMA
MORPHOLOGY
- **Storiform** proliferation of **plump spindled cells** with intermingled **giant cells**
- Scattered **hemosiderophages** and foamy macrophages
- **Necrosis may be present**, especially in a fracture
- Mitotic activity is low
- May have woven bone at the periphery

OTHER HIGH YIELD POINTS
- **Benign asymptomatic lesion** that usually occurs in the **first 2 decades of life**
- **Twice as common in males** than females
- Majority arise in the **metaphysis cortex** of long bones
  - ➢ **Distal femur**, proximal and distal tibia
- **Radiology**: Lucent lesion with sclerotic margin and trabeculations
- **Molecular**: KRAS, FGFR1, NF1 mutations → RAS-MAPK pathway activation

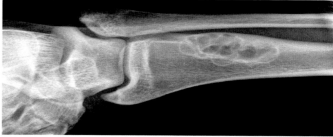

Radiograph courtesy of: Dr. Hellerhoff

 Path Presenter

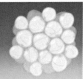
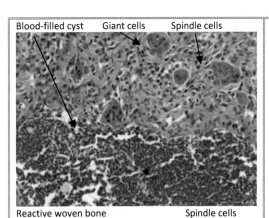

Blood-filled cyst   Giant cells   Spindle cells

Reactive woven bone   Spindle cells

ANEURYSMAL BONE CYST
MORPHOLOGY
- Cyst wall is composed of **plump** and **spindled fibroblasts**
- **Osteoclast-like giant cells**, **hemorrhage** and hemosiderin
- **Reactive woven bone** formation
- Mitoses are common, necrosis may be present if occurring at site of fracture
- **Solid type lacks blood-filled cystic** spaces

OTHER HIGH YIELD POINTS
- Most **common** in the **first two decades of life**, no sex predilection
- Presents with **pain** and **swelling** of the affected extremity
- Can arise in the metaphysis of long bones, vertebrae, hands and feet, or craniofacial skeleton
- **Radiology:** Circumscribed, lytic lesion with linear trabeculations and thin sclerotic borders
- **Molecular: CDH11-USP6** translocation → t(16;17)(q22;p13)
- **FISH: USP6 rearrangements**
- Lesions with **secondary ABC:** Giant cell tumor, chondroblastoma, osteoblastoma, fibrous dysplasia, and osteosarcoma

Path Presenter

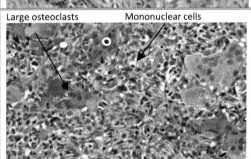

Large osteoclasts   Mononuclear cells

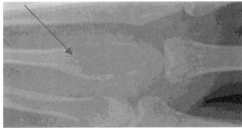

Giant cell tumor

Radiography courtesy of: Dr. James Heilman, MD

GIANT CELL TUMOR OF BONE
MORPHOLOGY
- Proliferation of numerous (reactive) **large osteoclasts** together with a **mononuclear neoplastic** component without atypia
- Mononuclear cells have oval nuclei, regular chromatin and ill-defined cytoplasm and grow in a syncytium
- Often associated with hemorrhage, **hemosiderin,** and macrophages
- Necrosis and vascular invasion can be seen

OTHER HIGH YIELD POINTS
- Usually seen in 3rd to 5th decade with slight female predominance
- Presents as swelling and pain in the affected bone
- Many arise in the **epiphyseal-metaphyseal region** of long tubular bones
  - Nearly half of cases occur in the knee area
- **Molecular:** Driver mutation in **H3F3A G34W**
- Other giant cell tumor of bone:
  - Chondroblastoma, Paget's disease of Bone, some osteosarcomas, Non-ossifying fibroma, aneurysmal bone cyst

Path Presenter

NOTOCHORDAL TUMORS

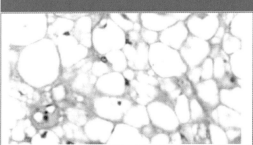

BENIGN NOTOCHORDAL TUMOR
MORPHOLOGY
- Polyhedral epithelioid cells with bland nuclei with fine chromatin, abundant clear to eosinophilic cytoplasm, and well-defined cell borders
- No extracellular myxoid matrix, vasculature, fibrous septae, or lobular architecture

OTHER HIGH YIELD POINTS
- Benign and usually in axial skeleton: Sacrum, coccyx, cervical spine, vertebrae
- IHC: Positive for Brachyury, S100, keratin, and EMA

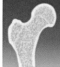

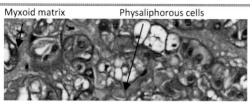

Myxoid matrix   Physaliphorous cells

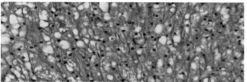

Cords

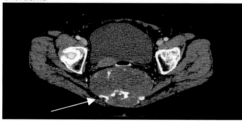

Chordoma

CT Scan courtesy of Dr. Hellerhoff

CHORDOMA
MORPHOLOGY
- **Large epithelioid cells** with eosinophilic to clear cytoplasm and may have bubbly **"physaliphorous"** cytoplasm
- Arranged in **cords** and **nests** embedded in **abundant myxoid matrix** or separated by **fibrous septae**
- **Variable pleomorphism** and mitotic activity

OTHER HIGH YIELD POINTS
- Usually seen in middle-aged to elderly patients with male predilection
  - ➤ If arising in **children**, usually is at **skull base**
- Presentation dependent on site of origin
  - ➤ **Skull base:** diplopia, headache, cranial nerve palsy
  - ➤ **Spine:** neurologic symptoms and pain
  - ➤ **Sacrum:** pain, incontinence, constipation, erectile dysfunction
- **Radiology:** destructive lytic mass and variable calcifications
- Prognosis: Depends on size, location, and dedifferentiation (poor)
- IHC: **(+)** for **brachyury, cytokeratin 8/19**
- Molecular: **T-box duplication (Brachyury)**, PI3K pathway, LYST, others
  - ➤ **Poorly differentiated chordoma:** loss of **SMARCB1**, and has scattered signet ring-like cells and rhabdoid areas

Path Presenter

MISCELLANOUS BONE LESIONS

Fibrous wall   Reactive bone formation

SIMPLE BONE CYST
MORPHOLOGY
- Cyst wall composed of **fibrous tissue** with **no true lining**
- May have reactive woven bone formation, chronic inflammation, multinucleated giant cells, fibrin, calcification, and cholesterol

OTHER HIGH YIELD POINTS
- Benign lesion seen in the proximal femur or humerus of young patient

Path Presenter

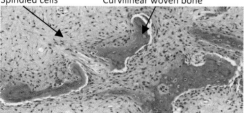

Spindled cells   Curvilinear woven bone

Normal   Fibrous Dysplasia   Shepherd's Crook

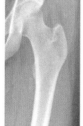

Radiography courtesy of Dr. Basmajoor

FIBROUS DYSPLASIA
MORPHOLOGY
- Fibrous tissue composed of **spindled cells** with **tapered nuclei** and **inconspicuous** cytoplasmic **borders**
- Bone trabeculae are composed of **curvilinear woven bone** and appear to "arise" from the fibrous tissue

OTHER HIGH YIELD POINTS
- Most commonly develops during childhood and may be associated with genetic syndromes
  - ➤ **Mazabraud syndrome:** Fibrous dysplasia and intramuscular myxomas
  - ➤ **McCune-Albright syndrome:** Fibrous dysplasia, café-au-lait macules, and endocrinopathies
- **Radiology:** Elongated intramedullary tumor with "rind-like" margins; severe cases have **"shepherd's crook"** appearance
- May be **monostotic** or **polyostotic** and involve many different sites
- Most **common extraskeletal manifestation** is **"café-au-lait"** macules
- **Molecular:** Activating **GNAS** missense mutations in polyostotic form

 Path Presenter

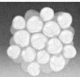
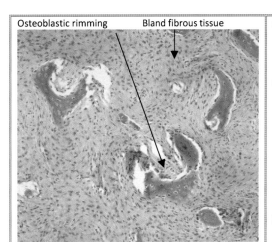

Osteoblastic rimming   Bland fibrous tissue

Image courtesy of Dr. Bonnie Balzer

OSTEOFIBROUS DYSPLASIA
MORPHOLOGY
- Woven bone with prominent **osteoblastic rimming** with intervening bland fibrous tissue

OTHER HIGH YIELD POINTS
- Benign lesion occurring in the first 2 decades of life
- Almost exclusively in **tibia or fibula anterior cortex** during childhood
- Presents as a pain, localized swelling, or fracture
- Radiology: Solitary lytic lesion with sclerotic borders
- IHC: **(+)** for **cytokeratin** which highlights scattered **single cells**
  - ➤ **If CK highlights clusters of cells, consider:** Osteofibrous dysplasia-like adamantinoma
- **Molecular:** Germline MET mutations (hereditary OFD); lacks GNAS mutations

Path Presenter

CHONDROMESENCYMAL HAMARTOMA OF CHEST WALL
MORPHOLOGY
- Composed of **nodules of hyaline cartilage**, admixed with blood-filled cystic spaces, reactive bone, bland spindled cells, and osteoclast-like giant cells

OTHER HIGH YIELD POINTS
- Benign
- Well-circumscribed mass arising from the rib, **presents at birth**

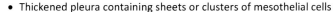

NON-NEOPLASTIC SEROSAL LESIONS

Mesothelial cells   Layering

Image courtesy of Dr. Bonnie Balzer

REACTIVE MESOTHELIAL HYPERPLASIA
MORPHOLOGY
- Thickened pleura containing sheets or clusters of mesothelial cells
- May have papillary excrescences
- Can have psammomatous calcifications
- May demonstrate layering of fibrous tissue and mesothelium
  - ➤ "Sedimentary-rock appearance"

OTHER HIGH YIELD POINTS
- Seen with recurrent pleural irritation, resolves when stimulus removed
- IHC: **(+)** for **calretinin**, **WT-1**, D2-40, CK5/6 and **retained BAP1** expression

Path Presenter

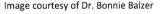

Hypocellular fibrous tissue deposition

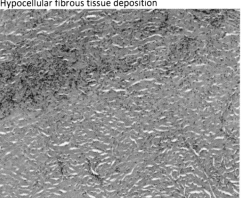

FIBROUS PLEURISY
MORPHOLOGY
- Deposition of **bland, hypocellular fibrous tissue** in the pleura
- Often involves the visceral pleura
- May produce **apical fibrous "capping"**

OTHER HIGH YIELD POINTS
- Often involves the **visceral pleura**
- Severe cases can obliterate the pleural space
- Can **mimic desmoplastic mesothelioma**
- May be **associated with a variety of conditions**
  - ➤ **Connective tissue disorders:** lupus erythematosus or rheumatoid arthritis
  - ➤ **Chronic infections**
  - ➤ **Asbestos exposure**

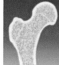

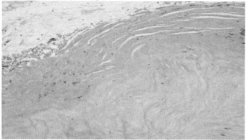

Dense hyalinized collagen

Image courtesy of Dr. Bonnie Balzer

PLEURAL PLAQUE (HYALINE PLEURAL PLAQUE)
MORPHOLOGY
- **Hypocellular, dense bundles** of **hyalinized collagen**, often with a "basket weave" arrangement
- Often dystrophic calcifications and variable chronic inflammation
OTHER HIGH YIELD POINTS
- Often on parietal pleura, particularly on diaphragm
- Often a **marker of asbestos exposure**, but **can be seen with other sources** of chronic pleural irritation

Path Presenter

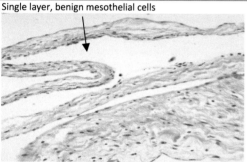

Single layer, benign mesothelial cells

Image courtesy of Dr. Bonnie Balzer

PERITONEAL INCLUSION CYST
MORPHOLOGY
- Single or multiple, **small, thin-walled, translucent, unilocular cysts**
- Attached or free in the peritoneal cavity
- Lined by a **single layer** of flattened, benign-appearing mesothelial cells
- Variable thickened septae within the cyst and eosinophilic fluid
OTHER HIGH YIELD POINTS
- Often discovered incidentally, more **common in women**
  - **Common** in **pelvic organs, upper abdominal cavity,** or **retroperitoneum**

Path Presenter

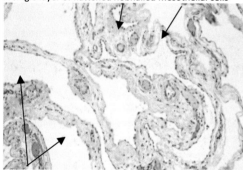

A single layer of flattened hobnailed mesothelial cells

Multilocular

BENIGN MULTICYSTIC PERITONEAL "MESOTHELIOMA"
MORPHOLOGY
- Grossly: often **large, multiple small, thin-walled, translucent,** unilocular **cysts** that may be attached or free floating
- Often fibrous tissue in septae with sparse inflammation
- Cysts are lined by a single layer of flattened to cuboidal mesothelial cells which occasionally have a "**hob-nail**" appearance
OTHER HIGH YIELD POINTS
- Occurs usually in **young to middle-aged women** in the **peritoneum or pelvis**
- Better name is "**multilocular peritoneal inclusion cysts**"
- Likely a hyperplastic reactive lesion (vs. a benign neoplasm)
- **Associated** with **previous abdominal surgery, pelvic inflammatory disease,** and **endometriosis**

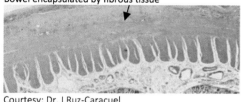

Bowel encapsulated by fibrous tissue

Courtesy: Dr. I Ruz-Caracuel

SCLEROSING PERITONITIS
MORPHOLOGY
- Encasement of the bowel by fibrous tissue
OTHER HIGH YIELD POINTS
- Rare, causes bowel obstruction from encasement →"Cacoon abdomen"
- Can be idiopathic, or seen with intraperitoneal dialysis, VP shunts, and fibrothecomas of the ovary

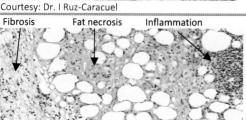

Fibrosis   Fat necrosis   Inflammation

SCLEROSING MESENTERITIS
MORPHOLOGY
- Varying degrees of fat necrosis, chronic inflammation, and fibrosis, usually involving the mesentery of the small bowel → forms a **distinct mass**
OTHER HIGH YIELD POINTS
- Rare, idiopathic, forms a distinct mass involving the small bowel mesentery

Path Presenter

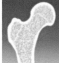

BENIGN/INDOLENT MESOTHELIAL TUMORS

Irregularly shaped microcystic spaces

Image courtesy of Dr. Bonnie Balzer

ADENOMATOID TUMOR
MORPHOLOGY
- **Irregularly shaped gland-like microcystic spaces** composed of flattened or cuboidal cells with associated fibrous stroma
- **Bland cytologic features**
- Helpful feature: "thread-like bridging strands"; Sometimes signet ring-like vacuolated cells

OTHER HIGH YIELD POINTS
- Solitary, localized lesion that occurs in both **males** and **females**
- Seen in young to middle-aged adults
- May be seen in **uterine** or **adnexal surfaces**, **testis**, or **spermatic cord**
- Presents as a firm painless mass

Path Presenter

Papillary architecture   Myxoid cores   No atypia

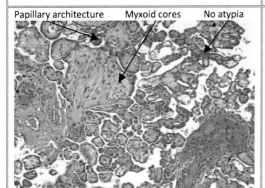

Image courtesy of Dr. Bonnie Balzer

WELL DIFFERENTIATED PAPILLARY MESOTHELIOMA
MORPHOLOGY
- **Prominent papillary architecture** with myxoid cores covered by a single layer of **flattened to cuboidal bland epithelioid cells**
- Epithelioid cells have small bland round **nuclei, without atypia**
- No inflammatory reaction is present

OTHER HIGH YIELD POINTS
- Rare indolent tumors, most cases cured by excision
- Average survival is ~75 months
- Gross examination: velvety appearance
- **IHC: (+)** for pancytokeratin, CK5/6, calretinin, D2-40, WT1, GLUT1
- **Molecular:** Somatic missense mutations in **TRAF7** or **CDC42**

Path Presenter

MALIGNANT MESOTHELIAL TUMORS

Eosinophilic cytoplasm in vesicular nuclei

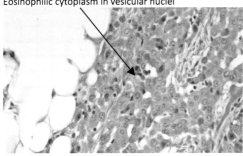

Invasion

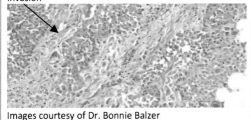

Images courtesy of Dr. Bonnie Balzer

EPITHELIOID MESOTHELIOMA
MORPHOLOGY
- **Malignant** proliferation of mesothelial cells with **epithelioid morphology**
- Cytologically bland with **eosinophilic cytoplasm** and **vesicular chromatin**
- Demonstration of tissue invasion (e.g., into chest wall or lung) is often key for diagnosis
  - ➢ However, when a substantial amount of solid, malignant tumor (i.e., a mass) is identified, the presence of invasion is not required for diagnosis
- **Common histologic patterns**: solid, tubulopapillary, trabecular
- **Rare patterns**: micropapillary, clear cell, deciduoid, adenomatoid, transitional, small cell, lymphohistiocytoid
- Can see psamomma bodies

OTHER HIGH YIELD POINTS
- Most common in **elderly males** and often **unilateral** at first
- Most common cause is **asbestos exposure**
- Often **insidious onset** with **chest pain** and/or **dyspnea**
- Prognosis depends on extent of involvment
  - ➢ Usually **diffuse** (**circumferential**, rind-like) → **Poor** prognosis
  - ➢ Rarely, **localized** (**solitary**, well-circumscribed) → **Better** prognosis

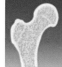
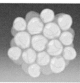
Pleural Thickening

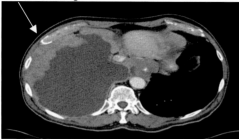

CT Scan courtesy of Dr. Thomas Dvorak, MD

- Clinical information (either from imaging or intraoperative findings) can be very helpful with diagnosis:
  - ➤ **Circumferential** pleural **thickening** is **highly suggestive** of **malignancy**
  - ➤ **Nodular pleural thickening** is also often **malignant**
- **IHC: (+)** for mesothelial markers; **loss of BAP1** or **MTAP** expression
- **FISH: CDKN2A (p16) deletion**
- **Molecular:** Often multiple chromosomal alterations
  - ➤ Frequent loss of tumor suppressors CDKN2A, BAP1, and NF2

Path Presenter

Haphazard spindle cells (sarcomatoid mesothelioma)

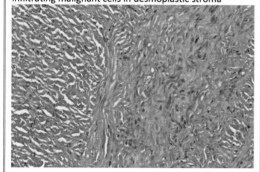

Infiltrating malignant cells in desmoplastic stroma

SARCOMATOID, DESMOPLASTIC, AND BIPHASIC MESOTHELIOMA

MORPHOLOGY

- **Sarcomatoid mesothelioma:**
  - ➤ **Spindle cell** appearance
  - ➤ Arranged in **fascicles** or **haphazardly**
  - ➤ Can see **heterologous elements** (e.g., rhabdomyosarcoma)
- **Desmoplastic mesothelioma:**
  - ➤ **Dense collagenized tissue** with malignant mesothelial cells
  - ➤ Either **patternless** or **storiform** pattern
  - ➤ Must be **≥50% of tumor**
  - ➤ **Invasion** into fat is most helpful feature to differentiate from organizing pleuritis
- **Biphasic mesothelioma:**
  - ➤ Contains BOTH epithelioid and sarcomatoid patterns, **each ≥10%**
  - ➤ Stromal invasion is often more difficult to recognize in these spindle cell proliferations as the invasive malignant cells are often deceptively bland → Use IHC liberally

OTHER HIGH YIELD POINTS

- Poorer prognosis than epithelioid mesotheliomas
  - ➤ **Desmoplastic mesothelioma** has a **particularly dismal prognosis** (often less than 6 months)
- **IHC:** Usually stain (at least focally **+**) with a broad spectrum pancytokeratin (can also help to demonstrate invasion)
  - ➤ **Loss of BAP1** is **very uncommon** in these types

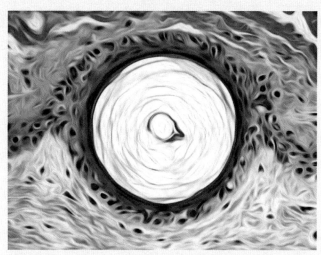

Skin appendage, H&E stain. Microscopic picture with digital filter applied for artistic effect, appearing as an "eye". Image courtesy: Ziad El-Zaatari, MD

CHAPTER 9: SKIN PATHOLOGY

Dinesh Pradhan, MD
Naomi Hardy, MD
Amandeep Kaur, MD
Akanksha Gupta, MD

NONNEOPLASTIC DERMATOPATHOLOGY
SPONGIOTIC DERMATOSES

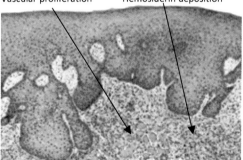

Spongiosis — Inflammation ± eosinophils

SPONGIOTIC DERMATITIS
MORPHOLOGY
- Intraepidermal intercellular edema (**spongiosis**)
- Presence of widened intercellular spaces between keratinocytes, with elongation of the intercellular bridges
- Superficial dermal inflammation ± **eosinophils** can be seen
- Acute (microvesicles), Chronic (acanthosis, psoriasiform hyperplasia, lichenification)

OTHER HIGH YIELD POINTS: ATOPIC DERMATITIS
- Clinically intensely pruritic vesicles, papules and plaques
- Aka **eczema or eczematous dermatitis**
- Histologically similar: atopic, contact, nummular dermatitis and Id reaction
- **Atopic Triad:** 1) Atopic dermatitis, 2) Seasonal allergies, 3) Asthma

Path Presenter

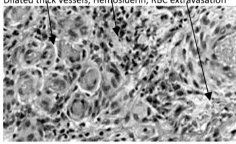

Vascular proliferation — Hemosiderin deposition

Dilated thick vessels, Hemosiderin, RBC extravasation

STASIS DERMATITIS
MORPHOLOGY
- Spongiotic dermatitis
- **Vascular proliferation,** dilated, thickened blood vessels in papillary dermis
- RBCs extravasation, **hemosiderin** deposition
- Can have chronic inflammation

OTHER HIGH YIELD POINTS
- Begins on **medial aspect on lower legs** but can become circumferential
- Clinically **mimics cellulitis**
- Prussian blue (iron stain) positive

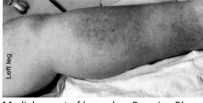
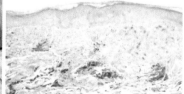

Medial aspect of lower leg; Prussian Blue stain, Credit: Jose Candido, MD

Path Presenter

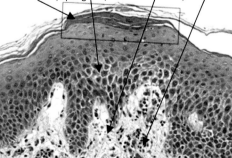

Parakeratosis, spongiosis, extravasated RBC, infiltrate

PITYRIASIS ROSEA
MORPHOLOGY
- Spongiotic dermatitis
- **Mounds of parakeratosis**
- Extravasated RBC.
- Superficial perivascular lymphohistiocytic infiltrate

OTHER HIGH YIELD POINTS
- Flu-like prodrome 2-3 weeks before eruption
- Clinically starts with **Herald patch** (salmon-colored plaque)
- The Herald patch increases in size over 48 hours.
- Eventually a **Christmas tree pattern** develops

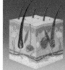

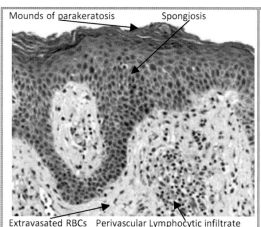

Mounds of parakeratosis — Spongiosis

Extravasated RBCs — Perivascular Lymphocytic infiltrate

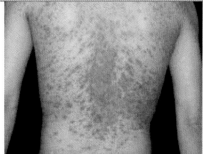

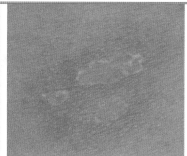

Herald's Patch and Christmas tree pattern, collarette scaling at the periphery of the lesion

Path Presenter

PSORIASIFORM DERMATOSES

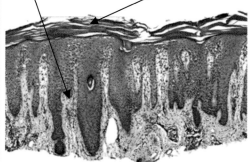

Regular psoriasiform hyperplasia Confluent parakeratosis

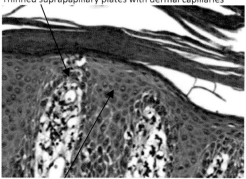

Thinned suprapapillary plates with dermal capillaries

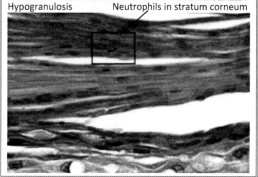

Hypogranulosis   Neutrophils in stratum corneum

PSORIASIS

MORPHOLOGY

- Regular **psoriasiform hyperplasia**
- **Confluent parakeratosis**
- Hypogranulosis
- Neutrophils in the stratum corneum/epidermis
- Suprapapillary plates are **thinned** beneath which are **dilated tortuous capillaries** within the dermal papillae

OTHER HIGH YIELD POINTS

- Clinically erythematous plaques and **silvery white scale**
- Mostly on **extensor** surfaces
- **Auspitz sign**: Pinpoint bleeding when scale is removed
- **Munro microabscess**: Neutrophil collection in corneal layer
- **Spongiform pustules of Kogoj**: Neutrophil collection in spinous layer
- Variants: Guttate, pustular, inverse, nail and erythrodermic psoriasis
- **Reiter Syndrome**: Conjunctivitis, Urethritis, Arthritis with psoriasiform skin lesions
- **Erythroderma - SCALP-ID** - Sezary syndrome, Contact dermatitis, Atopic dermatitis, Lymphoma/Leukemia, Psoriasis, Idiopathic, Drug

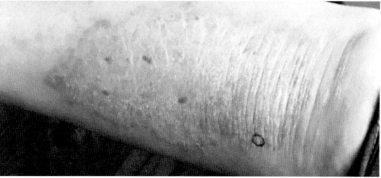

Silvery white scale

Path Presenter

LICHENOID AND INTERFACE DERMATOSES

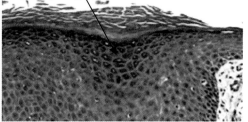

Saw tooth rete ridges   Lichenoid interface dermatitis

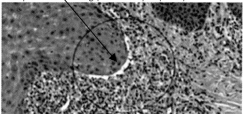

Wedge-shaped hypergranulosis

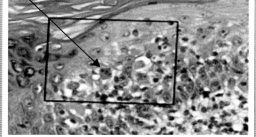

Subepidermal clefting ("Max Joseph space")

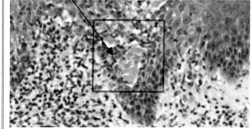

Civatte bodies

Basal keratinocyte liquefactive degeneration

LICHEN PLANUS
MORPHOLOGY
- **Lichenoid interface dermatitis** - Band-like inflammatory Infiltrate at dermoepidermal junction
- Compact hyperkeratosis without parakeratosis, compact hyperorthokeratosis
- Wedge-shaped hypergranulosis
- "**Saw-tooth**" rete ridges
- Basal keratinocyte liquefactive degeneration
- Subepidermal clefting ("Max Joseph space")
- **Civatte bodies** and **Colloid bodies** (necrotic keratinocytes in epidermis and dermis, respectively)

OTHER HIGH YIELD POINTS
- Clinically **p**ruritic, **p**urple, **p**lanar, and **p**olygonal **p**apules (5Ps)
- Distribution over flexural wrists, ankles, arms, legs, trunks, genitalia, and oral mucosa. The face is rarely affected
- Wickham striae: reticulate network of lacy white scaling
- Main differential - Benign Lichenoid Keratosis (single lesion on trunk)
- Direct immunofluorescence (DIF) - Predominantly IgM and fibrin staining of colloid bodies

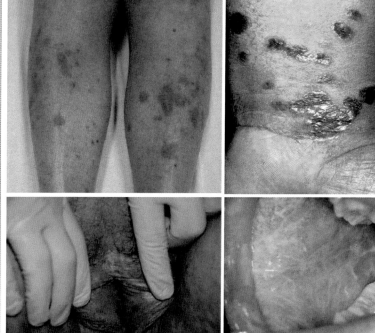

Path Presenter

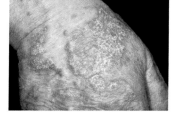

9. SKIN PATHOLOGY

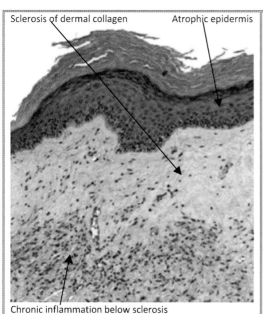

Sclerosis of dermal collagen — Atrophic epidermis

Chronic inflammation below sclerosis

LICHEN SCLEROSUS ET ATROPHICUS
MORPHOLOGY
- Homogenization/ **sclerosis of dermal collagen**
- Chronic inflammation below edema and homogenization
- Atrophic epidermis
- Early lesions - lichenoid interface dermatitis

OTHER HIGH YIELD POINTS
- Aka lichen sclerosus or **balanitis xerotica** obliterans (glans penis)
- Predilection for anogenital skin
- Clinically ivory white plaques with **cigarette paper**-like appearance

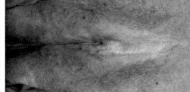

Courtesy: Mikael Häggström, MD

Path Presenter

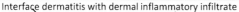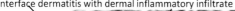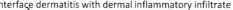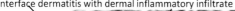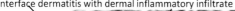

Interface dermatitis with dermal inflammatory infiltrate

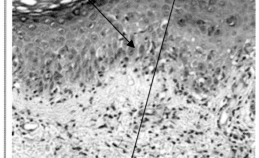

Epidermal necrosis — Subepidermal bullae

ERYTHEMA MULTIFORME
MORPHOLOGY
- **Erythema multiforme (EM)** - **Interface dermatitis** with necrotic keratinocytes
- Stevens-Johnson syndrome/toxic epidermal necrolysis (SJS/TEN) - **Full-thickness epidermal necrosis**
- **Subepidermal bullae** with basement membrane in bullae roof due to dermal edema
- Severe **dermal perivascular inflammatory infiltrate** (lymphocytes)
- Eosinophils may be present, but neutrophils are sparse or absent
- Overlying epidermis often demonstrates **liquefactive necrosis** and degeneration, **dyskeratotic keratinocytes**
- May also have dermoepidermal bullae with basal lamina at floor of bullae
- No leukocytoclasis, no microabscesses, no festooning of dermal papillae

OTHER HIGH YIELD POINTS
- On spectrum with SJS/TEN
- Reactive in nature (mainly due to **HSV, Mycoplasma, or Drug**)
- SJS/TEN - Serious, life-threatening reaction
- EM - Acute, self-limited disease
- Clinically, targetoid dusky lesions on acral sites and face

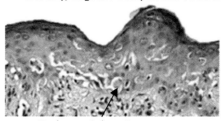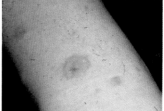

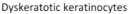

Dyskeratotic keratinocytes   Targetoid dusky lesion

Path Presenter

CONNECTIVE TISSUE/SOFT TISSUE DISEASES

Vacuolar interface dermatitis   Increased dermal mucin

Superficial & deep perivascular & periadnexal infiltrate

Path Presenter

LUPUS ERYTHEMATOSUS (LE)
MORPHOLOGY
- **Vacuolar interface dermatitis** with dyskeratotic keratinocytes
- Thickened basement membrane
- **Superficial and deep** perivascular and periadnexal lymphohistiocytic infiltrate
- Increased **dermal mucin**

OTHER HIGH YIELD POINTS
- Acute and subacute cutaneous LE: Associated with systemic diseases
- Chronic cutaneous LE /discoid LE (DLE)-usually only limited to the skin
- Immunofluorescence: IgM, IgG, C3 - granular BM deposition
- Tumid LE - No interface dermatitis

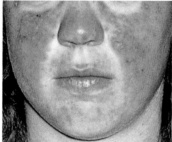
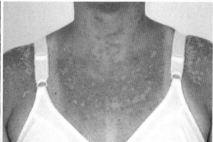

GRANULOMATOUS DISEASES

Central mucin with palisaded histiocytes

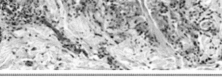

Classic granuloma annulare

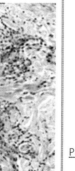

GRANULOMA ANNULARE (GA)
MORPHOLOGY
- **Central mucin** with surrounding palisaded histiocytes
- Mucin can be stained with **Alcian blue** or **colloidal iron**
- Histologic variants include classic (or palisading) GA, interstitial GA, deep (or subcutaneous) GA, and perforating GA
- Deep GA - in subcutaneous tissues
- Interstitial pattern - Interstitial histiocytes

OTHER HIGH YIELD POINTS
- Clinically rashes are often **annular** (round) or arcuate non-scaly red-brown plaques with **central clearing**
- Most commonly on **arms/legs** or **back of hands/feet**
- **Self-limited** dermatoses
- Unknown etiology

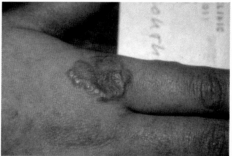
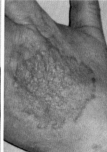

Annular / arcuate red brown plaque

Path Presenter

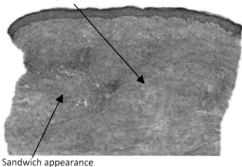

Altered collagen (necrobiosis)

Sandwich appearance

NECROBIOSIS LIPOIDICA
MORPHOLOGY
- **Layers of altered collagen (necrobiosis)** alternating with layers of inflammation (**sandwich appearance**)
- Epithelioid granulomas or cholesterol clefts may be seen

OTHER HIGH YIELD POINTS
- Often involves **bilateral shins**
- Differential diagnosis - Granuloma Annulare, Rheumatoid nodule
- Associated with diabetes - aka Necrobiosis lipoidica diabeticorum (NLD)

Path Presenter

VESICULOBULLOUS DERMATOSES

Intraepidermal vesicle

Suprabasilar acantholysis ("tombstoning")

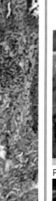

Perivascular and interstitial infiltrate

Follicular extension of acantholysis

Path Presenter

PEMPHIGUS VULGARIS
MORPHOLOGY
- May show **intraepidermal vesicles** with **eosinophilic spongiosis** in early stages
- Well-developed lesions show **intraepidermal split** immediately above basal layer leaving a **tombstone** row of basal keratinocytes
- **Follicular extension** of acantholysis
- Superficial **perivascular and interstitial** lymphocytes and eosinophils

OTHER HIGH YIELD POINTS
- Clinically **painful flaccid blisters and erosions** – involving the skin as well as **mucosa**, including **oral mucosa**, esophagus, conjunctiva, nasal mucosa, vagina, labia, anus.
- Positive **Nikolsky sign**: extension of the epidermis laterally with slight pressure/rubbing.
- Most common type of pemphigus
- Autoantibodies directed against **desmoglein 1 and/or 3**
- Direct immunofluorescence - IgG and C3 in a **chicken-wire/net-like pattern**
- IIF and ELISA detect antibodies.

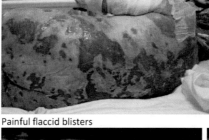

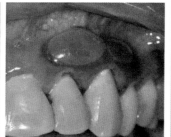

Painful flaccid blisters

Almost always involves oral mucosa

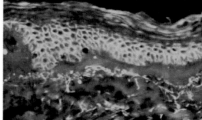

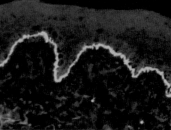

PV: Direct DIF- net-like pattern with IgG and C3

Bullous Pemphigoid: Linear IgG in DEJ

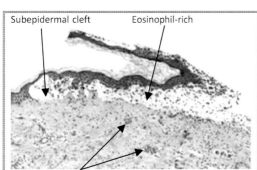

Subepidermal cleft · Eosinophil-rich

Inflammatory infiltrate
Eosinophilic spongiosis

Subepidermal split with eosinophils

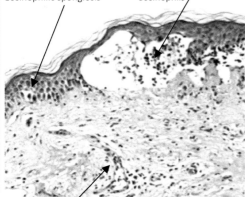

Superficial perivascular and interstitial inflammatory infiltrate of lymphocytes and eosinophils

Immunoflorescence:
A. Bullous Pemphigoid: Linear staining of IgG at DEJ
B. Pemphigus Vulgaris: IgG and C3 in a chicken-wire / net-like pattern
C. Dermatitis Herpetiformis: Granular IgA in dermal papillae on DIF
D. Linear IgA: Linear IgA at DEJ (not shown)

BULLOUS PEMPHIGOID (BP)
MORPHOLOGY
- **Subepidermal blister** with **eosinophils**
- At the edge of the blister, **eosinophilic spongiosis** is often seen
- A superficial **perivascular and interstitial** inflammatory infiltrate of lymphocytes and eosinophils is present in the dermis
- The **urticarial** variant clinically of BP may only demonstrate eosinophilic spongiosis on biopsy

OTHER HIGH YIELD POINTS
- Clinically, symmetric, **tense bullae, exquisitely pruritic, crusting erosions**
- Usually affects **older adults**
- Direct **immunofluorescence shows linear deposition** of IgG and C3 at dermoepidermal junction (DEJ) In the perilesional skin
- Autoantibodies to **BPAG1 and BPAG2 on hemidesmosomes** at DEJ
- Drug-induced pemphigoid: diuretics (furosemide), captopril, amoxicillin etc.
- Salt-split skin distinguishes between BP and epidermolysis bullosa acquisita

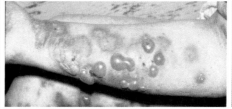
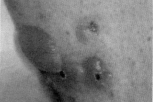

Bullous Pemphigoid: Pruritic tense bullae, with crusting erosions

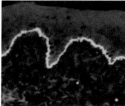
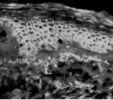
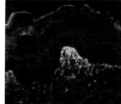

A: Bullous Pemphigoid   B: Pemphigus Vulgaris   C. Dermatitis Herpetiformis

Path Presenter

Subepidermal split with neutrophils

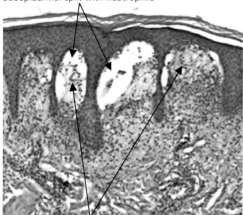

Papillary dermal microabscesses

DERMATITIS HERPETIFORMIS
MORPHOLOGY
- Subepidermal split with numerous neutrophils, and rare eosinophils
- **Papillary dermal microabscesses**

OTHER HIGH YIELD POINTS
- Clinically, symmetrically involves elbows, knees, back of neck, sacrum, posterior scalp, with urticarial papules/plaques
- intense **pruritus**, excoriations/erosions
- Highly associated with **Celiac disease**/ gluten-sensitive enteropathy
- **Granular IgA** in dermal papillae on DIF
- **IgA** antibodies to gluten-**tissue transglutaminase** (t-TG), which is found in the gut.

Path Presenter

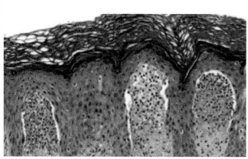

Papillary dermal microabscesses, numerous neutrophils

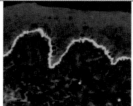 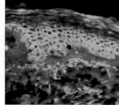 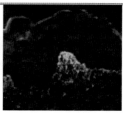

A: Bullous Pemphigoid   B: Pemphigus Vulgaris   C. Dermatitis Herpetiformis

A. Bullous Pemphigoid: Linear staining of IgG at DEJ
B. Pemphigus Vulgaris: IgG and C3 in a chicken-wire / net-like pattern
C. Dermatitis Herpetiformis: Granular IgA in dermal papillae on DIF

VASCULITIS AND VASCULOPATHY

Papillary dermal edema

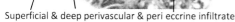

Superficial & deep perivascular & peri eccrine infiltrate

Path Presenter

PERNIO
MORPHOLOGY

- Superficial and deep perivascular infiltrate of lymphocytes
- Prominent peri eccrine inflammatory infiltrates
- **Papillary dermal edema**

OTHER HIGH YIELD POINTS

- aka chilblains
- Caused by **exposure to cold**, damp conditions
- Tender violaceous papules mostly on **acral skin**, ears, and nose
- Most common association is with systemic lupus erythematosus

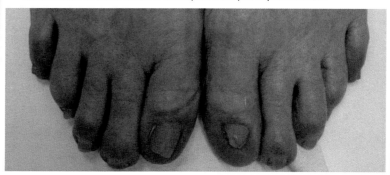

Perivascular neutrophils, fibrinoid necrosis, Karyorrhexis

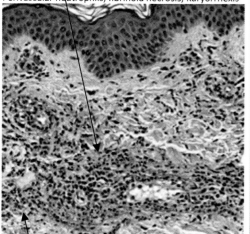

RBCs extravasation

LEUKOCYTOCLASTIC VASCULITIS
MORPHOLOGY

- **Fibrinoid necrosis** of vessel walls
- Endothelial cell swelling
- Perivascular neutrophilic infiltrate
- **Karyorrhexis (leukocytoclasia**, nuclear dust)
- RBCs extravasation

OTHER HIGH YIELD POINTS

- Clinically, non-blanching **palpable purpura**, mostly on **lower legs**
- Immune complexes deposition in blood vessel walls
- Differential diagnosis – Atrophie blanche/ livedoid vasculopathy

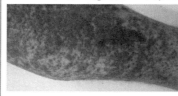

Path Presenter

PANNICULITIDES

Septal Panniculitis with thickened fibrous septa

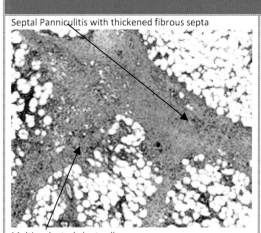

Multinucleated giant cells

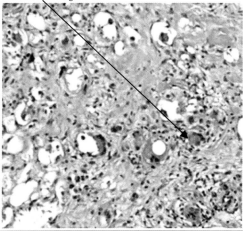

ERYTHEMA NODOSUM
MORPHOLOGY
- **Septal Panniculitis**
- **Thickening** of fibrous septa, with lymphohistiocytic infiltrate
- Multinucleated **giant cells**, granulomas/lipogranulomas/**Miescher radial granulomas**

OTHER HIGH YIELD POINTS
- Clinically, red, **tender nodules on the pretibial area**
- Most often in young to middle-aged females
- Associated with **infection as well as drugs**
- Systemic symptoms may be present
- Differential diagnosis – erythema induratum (lobular panniculitis)

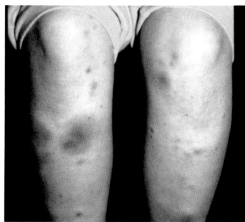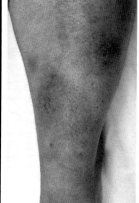

Path Presenter

BACTERIAL INFECTIONS

Subcorneal splitting

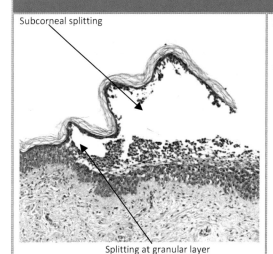

Splitting at granular layer

Path Presenter

STAPHYLOCOCCAL SCALDED SKIN SYNDROME
MORPHOLOGY
- **Subcorneal splitting** of epidermis at granular layer

OTHER HIGH YIELD POINTS
- Extremely tender flaccid blisters in infants and young children
- Usually resolves spontaneously
- Due to **exfoliatin A and B from strains of Staphylococcus aureus**
- Differential diagnosis-
  - Bullous Impetigo – direct infection, cocci present
  - Toxic Epidermal Necrolysis – subepidermal split
  - Pemphigus Foliaceous – DIF positive

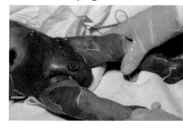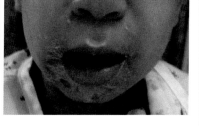

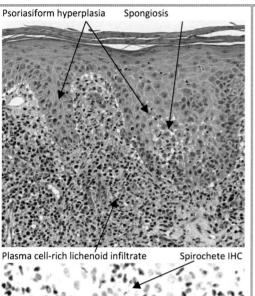

Psoriasiform hyperplasia   Spongiosis

Plasma cell-rich lichenoid infiltrate   Spirochete IHC

SYPHILIS
MORPHOLOGY
- Great mimicker - variable histology
- Usually **psoriasiform hyperplasia, spongiosis, and interface changes**
- **Plasma cell-rich infiltrate,** sometimes **lichenoid**

OTHER HIGH YIELD POINTS
- Secondary syphilis (SS) occurs 1-2 months after primary chancre
- Maculopapular patches or plaques usually involving **palms and soles**
- **Spirochete immunostain is positive**
- Warthin-Starry silver stains and PCR – less sensitive

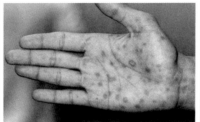
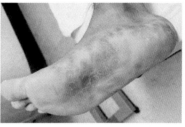

Path Presenter

VIRAL INFECTIONS

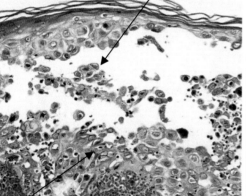

Intraepidermal vesicle with acantholysis

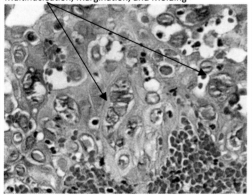

Multinucleation, Margination, and Molding

HERPESVIRUS/ HERPES ZOSTER/ VARICELLA
MORPHOLOGY
- **Intraepidermal vesicle** with acantholysis and ballooning of keratinocytes
- **3M - Multinucleation, Margination, and Molding** of nucleus

OTHER HIGH YIELD POINTS
- HSV – **Clear, fluid-filled vesicles**
- Herpes Zoster – fever and malaise followed by **grouped vesicles** in dermatome distribution
- Varicella – vesicles at different stages
- **HSV-1, HSV-2, or VZV** immunostain **(+)**
- DIF, In-situ hybridization, serologic testing and PCR can be done

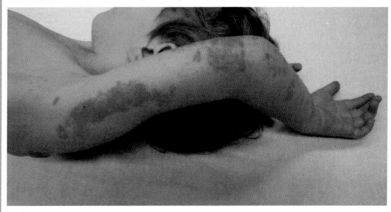

Path Presenter

Mounds of parakeratosis   Papillomatosis

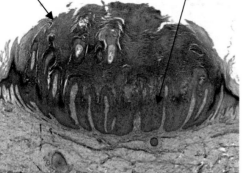

Keratohyalin granules and Koilocytes

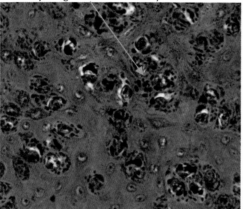

VERRUCA VULGARIS (VV)
MORPHOLOGY
- Cup shaped papillomatosis
- Mounds of parakeratosis (**church spires**)
- Prominent keratohyalin granules and **koilocytes**

OTHER HIGH YIELD POINTS
- Mostly involves fingers and dorsal hands (VV), and palms and soles (palmoplantar wart) of children
- Variants – Common wart (VV), Palmoplantar wart (Myrmecia) and Flat wart (verruca plana)
- Due to HPV – most common types include 1, 2, 3, 4, 7, and 10
- **Condyloma acuminatum** – Other HPV related lesion (**HPV 6,11**) involving genitalia

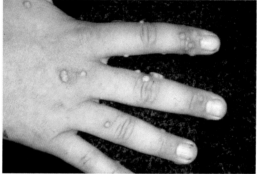

Path Presenter

Lobulated lesion, epidermal acanthosis, cup-like

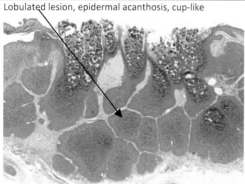

Molluscum bodies / Henderson-Patterson bodies

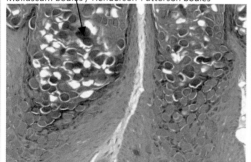

MOLLUSCUM CONTAGIOSUM
MORPHOLOGY
- Crater with distinct **Molluscum bodies/Henderson-Patterson bodies** (eosinophilic to basophilic large intracytoplasmic inclusions)
- Epidermal acanthosis with **cup-shaped lesion**
- Low power: **lobulated**, well-circumscribed, somewhat crateriform intradermal pseudotumor-like lesion

OTHER HIGH YIELD POINTS
- Clinically, pearly papules with **central umbilication** in young children
- Caused by **Molluscum contagiosum virus (Poxvirus)**

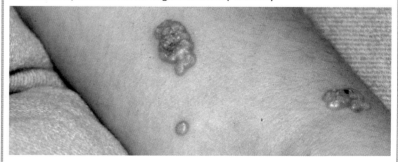

Path Presenter

FUNGAL INFECTIONS

Fungal hyphae in stratum corneum

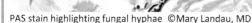

Courtesy: Dutch Berry, MD

PAS stain highlighting fungal hyphae ©Mary Landau, MD

DERMATOPHYTOSIS/TINEA
MORPHOLOGY
- **Hyphae in stratum corneum**
- Psoriasiform hyperplasia and/or spongiosis
- Mild to moderate inflammation usually with some **neutrophils**
- Neutrophils in the cornified layer
- **Sandwich sign**: neutrophils between layers of orthokeratosis or parakeratosis

OTHER HIGH YIELD POINTS
- Clinically, annular plaque with scale at border
- **PAS or GMS highlights hyphae**
- Infection by dermatophytes – Trichophyton, Epidermophyton, and Microsporum
- **Majocchi granuloma** – Fungal hyphae extending into hair follicles'

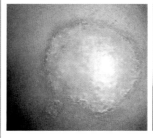
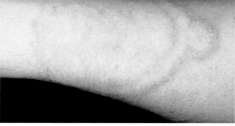

Path Presenter

ARTHROPODS

Wedge-shaped infiltrate rich in eosinophils

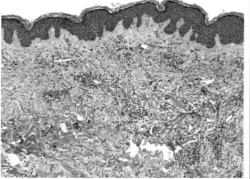

Perivascular infiltrate with lymphocytes and eosinophils

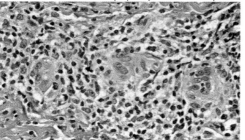

ARTHROPOD BITE REACTION
MORPHOLOGY
- **Wedge-shaped** perivascular lymphocytic **infiltrate with eosinophils**
- **Insect bites** - prominent papillary dermal edema, spongiosis, blister, epidermal necrosis
- **Tick bite** - mouth part may be seen
- **Spider bites** - more neutrophils

OTHER HIGH YIELD POINTS
- Clinically variable presentations - erythematous papule, plaque, nodule, vesicle, or bulla
- Hypersensitivity reaction

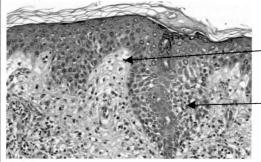

Papillary dermal edema

Spongiosis

Path Presenter

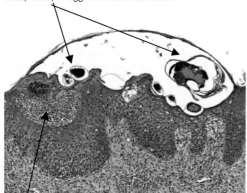

Mite, feces, or eggs in stratum corneum

Eosinophilic Spongiosis

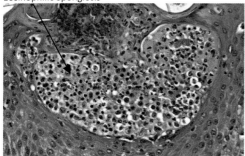

Eosinophil – rich infiltrate

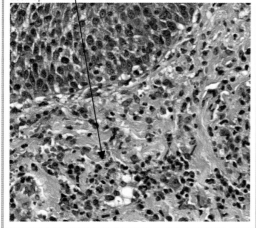

SCABIES

MORPHOLOGY

- Scabies mite, ova or scybala is found within the stratum corneum
- Spongiosis and eosinophilic spongiosis may be present to varying degrees within the epidermis
- In the dermis, a superficial and deep perivascular and interstitial inflammatory infiltrate is present with prominent numbers of eosinophils

OTHER HIGH YIELD POINTS

- Usually involves interdigital areas, flexures, and intergluteal folds
- Papulovesicular, nodules or Norwegian (crusted)
- Caused by **Sarcoptes scabiei**

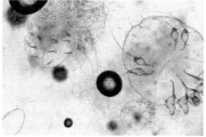

Scabies mite   Flexural papulovesicular rashes

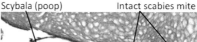

Scybala (poop)   Intact scabies mite

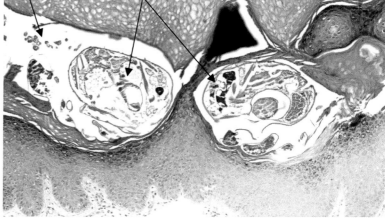

Path Presenter

NEOPLASTIC DERMATOPATHOLOGY

WHO CLASSIFICATION OF SKIN TUMORS

- Keratinocytic tumors
- Appendageal tumors
- Melanocytic tumors
- Other (soft tissue tumors and tumors of hematopoietic and lymphoid origin)

KERATINOCYTIC TUMORS/LESIONS AND CYSTS

- Seborrheic keratosis
- Solar lentigo
- Epidermal inclusion cyst (EIC)
- Dermoid cyst
- Pilar/Trichilemmal cyst
- Verruca vulgaris
- Actinic keratosis
- Squamous cell carcinoma in situ (SCCIS, Bowen disease)
- Squamous cell carcinoma (SCC)

	• Basal cell carcinoma (BCC) • Merkel cell carcinoma

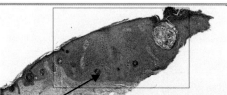

Acanthosis with hyperkeratosis   Horn cysts

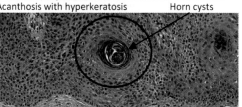

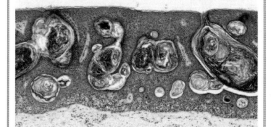

SEBORRHEIC KERATOSIS

MORPHOLOGY

- Clinical: Brown, waxy "stuck-on" papule
- Microscopy: **Acanthosis with hyperkeratosis** and hyperpigmentation, anastomosing rete, **horn cysts** with lamellated keratin, and without atypia

OTHER HIGH YIELD POINTS

- Intraepidermal basaloid keratinocytic proliferation with multiple variants (no clinical or prognostic significance)
- Common in the middle-aged and elderly with incidence increasing with age
- Leser-Trélat sign: Paraneoplastic phenomenon of rapid growth of multiple seborrheic keratoses associated with gastrointestinal adenocarcinoma

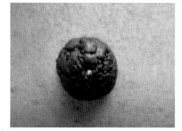
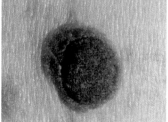

Path Presenter

SOLAR LENTIGO

MORPHOLOGY

- Clinical: **Hyperpigmented macule**
- Microscopy: **"Dirty feet"** or finger-like proliferation of hyperpigmented rete growing down from the epidermis

OTHER HIGH YIELD POINTS

- Accumulation of melanin in keratinocytes due to sun exposure
- Also known as age spot and found on sun-exposed skin of the elderly
- Pigmentation may be irregular, and there may be solar elastosis and some chronic inflammation in the dermis

Path Presenter

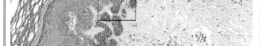

Hyperpigmented macule   "Dirty feet"

Squamous-lined cyst with granular layer and containing laminated keratin

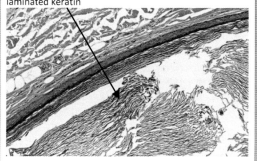

EPIDERMAL INCLUSION CYST (EIC)

MORPHOLOGY

- Gross: Subcutaneous cyst filled with thick yellow keratinaceous debris
- Microscopy: Lined by **squamous epithelium with granular layer and containing laminated (basket weave) keratin**

OTHER HIGH YIELD POINTS

- Acquired unilocular cyst due to trauma
- May rupture and become inflamed

Path Presenter

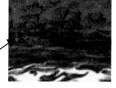

Granular layer

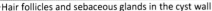

Hair follicles and sebaceous glands in the cyst wall

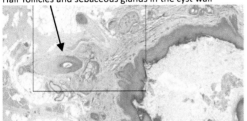

DERMOID CYST
MORPHOLOGY
- Like EIC, but with **hair follicles and sebaceous glands**

OTHER HIGH YIELD POINTS
- Present at birth

Path Presenter

Dense "wet" keratin with absent granular layer

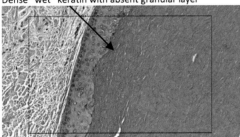

PILAR/TRICHILEMMAL CYST
MORPHOLOGY
- Filled with **dense, "wet" eosinophilic keratin**
- Stratified squamous epithelium with an **absent granular layer**

OTHER HIGH YIELD POINTS
- Scalp/head and neck location

Path Presenter

"Church spire" papillae

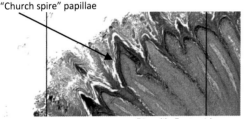

"Cup-like" rete ridges

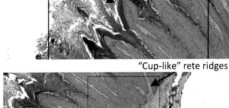

VERRUCA VULGARIS
MORPHOLOGY
- Clinical: Flesh-colored papule with a rough surface
- Microscopy: **"Church spire" papillae,** tiered parakeratosis, **"Cup-like" rete** with inward bending of rete at the base of the lesion, and increased vasculature in the papillary dermis (bleeds easily)

OTHER HIGH YIELD POINTS
- HPV-induced, circumscribed lesion
- Koilocytes or vacuolated keratinocytes with raisin-like nuclei may be variably present
- Verruca plana = flat wart

Path Presenter

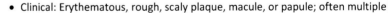

ACTINIC KERATOSIS
MORPHOLOGY
- Clinical: Erythematous, rough, scaly plaque, macule, or papule; often multiple
- Microscopy: **Basal atypia** limited to the lower third of the epidermis with **"Flag sign"** of alternating orthokeratosis and parakeratosis and solar elastosis in the dermis

OTHER HIGH YIELD POINTS
- Intraepidermal keratinocytic lesion due to sun damage
- Precancerous, risk of malignancy (progression to SCC) is ~8-20% per year
- Sparing of cutaneous adnexa in most circumstances, if extending down the hair follicle and sweat duct -> proliferative actinic keratosis

Path Presenter

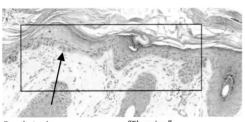

Basal atypia   "Flag sign"

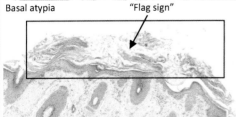

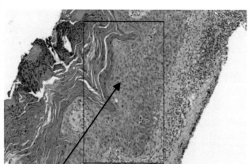

Full thickness dysplasia with loss of the granular layer; can have a pagetoid appearance

SQUAMOUS CELL CARCINOMA IN-SITU (SCCIS OR BOWEN DISEASE)

MORPHOLOGY

- **Full thickness dysplasia** of the epidermis without invasion -> Loss of granular layer
- Can have a **pagetoid appearance**

OTHER HIGH YIELD POINTS

- No epidermal maturation
- Epidermis appears disorganized
- Important differential is Paget disease and melanoma

Path Presenter

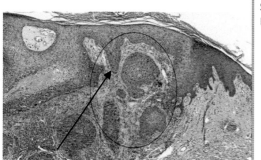

Squamous nests arising from the epidermis and invading the dermis

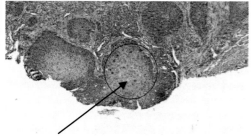

Deep keratinization

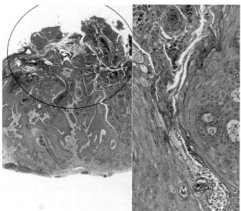

Keratoacanthoma type with crateriform architecture (circled, left) and glassy, pale pink cytoplasm (right)

SQUAMOUS CELL CARCINOMA (SCC)

MORPHOLOGY

- Nests of atypical squamous cells arise from the epidermis and **invade the dermis**
- Findings that suggest invasion
  - ➤ Jagged interface with dermis
  - ➤ Aberrant **deep keratinization**
  - ➤ Single cell invasion
- Evidence of squamous differentiation (keratinization and intercellular bridges)
  - ➤ Dyskeratotic cells = squamous differentiation
- Often associated with AK or SCCIS

OTHER HIGH YIELD POINTS

- Second most common form of skin cancer (20% of cutaneous malignancies)
- Locally destructive; metastatic potential
  - ➤ Risk factors for metastasis (high risk): location (ear, lip), size (>2cm), depth, evidence of perineural invasion, evidence of desmoplastic features
- Tx: Depends on size, location, and depth of invasion: Excision, Mohs micrographic surgery, Radiation
- Variants:
  - ➤ *Keratoacanthoma* - well-differentiated variant of SCC that spontaneously regresses in most cases. Typically composed of large, **crateriform** (cup-like) lesion filled with abundant keratin debris and composed of cells with **glassy, pale pink cytoplasm**
  - ➤ *Acantholytic SCC* – acantholysis with large epithelioid cells with dense eosinophilic cytoplasm and scattered dyskeratotic (apoptotic) cells
  - ➤ *Verrucous SCC* – Extremely well-differentiated, low-risk with pushing border and acanthotic papilla. NO infiltrative growth. Associated inflammation at base.
  - ➤ *Desmoplastic SCC* – tumor cells become spindled/sarcomatoid

- *HMWCKs, p63, and p40 are the most sensitive markers for poorly differentiated and spindle cell/sarcomatoid SCC (Pankeratin can be lost in poorly differentiated and spindle cell tumors)

Path Presenter

Pearly pink/tan papule

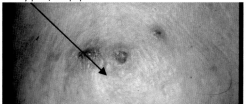

Basaloid cells with retraction and peripheral palisading (nodular type)

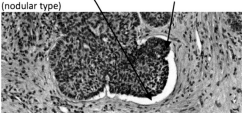

Infiltrative type

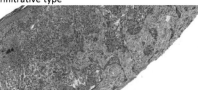

Fibroepithelioma of Pinkus

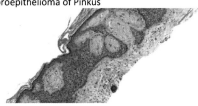

BASAL CELL CARCINOMA

MORPHOLOGY

- Clinical: Nodular variant presents as a pearly papule, often with telangiectasia and/or ulceration
- Microscopy: Basaloid appearance at low power (high N:C ratio) often with an epidermal connection, **peripheral palisading, and retraction from the surrounding stroma**
- Many subtypes that vary in morphology
  - ➢ Nodular – Large, rounded nests
  - ➢ Micronodular* – smaller nests
  - ➢ Superficial – superficial nests separated by uninvolved areas
  - ➢ Infiltrative*- small infiltrative cords
  - ➢ Sclerosing/morpheic* - infiltrative nests with desmoplastic stroma
  - ➢ Basosquamous* - Prominent areas of squamous differentiation
  - ➢ Infundibulocystic – resemble hair follicle
  - ➢ Fibroepithelioma of Pinkus – anastomosing cords

*Aggressive variants

OTHER HIGH YIELD POINTS

- Most common malignancy in humans
- Locally aggressive and destructive behavior
- Very low metastatic potential (< 0.1%)
- Pediatric BCC? -> consider Gorlin's Syndrome
- Note: Some focal keratinization may be present
- May mimic adnexal structures, making margins challenging. However, basal cell carcinoma tumor cells should have darker chromatin, more apoptosis and mitoses, and paler cytoplasm than the hair follicles.
- IHC: BerEP4 will stain **BCC** but **not SCC**

Path Presenter

Dermal tumor composed of basaloid islands of cells

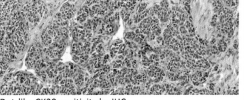

Dot-like CK20 positivity by IHC

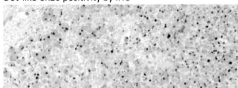

MERKEL CELL CARCINOMA

MORPHOLOGY

- Cutaneous neuroendocrine carcinoma
- Dermal-based tumor with **basaloid islands in the dermis**
- Can resemble BCC on low power
- Composed of cells with salt and pepper chromatin

OTHER HIGH YIELD POINTS

- High mitotic rate and apoptotic index
- **Dot-like CK20 positivity**
- **P63**+ have a worse prognosis

Path Presenter

APPENDAGEAL TUMORS

SEBACEOUS, FOLLICULAR, AND APOCRINE/ECCRINE TUMORS	
- Sebaceous hyperplasia - Sebaceous adenoma - Sebaceous carcinoma - Nevus sebaceus of Jadassohn - Trichofolliculoma	- Chondroid syringoma - Eccrine poroma - Hidradenoma papilliferum - Syringocystadenoma papilliferum - Acrospiroma - Spiradenoma

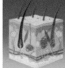

• Trichilemmoma • Pilomatrixoma (Calcifying Epithelioma of Malherbe) • Tumor of follicular infundibulum • Trichoepithelioma • Fibrofolliculoma/Trichodiscoma	• Cylindroma • Syringoma • Microcystic adnexal carcinoma • Extramammary Paget's disease (EMPD)

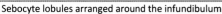

Sebocyte lobules arranged around the infundibulum

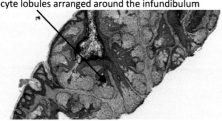

No thickening of the peripheral germinative layer

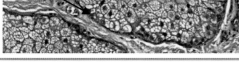

SEBACEOUS HYPERPLASIA
MORPHOLOGY
- Clinical: yellow papule with a central dimple
- Microscopic: Lobules of sebocytes are arranged around the infundibulum of a **central hair follicle without thickening of the peripheral germinative layer**

OTHER HIGH YIELD POINTS
- Nose or cheeks of the elderly
- Umbilicated yellowish papules
- No cytologic atypia

Path Presenter

Ulcerated papule

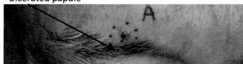

multilobulated proliferation of sebaceous glands

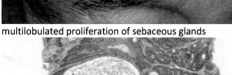

Expansion of the peripheral germinative layer (<50%)

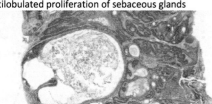

SEBACEOUS ADENOMA
MORPHOLOGY
- Clinical: **ulcerated papule,** mostly in the **head and neck,** particularly on the **face and scalp**
- Microscopic: well-circumscribed, **multilobulated proliferation of sebaceous glands with expansion of the peripheral germinative layer of more than 2 layers (<50%)**

OTHER HIGH YIELD POINTS
- Similar low power look to sebaceous hyperplasia but larger nodular aggregates with downward growth from epidermis
- Predominance (> 50%) of sebocytes. Cytologic atypia not prominent
  ➤ Composed of > 50% germinative/basaloid cells -> Sebaceoma (still has a well-circumscribed lobulated appearance)
- Associated with **Muir Torre** if multiple in younger patients <50 yo
  ➤ AD form of Lynch syndrome
  ➤ Mutations in one of the DNA mismatch repair genes, MLH1, MSH2, MSH6
  ➤ Associated with gastrointestinal carcinomas and KAs of skin

Path Presenter

Infiltrative appearance

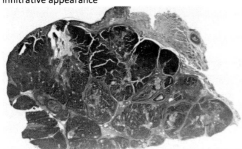

SEBACEOUS CARCINOMA
MORPHOLOGY
- Microscopic: **>50% expansion** of the peripheral germinative layer with necrosis and a more infiltrative appearance
- Clear cells often present but vary greatly in number
- Show prominent **cytologic atypia and pleomorphism**
- Mitotic figures, including atypical forms, are usually abundant
- IHC: May stain **(+)** with Adipophilin, AR, EMA, and Factor XIIIa

OTHER HIGH YIELD POINTS
- Aggressive tumors with a high incidence of metastasis (> 30%)
- Strong association with Muir-Torre syndrome if patients have multiple

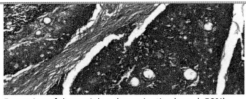

Expansion of the peripheral germinative layer (>50%)

- Sebaceous tumors (Genes implicated include MLH1, MSH2, MSH6, PMS2)
- Eyelids are the most common site (~ 75% of cases)
- Periocular or extraocular

Path Presenter

"Cobblestone" lesion

Hamartoma of excess sebaceous glands high in the dermis with overlying alopecia

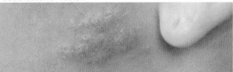

NEVUS SEBACEUS OF JADASSOHN (ORGANOID NEVUS)
MORPHOLOGY
- Clinical: **"Cobblestone" greasy-appearing lesion**
- Microscopic: **Hamartoma of excess sebaceous glands,** absent or abortive hair follicles, and **dilated ectopic apocrine glands**

OTHER HIGH YIELD POINTS
- Present at birth on the head and neck
- Cerebriform looking initially, then more verrucoid during puberty
- In older adults, you can see other tumors arising in them like syringocystadenoma papilliferum, trichilemmoma, and basal cell carcinoma

Path Presenter

Centrally dilated hair follicle with primitive smaller hair follicles in the periphery

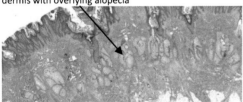

TRICHOFOLLICULOMA
MORPHOLOGY
- **Centrally dilated hair follicle filled with keratinaceous debris** and lined by squamous epithelium with a thin granular layer and dilated hair follicles that have several **radiating primitive smaller hair follicles in the periphery**

OTHER HIGH YIELD POINTS
- Communicates with the epidermis

Path Presenter

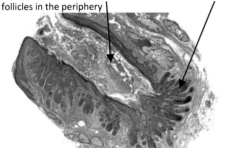

Pale to clear-staining cytoplasm, peripheral palisading of basaloid cells, and thickened pink basement membrane in the periphery

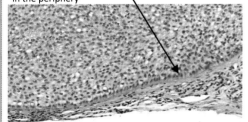

TRICHILEMMOMA
MORPHOLOGY
- Overall circumscribed looking lobular proliferation of **mature squamoid cells with pale to clear-staining cytoplasm, peripheral palisading of basaloid cells, and thickened pink basement membrane in the periphery**

OTHER HIGH YIELD POINTS
- Almost exclusively on the face
- Multiple broad connections to epidermis and follicles
- Associated with Cowden's Syndrome:
  - ➤ COWden's Syndrome
  - ➤ PTEN mutation (tumor suppressor) on chromosome 10
  - ➤ Multiple hamartomas (mouth, GIT)
  - ➤ Thyroid carcinoma (usually Follicular)
  - ➤ Breast Cancer (very high risk)
  - ➤ Endometrial Cancer
  - ➤ Macrocephaly
  - ➤ TrichileMMOOOOmas

Path Presenter

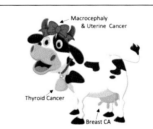

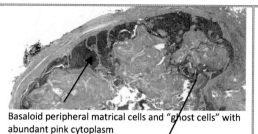

Basaloid peripheral matrical cells and "ghost cells" with abundant pink cytoplasm

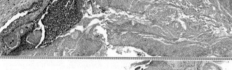
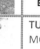

PILOMATRICOMA (CALCIFYING EPITHELIOMA OF MALHERBE)
MORPHOLOGY
- Sharply circumscribed dermal mass with **basaloid peripheral matrical cells and "ghost cells" with abundant pink cytoplasm** and no nucleus

OTHER HIGH YIELD POINTS
- Benign tumor arising from hair matrix
- Usually, children and young adults in head, neck or upper extremities
- Dystrophic calcification is frequently seen
- Foreign-body giant cell reaction surrounding the tumor is common
- Aggressive pilomatrixoma: Benign tumor arising from hair matrix
- Infiltrative, prominent nucleoli, necrosis, mitoses, sarcomatoid features, transition to squamous -> Pilomatrical Carcinoma

Path Presenter

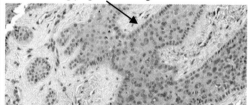

Reticulated cords and nests of pale pink staining, monotonous glycogen-containing cells

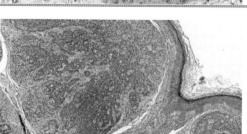

TUMOR OF FOLLICULAR INFUNDIBULUM
MORPHOLOGY
- **Acanthoma** composed of pale pink cells and sometimes clear cells
- The tumour forms **anastomosing narrow strands** that run parallel to the epidermis. These strands have **peripheral palisading of basaloid cells**
- Subepidermal tumor of **reticulated cords and nests of pale pink staining, monotonous glycogen containing cells**

OTHER HIGH YIELD POINTS
- Arise in the head and neck, and clinically resemble superficial basal cell carcinoma
- Can mimic Fibroepithelioma of Pinkus (those are basaloid, these are pink)
- No significant atypia or pleomorphism

Path Presenter

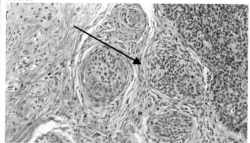

Basaloid islands of cells with papillary mesenchymal bodies

TRICHOEPITHELIOMA
MORPHOLOGY
- Dermal tumor of **basaloid islands of cells** with fibroblastic looking stroma known as **papillary mesenchymal bodies**/rudimentary hair follicles (aggregates of abortive attempts to form papillary mesenchyme)

OTHER HIGH YIELD POINTS
- Desmoplastic variant can look like microcystic adnexal carcinoma but as a papule with a central dell as opposed to MAC which is a plaque
- **Another mimic is infiltrative basal cell carcinoma**, but there is retraction and cellular atypia in basal cell carcinoma (IHC for BCL2 would be positive in BCCs and the basal layer of trichoepithelioma, and CD34 would be positive in the spindle-shaped cells around the basaloid islands of desmoplastic trichoepithelioma)
- Association with **Brooke Spiegler Syndrome**: Multiple cylindromas, trichoepitheliomas, spiradenomas, milia
- **Multiple familial trichoepitheliomas**: Multiple trichoepitheliomas only

Path Presenter

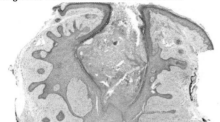
Radiating cords from a central follicular structure

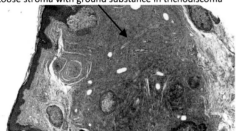
Loose stroma with ground substance in trichodiscoma

FIBROFOLLICULOMA/TIRCHODISCOMA
MORPHOLOGY
- **Radiating cords from a central follicular structure** with surrounding well-circumscribed proliferation of loose stroma and delicate spindle cells
- Trichodiscoma is on a spectrum from fibrofolliculoma, with the former consisting of just **loose stroma with mucin/ground substance**

OTHER HIGH YIELD POINTS
- Considered a hamartoma of hair follicle
- Multiple skin-colored papules
- Associated with **Birt-Hogg-Dubé syndrome**:
  - ➢ Autosomal dominant, mutation in the FLCN (BD) gene on chromosome 17p11.2 encoding folliculin protein
  - ➢ Cutaneous fibrofolliculomas, oncocytic neoplasm, and chromophobe renal cell carcinoma
  - ➢ Lung cysts and spontaneous pneumothorax

Path Presenter

CHONDROID SYRINGOMA (CUTANEOUS MIXED TUMOR)
MORPHOLOGY
- Well circumscribed mixture of epithelial cells in **cords and nests with cartilaginous matrix** that varies depending on the degree of mesenchymal versus epithelial components

OTHER HIGH YIELD POINTS
- **Essentially a pleomorphic adenoma**, but primary to the skin
- Ducts of variable size and shape are lined by two layers of cuboidal cells and a peripheral layer of myoepithelial cells

Path Presenter

Well circumscribed, mixture of epithelial cells embedded in myxoid, cartilaginous, or fibrous stroma

ECCRINE POROMA
MORPHOLOGY
- Acanthotic lesion connecting to the epidermis that resembles an endophytic seborrheic keratosis (downward growth) with **monotonous, evenly spaced cells with occasional duct formation**

OTHER HIGH YIELD POINTS
- Duct formation will be EMA/CEA positive
- If purely intraepidermal -> hidroacanthoma simplex

Path Presenter

Downward growth of monotonous, evenly spaced cells with occasional duct formation

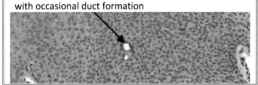
Arborizing network of cuboidal cells

HIDRADENOMA PAPILLIFERUM
MORPHOLOGY
- Dermal papillary and **arborizing network of cuboidal cells** that connect to the epidermis

OTHER HIGH YIELD POINTS
- Solid, skin colored papule, usually < 1 - 2 cm
- Neoplasm of sweat glands in the vulva and perianal regions

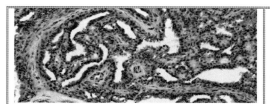

- Usually solitary and <1cm in middle-aged females
- Partially cystic, glandular, and papillary areas
- IHC: (+) CK7, EMA, CEA, GCDFP-15, ER, PR, androgen receptor

Path Presenter

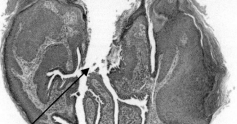

Cystic invagination   Apocrine-lined, double-layered
papillae with stromal plasma cell

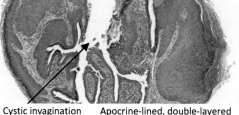

SYRINGOCYSTADENOMA PAPILLIFERUM
MORPHOLOGY
- **Cystic invagination** from the epithelium into the underlying dermis of **apocrine-lined, double-layered papillae with stromal plasma cells**
- Innermost layer is composed of columnar cells with decapitation secretion
- Outermost layer is composed of cuboidal cells with papillary projections

OTHER HIGH YIELD POINTS
- Benign, hamartomatous, adnexal tumor
- Most commonly occurring in the head and neck in early childhood
- **SCAP**: **S**calp location, **C**ommunicate**s** with the epidermis, **A**ssociated with Nevus Sebaceous (in 1/3 of cases), **P**lasma cells within papillae
- Looks similar to hidradenoma papilliferum but in the head and neck

Path Presenter

Monotonous cells that resemble poroma cells

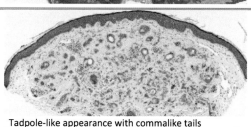

ACROSPIROMA
MORPHOLOGY
- Dermal tumor consisting of **monotonous cells that resemble poroma cells** but deeper down

OTHER HIGH YIELD POINTS
- Include nodular hidradenoma and clear cell hidradenoma
- Evidence of ductal differentiation
- Pink squamous-looking cells or clear cell change can be present

Path Presenter

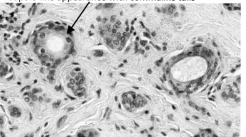

Tadpole-like appearance with commalike tails

SYRINGOMA
MORPHOLOGY
- Clinical: papule in cheek or lower eyelid
- Microscopic: Small ducts, nests, cords, and cysts in the superficial dermis lined by 1-2 layers of small, bland cuboidal cells that frequently have a **tadpole-like appearance with commalike tails (like paisley)**

OTHER HIGH YIELD POINTS
- Most common in the head/neck, especially eyelids
- Dilated ducts may contain eosinophilic contents
- Nests, cords, and cysts are EMA positive
- If deep/perineural invasion -> consider Microcystic Adnexal Carcinoma (MAC)

Path Presenter

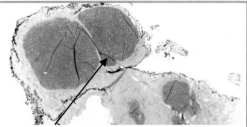

"Blue cannonballs" composed of 2 cell types:

SPIRADENOMA
MORPHOLOGY
- Dermal tumor consisting of **"blue cannonballs" or basophilic tumor nodules**

OTHER HIGH YIELD POINTS
- Tumor lobules may be partially encapsulated
- Biphasic appearance with **2 cell types:**
  - ➢ Peripheral small cells with scant cytoplasm and small hyperchromatic nuclei
  - ➢ Central larger cells with eosinophilic cytoplasm and oval, vesicular nuclei
- Stroma can have prominent vessels +/- hemorrhage
- Tumor lobules are sometimes surrounded by thickened basement membrane, similar to cylindroma
- Associated with Brooke Spiegler Syndrome
  - ➢ Mutations in CYLD gene on chromosome 16q12-q13
  - ➢ Multiple trichoepitheliomas, multiple cylindromas, sometimes spiradenoma or spiradenoma/cylindroma overlap lesions

Path Presenter

Basaloid nests with a "jigsaw puzzle" look and dense eosinophilic basement membrane surrounding each nest

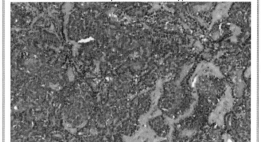

CYLINDROMA
MORPHOLOGY
- Basaloid nests with a **"jigsaw puzzle"** look and **dense eosinophilic basement membrane surrounding each nest**

OTHER HIGH YIELD POINTS
- Tumor lobules have a complex pattern and can resemble spiradenoma but do not contain the two cell types of a spiradenoma

Path Presenter

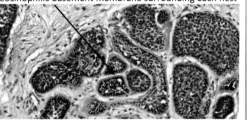

Buckshot growth of neoplastic cells in the epidermis

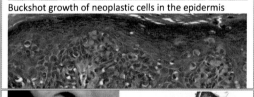

EXTRAMAMMARY PAGET'S DISEASE (EMPD)
MORPHOLOGY
- **Buckshot growth of neoplastic cells in the epidermis**

OTHER HIGH YIELD POINTS
- Rarely with underlying dermal involvement
- Usually not right at the dermal-epidermal junction as opposed to melanoma
- IHC: **(+)** CK7, EMA

Path Presenter

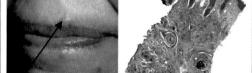

Plaque   Comma-shaped ducts with keratin-filled cysts that infiltrate down to the subcutis

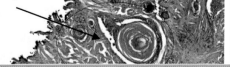

MICROCYSTIC ADNEXAL CARCINOMA
MORPHOLOGY
- Clinical: **plaque**
- Microscopic: **comma-shaped, dilated ducts** with keratin-filled cysts that **infiltrate down to the subcutis**

OTHER HIGH YIELD POINTS
- Resembles desmoplastic trichoepithelioma and syringoma histologically, but clinical appearance varies (plaque in MAC, papule in trichoepithelioma and syringoma)

Path Presenter

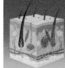

9. SKIN PATHOLOGY

MELANOCYTIC TUMORS	
BENIGN AND MALIGNANT NEVI • Nevi • Spitz nevus	• Blue nevus • Clark's dysplastic nevus • Melanoma

Compound nevus with absent shoulder and normal maturation from top to bottom

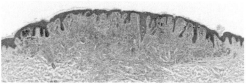

Intradermal nevus

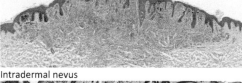

NEVI
MORPHOLOGY
• Common Types:
  ➤ **Junctional nevus:** Nevus cells limited to the epidermis
  ➤ **Compound nevus:** Few nests in the epidermis and dermis
  ➤ **Intradermal nevus:** Dermal component only
OTHER HIGH YIELD POINTS
• Signs of a benign nevus: absence of a "shoulder" or junctional component extending past the dermal component and normal maturation or reduction in size and shape from the top to the bottom of the dermis

Path Presenter

Epithelioid or spindled cells with epidermal hyperplasia and eosinophilic globules (Kamino bodies)

Path Presenter

SPITZ NEVUS
MORPHOLOGY
• Well-circumscribed nest of epithelioid or spindled cells with epidermal hyperplasia of the rete ridges and **no "shoulder"**
• Melanocytes are **large, spindled,** or epithelioid
• Junctional nests often show **separation artifacts (clefting)** to the surrounding epidermis and are **oriented perpendicularly to the epidermis**
• **Pagetoid** melanocytes centrally
• **PAS positive eosinophilic hyaline globules (Kamino bodies)** at the DEJ
OTHER HIGH YIELD POINTS
• Child or young adult with a pink smooth, dome-shaped firm papule or nodule on the face, trunk, or extremities
• Maturation of the dermal component

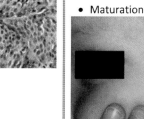

Pink, dome shaped papule   Vertically oriented nests of epithelioid and spindled cells

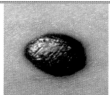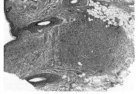

Blue/black papule. melanocytes with abundant melanin

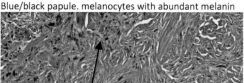

Bipolar spindled dendritic melanocytes

BLUE NEVUS
MORPHOLOGY
• Clinical: **blue or black macule, papule, or nodule**
• Microscopic: **dermal melanocytes with abundant melanin**
OTHER HIGH YIELD POINTS
• Common blue nevus has **bipolar spindled dendritic melanocytes embedded in dense collagenous stroma,** whereas cellular blue nevus is composed of these cells plus ovoid cells with clear cytoplasm arranged in nests
• Lack high mitotic activity, marked cytologic atypia, or necrosis

Path Presenter

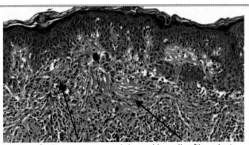

Fusion of adjacent nests and dermal lamellar fibroplasia

CLARK'S DYSPLASTIC NEVUS
MORPHOLOGY
- Melanocytes show nuclear enlargement and pleomorphism with **fusion of adjacent nests**, upward pagetoid spread, and **dermal lamellar fibroplasia** or darker, wavy stroma below nevus cells

OTHER HIGH YIELD POINTS
- Asymmetric distribution and/or shoulder present

Path Presenter

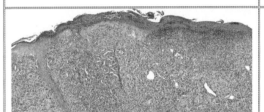

Ulcerated nodular type melanoma composed of cytologically atypical melanocytic nests

Desmoplastic type melanoma (below)

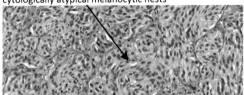

Malignant Melanoma, Superficial Spreading Type

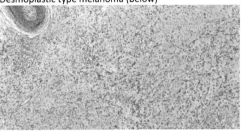

Nodular Melanoma

Spindle cell Melanoma

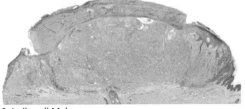
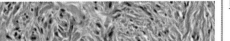

MELANOMA
MORPHOLOGY
- Clinical: **ABCDE** (**A**symmetry, irregular **B**order, variegated **C**olor, **D**iameter >5 mm, **E**volving/changing)
- Microscopic: Asymmetric, poorly circumscribed lesion composed of **cytologically atypical melanocytic nests**. *The great mimicker – can mimic almost any malignancy in appearance cytologically
- IHC: **(+)** S100 (nuclear and cytoplasmic), SOX10 (nuclear), MelanA / MART1 (cytoplasmic), HMB45 (cytoplasmic), Tyrosinase (cytoplasmic), MiTF (nuclear), PRAME (nuclear)

OTHER HIGH YIELD POINTS
- Accounts for the majority of skin cancer mortality
- Can occur de novo or in a pre-existing nevus
- Risk factors include high sun exposure, fair skin, personal or family history, increased number of nevi (particularly if dysplastic), germline mutations, immunosuppression
- Prognosis most dependent on Breslow depth
- In higher stage disease, BRAF mutation testing is recommended
- **Desmoplastic type**
  - Spindled cells-not circumscribed, scar like, with lymphoid aggregates
  - Can look as bland as neurofibroma
  - May not retain melanocytic markers except SOX10 and S100
- **Other** types of Melanomas:
  - Malignant Melanoma, **Superficial Spreading** Type: Most common subtype, radial growth with pagetoid spread
  - Malignant Melanoma, **Lentigo Maligna** Type: Elderly patients on chronic sun damaged skin
  - **Nodular Melanoma**: Vertical growth phase
  - **Nevoid Melanoma**: Verrucous or doom shaped silhouette
  - **Acral Melanoma**: Acral location (palms, soles and subungual)
  - **Spindle Cell Melanoma**: Prominent spindle cell morphology
  - **Spitzoid Melanoma**: Mimics spitz nevus, with confluent growth pattern
  - **Melanoma Arising in Cellular Blue Nevus**: Presence of a pre-existing blue nevus at the periphery
  - **Melanoma Of Soft Parts**: Multilobulated lesion with nests and fascicles of oval to fusiform cells, separated by fibrous trabeculae
  - **Metastatic Melanoma**: Well-circumscribed nodule in the upper dermis with collarette formation, stromal fibrosis

Path Presenter

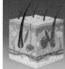

CUTANEOUS SOFT TISSUE TUMORS AND TUMORS OF HEMATOPOIETIC AND LYMPHOID ORIGIN	
• Palisaded encapsulated neuroma • Neurofibroma • Granular cell tumor • Neurothekeoma • Hemangioma • Glomus tumor • Papillary endothelial hyperplasia (Masson's tumor) • Kaposi sarcoma • Angiosarcoma • Atypical fibroxanthoma (AFX) • Dermatofibroma (Benign fibrous histiocytoma)	• Dermatofibrosarcoma protuberans (DFSP) • Fibrous hamartoma of infancy • Fibroepithelial polyp (Acrochordon) • Angiofibroma • Sclerotic fibroma • Scar • Leiomyoma • Mycosis fungoides • Lymphomatoid papulosis • Primary cutaneous anaplastic large cell lymphoma

Delicate spindle cells with palisading

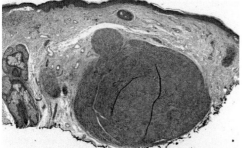

PALISADED ENCAPSULATED NEUROMA
MORPHOLOGY
- Dermal nodule made up of **delicate spindle cells with palisading**

OTHER HIGH YIELD POINTS
- 90% on the face of elderly individual
- Not truly encapsulated and fascicles are separated by clefts
- IHC: S100 (+) and EMA (+) peripherally (around "capsule"), GFAP (-)

Path Presenter

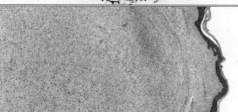

NEUROFIBROMA
MORPHOLOGY
- Dermal lesion composed of **delicate spindle cells** (Schwann cells, fibroblasts, perineural-like cells, and residual nerve axons) **in a sclerotic or mucinous stroma**

OTHER HIGH YIELD POINTS
- Frequently multiple
- Sporadic in ~ 90% of cases; others are syndromic with NF1
- Loosely arranged spindle cells in haphazard arrangement
- Poorly defined cytoplasmic borders/processes–Small, hyperchromatic, wavy, or buckled nuclei
- IHC: **(+)** S100 in ~ 50% of total cells (Schwann cells) & CD34
- Admixed spindled fibroblasts; Neurofilament protein highlights intratumoral axons

Path Presenter

Delicate spindle cells in a sclerotic or mucinous stroma

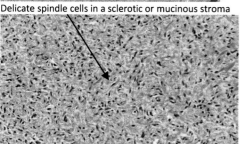

Abundant granular cytoplasm

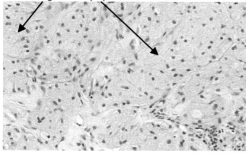

GRANULAR CELL TUMOR
MORPHOLOGY
- Cells with **abundant granular cytoplasm and frequently overlying pseudoepitheliomatous hyperplasia** (epidermal change can mimic SCC)

OTHER HIGH YIELD POINTS
- Benign tumor of putative schwannian origin
- IHC: PAS-D (+) granules; Strong, diffuse **(+)** S100, SOX10, Calretinin, CD68

Path Presenter

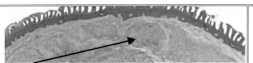

Nests of cells with abundant pale eosinophilic cytoplasm in a myxomatous background

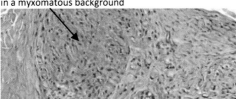

NEUROTHEKEOMA
MORPHOLOGY
- Epithelioid to spindled cells **with abundant pale eosinophilic cytoplasm** arranged in multiple nests divided by **dense fibrous septa**
- **Myxoid variant** shows variable gray blue myxomatous change

OTHER HIGH YIELD POINTS
- Rare dermal tumor of uncertain histogenesis
- IHC: Often **(+)** for variety of nonspecific markers, including NKI/C3, NSE, PGP9.5

Path Presenter

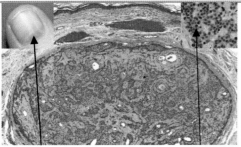

Red painful nodule (left upper inset)   Round cells with central nuclei (right upper inset)

GLOMUS TUMOR
MORPHOLOGY
- Clinical: **small, red, painful nodule**
- Microscopy: Solid nests of **round cells with uniform, central nuclei** closely associated with variably sized blood vessels

OTHER HIGH YIELD POINTS
- Most common in distal extremities, particularly nail bed
- IHC: **(+)** SMA

Path Presenter

Pyogenic Granuloma

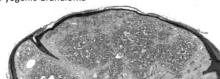

Cavernous Hemangioma

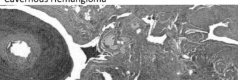

Infantile (Juvenile) Hemangioma

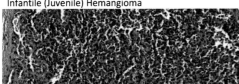

HEMANGIOMA
MORPHOLOGY
- Benign vascular tumors composed of blood vessels lined by plump to flattened endothelial cells with no atypia

OTHER HIGH YIELD POINTS
- **Lobular Capillary Hemangioma (Pyogenic Granuloma):** exophytic with collarette, numerous small capillaries radiating out from larger central vessels, may be ulcerated
- **Cavernous Hemangioma:** non-lobular, poorly demarcated proliferation of large cystically dilated vessels filled with blood
- **Infantile (Juvenile) Hemangioma:** tightly packed small to medium-sized vessels; onset during infancy with rapid growth and spontaneous involution, appearance changes over time; unique immunoprofile of placental vasculature with GLUT1 **(+)**

(From L to R: Pyogenic Granuloma, Cavernous Hemangioma, Infantile Hemangioma)

Link   Link   Link

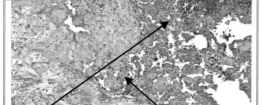

Fibrin thrombus with associated papillary structures lined by a single layer of endothelium

PAPILLARY ENDOTHELIAL HYPERPLASIA (MASSON'S TUMOR)
MORPHOLOGY
- Circumscribed, intravascular endothelial proliferation
- **Fibrin thrombus** with associated **papillary structures lined by a single layer of endothelium** that may form an anastomosing network

OTHER HIGH YIELD POINTS
- Reactive process

Jagged interconnected slit-like vascular channels and extravasated erythrocytes 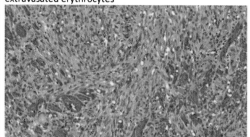	**KAPOSI SARCOMA** MORPHOLOGY <ul><li>Dermal spindle cell tumor with **jagged interconnected slit-like vascular channels and extravasated erythrocytes**</li><li>"Promontory sign" of a blood vessel forming inside another blood vessel</li></ul>OTHER HIGH YIELD POINTS <ul><li>Vascular neoplasm caused by HHV8</li><li>Often AIDS-associated</li></ul>Path Presenter
Infiltrative & poorly circumscribed malignant neoplasm 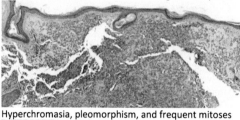 Hyperchromasia, pleomorphism, and frequent mitoses	**ANGIOSARCOMA** MORPHOLOGY <ul><li>**Infiltrative and poorly circumscribed malignant neoplasm** showing morphologic and/or immunophenotype evidence of vascular/endothelial differentiation</li></ul>OTHER HIGH YIELD POINTS <ul><li>Most often scalp/face in elderly (sun-exposed) or breast s/p radiation</li><li>Aggressive tumor treated surgically</li><li>Variable vascular formation</li><li>Often cytologic atypia (hyperchromasia, nuclear pleomorphism) and mitoses</li><li>IHC: **(+)** CD31, CD34, ERG, FLI1; Epithelioid angiosarcomas may be CK **(+)**</li></ul>Path Presenter
  Dermal-based proliferation of spindled to epithelioid cells with scattered large, bizarre multinucleated cells 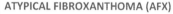	**ATYPICAL FIBROXANTHOMA (AFX)** MORPHOLOGY <ul><li>Highly atypical and pleomorphic **dermal-based proliferation of spindled to epithelioid cells often with scattered large, bizarre multinucleated cells**</li></ul>OTHER HIGH YIELD POINTS <ul><li>Mesenchymal neoplasm of no specific lineage of differentiation (can mimic a SCC or melanoma), usually H&N location</li><li>Numerous mitoses, including atypical forms</li><li>Diagnosis of exclusion:<ul><li>**(-)** for melanocytic markers, cytokeratins (especially HMWCKs), p63, muscle (except for SMA), and vascular markers</li><li>**(+)** for nonspecific markers like CD10, CD68, CD99, and vimentin</li></ul></li><li>If it's unclear how deep it extends, should give a differential of dermal pleomorphic sarcoma</li></ul>Path Presenter
Tabling of the rete ridges 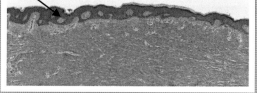	**DERMATOFIBROMA (BENIGN FIBROUS HISTIOCYTOMA)** MORPHOLOGY <ul><li>Dermal-based proliferation of bland, spindled to histiocytoid-appearing cells with **collagen trapping at the periphery**</li><li>Overlying epithelial basilar induction (**"tabling" of the rete ridges**) with hyperpigmentation (may mimic BCC)</li></ul>

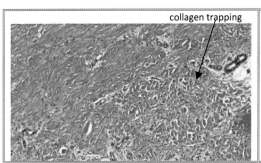
collagen trapping

OTHER HIGH YIELD POINTS
- Tumors are grossly circumscribed but microscopically have irregular, often jagged borders
- Evidence supports both neoplastic & reactive etiologies
- Many variants: Epithelioid, Cellular, with "monster cells"
- IHC: **(+)** FXIIIA, CD163, CD68; **(-)** CD34

Path Presenter

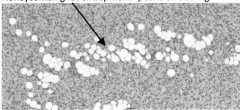
Honeycombing fat entrapment "pearls on a string"

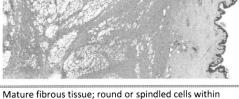
Infiltrating the deep dermis and subcutis

DERMATOFIBROSARCOMA PROTUBERANS (DFSP)
MORPHOLOGY
- Dermal, cellular **spindle cell proliferation** of monomorphic cells in a **storiform or cartwheel arrangement infiltrating the deep dermis and subcutis**
- Subcutaneous areas typically show **honeycombing fat entrapment ("pearls on a string")**

OTHER HIGH YIELD POINTS
- Defined by t(17;22): Rearrangement of COL1A1 with PDGFB
- Lesional cells typically lack significant atypia and pleomorphism
- If loses storiform pattern -> herringbone pattern -> consider malignant transformation to fibrosarcoma
- IHC: Strong, diffuse **(+)** CD34; **(-)** Factor XIIIA

Path Presenter

Mature fibrous tissue; round or spindled cells within loose stroma and interspersed mature fat
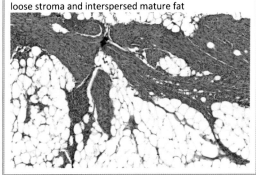

FIBROUS HAMARTOMA OF INFANCY
MORPHOLOGY
- 3 components:
  - ➢ **Intersecting bands of mature fibrous tissue**, comprising spindle-shaped myofibroblasts and fibroblasts
  - ➢ Nests of immature **round, ovoid, or spindled cells within loose stroma**
  - ➢ **Interspersed mature fat**

OTHER HIGH YIELD POINTS
- Benign superficial fibrous lesion occurring in the first 2 years of life

Path Presenter

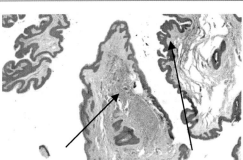

Mildly cellular fibrovascular core, hyperplastic or papillomatous epithelium

FIBROEPITHELIAL POLYP (ACROCHORDON)
MORPHOLOGY
- Clinical: sessile or pedunculated skin-colored polyp
- Microscopic: **Mildly cellular fibrovascular core** with **loose stroma** and **abundant small vessels**, **no adnexa**, and lined by **hyperplastic or papillomatous epithelium**

OTHER HIGH YIELD POINTS
- Common benign tumors often secondary to trauma
- No dysplasia

Path Presenter

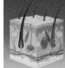
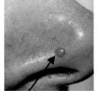
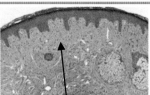

Dome-shaped papule   Spindled to stellate, and multinucleated fibroblasts in dense collagenous stroma with ectatic thin-walled blood vessels

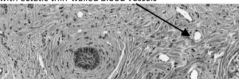

FIBROUS PAPULE
MORPHOLOGY
- Clinical: solitary, dome-shaped flesh-colored papule on the nose or central face
- Microscopic: **Scattered bland, spindled to stellate, and multinucleated fibroblasts in dense collagenous stroma with ectatic thin-walled blood vessels**

OTHER HIGH YIELD POINTS
- Type of angiofibroma
- If enlarged, hyperchromatic nuclei with small nucleoli and scant amounts of eosinophilic cytoplasm -> consider pleomorphic fibroma

Path Presenter

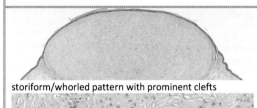

storiform/whorled pattern with prominent clefts

SCLEROTIC FIBROMA
MORPHOLOGY
- Circumscribed, unencapsulated dermal nodule composed of **thickened, hyaline-appearing collagen bundles in a storiform/whorled pattern with prominent clefts**

OTHER HIGH YIELD POINTS
- Sometimes an association with Cowden disease
- IHC: **(+)** CD34

Path Presenter

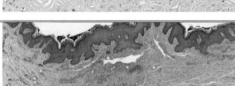

Scar with small, perpendicularly oriented vessels

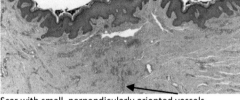

Keloid with thickened, hyalinized collagen

SCAR
MORPHOLOGY
- Scar:
  - ➤ **Dense** collagen fibers that run parallel to the surface
  - ➤ **Small, perpendicularly oriented vessels**
  - ➤ Loss of adnexal structures
- Keloid
  - ➤ Dense proliferation of **thickened, hyalinized collagen** bundles
  - ➤ Decreased vessels compared to conventional and hypertrophic scars

OTHER HIGH YIELD POINTS
- Keloidal collagen can appear edematous due to increased dermal mucosubstances
- IHC: **(+)** SMA

Path Presenter

Pilar leiomyoma -fascicles dissecting between collagen

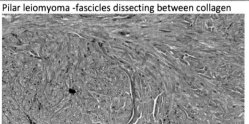

LEIOMYOMA
MORPHOLOGY
- Pilar leiomyoma:
  - ➤ Ill-defined dermal nodule composed of haphazardly arranged smooth muscle bundles/fascicles
  - ➤ **Fascicles often dissect between dermal collagen**
- Angioleiomyoma
  - ➤ Well-circumscribed neoplasm composed of mature smooth muscle cells arranged around prominent blood vessels

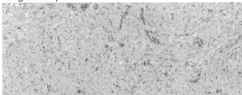

Angioleiomyoma

OTHER HIGH YIELD POINTS
- Benign smooth muscle tumor that is often painful (especially pilar type)
- If there are numerous mitoses, diffuse/marked cytologic atypia, or necrosis -> consider leiomyosarcoma

Path Presenter
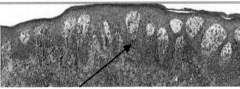

Lymphocytes lining up at the dermal-epidermal junction with a Pautrier's microabscess

MYCOSIS FUNGOIDES
MORPHOLOGY
- Atypical lymphoid infiltrate with epidermotropism or lymphocytes in the epidermis without spongiosis as well as **lymphocytes lining up like "birds on a wire" at the dermal epidermal junction**
- **Pautrier's microabscess** or solid intraepidermal nodule made up of malignant lymphocytes
- Morphology varies depending on the stage of tumor (patch, plaque, tumor)

OTHER HIGH YIELD POINTS
- Patch stage shows irregular patches in sun-protected sites
- Neoplastic cells are CD4+ T-lymphocytes, clonal TCR gene rearrangement

Path Presenter
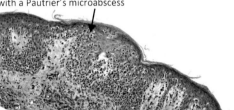

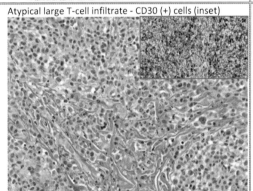

Atypical large T-cell infiltrate - CD30 (+) cells (inset)

LYMPHOMATOID PAPULOSIS (LyP)
MORPHOLOGY
- **Wedge-shaped atypical large CD30 (+) T-cell infiltrate**
- Multiple variants with different morphology and immunoprofiles that can mimic other entities such as mycosis fungoides and anaplastic large cell lymphoma

OTHER HIGH YIELD POINTS
- Crops of papules and nodules usually at different stages of development
- Difference between this and mycosis fungoides is the clinical -> if lesions appear and spontaneously regress after weeks or months, consider LyP

Path Presenter

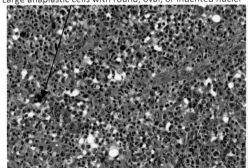

Large anaplastic cells with round, oval, or indented nuclei

PRIMARY CUTANEOUS ANAPLASTIC LARGE CELL LYMPHOMA (ALCL)
MORPHOLOGY
- Confluent sheet of **large anaplastic cells with round, oval, or indented nuclei**

OTHER HIGH YIELD POINTS
- Solitary or localized papules or masses
- >75% malignant cells positive for CD30
- Unlike primary systemic ALCL, cutaneous ALCL is usually ALK **(-)** -> if **(+)**, consider cutaneous spread of primary systemic ALCL

Path Presenter

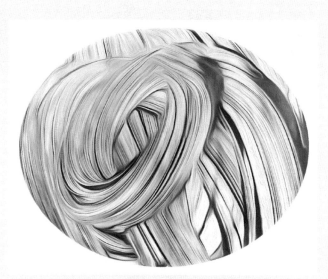

Who knew a "dot under a microscope" might constitute for a Path Art! Image courtesy: Ziad El-Zaatari, MD

CHAPTER 10: LYMPH NODE PATHOLOGY

Mayuri Shende, MD
Akanksha Gupta, MD

REACTIVE LYMPHADENOPATHIES	

Enlarged follicles (4-5X of reactive follicles)

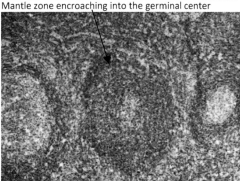

Mantle zone encroaching into the germinal center

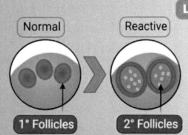

PROGRESSIVE TRANSFORMATION OF GERMINAL CENTERS

MORPHOLOGY

- **Enlarged (4-5x normal) follicles** with **hyperplastic germinal centers** (GCs), **disruption** of GCs due to **infiltration by a mantle zone**
- PTGC is associated with reactive follicular hyperplasia
- Germinal center cells: CD10(+), Bcl-6(+), Bcl-2(-)
- Mantle zone cells: IgD (+), Bcl-2(+), CD10(-), Bcl-6(-)

OTHER HIGH YIELD POINTS

- Young patients, M > F, usually asymptomatic, **single enlarged lymph node**
- Generalized lymphadenopathy with florid PTGC can occur in adolescents and patients with autoimmune diseases
- PTGC may precede, coexist with, or follow lymphoma, most commonly NLPHL
- Treatment and Prognosis: Usually resolves spontaneously and carries a good prognosis
- Differential Diagnosis: Nodular lymphocyte-predominant Hodgkin lymphoma, lymphocyte-rich classic Hodgkin lymphoma - nodular variant, follicular lymphoma - floral variant, HIV-associated lymphadenopathy, reactive follicular hyperplasia

Path Presenter

Progressive Transformation of Germinal Centers (PTGC)

Lymph Node

Normal | Reactive | PTGC | Germinal Centers (GCs)

1° Follicles | 2° Follicles

Clear germinal center (GC)
Tingible body macrophages
Expanded mantle zone

- GCs are 3-5x larger than normal
- Indistinct margins
- Tingible body macrophages present
- B-cells express GC markers: CD10, Bcl-6

- Composed of follicular mantle B-cells encroaching germinal centers with increased follicular dendritic cells

Mantle Zone

- Focal disruption of GCs by ingrowth of follicular mantle cells
- B-cell express: Bcl-2, IgD

Presents as a **nodule**

Differences between PTGC and Nodular Lymphocyte-Predominant Hodgkin Lymphoma (NLPHL)

NLPHL

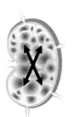

- Diffuse involvement
- Irregular nodules, moth-eaten appearence
- Scattered clonal cells (termed LP cells)
- Background of lymphocytes and histiocytes
- LP cells: CD20+, BOB1+, OCT2+
- T-cell rosettes around LP: CD3+, CD57+, PD1+

PTGC

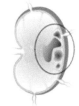

- Focal involvement
- Partial preservation of nodal architecture
- No LP cells
- No rosettes of T-cells
- Follicles composed of B-cells
- CD3: background follicular hyperplasia

PTGC may precede, coexist or follow NLPHL.

Dilatation of sinuses

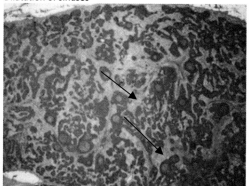

Dilatation of sinuses

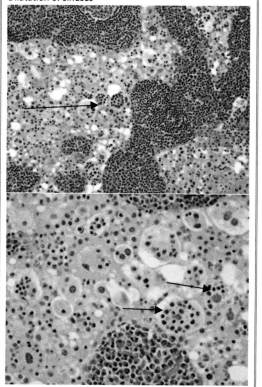

Emperipolesis

ROSAI-DORFMAN DISEASE

MORPHOLOGY Lymph Node

- Lymph node **architecture distorted by dilatation of sinuses** containing proliferation **of large histiocytes, small lymphocytes, and plasma cells**.
- Large **histiocytes** with distinct cell borders, central nuclei, and prominent nucleoli, and **abundant eosinophilic cytoplasm containing intact lymphocytes or RBCs** (**emperipolesis**, a pathognomonic feature).
- RDD histiocytes are **S100+, CD68+, and CD1a-**.

OTHER HIGH YIELD POINTS

- Affects lymph nodes, extra-nodal sites in 20% cases, usually presents with massive lymphadenopathy.
- **Regress spontaneously** in most cases with an excellent prognosis.

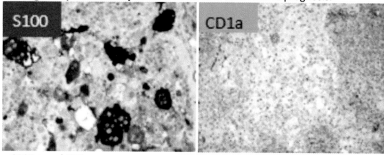

S100 + and CD1a -

Rosai-Dorfman disease	Langerhans Cell Histiocytosis	Metastatic Melanoma	Sinus Histiocytosis
LN architecture distorted by dilatation of sinuses containing large histiocytes, lymphocytes, and plasma cells	Sinusoidal pattern with **eosinophils and necrosis**	Sinusoidal involvement by metastasis to lymph nodes	**Nonspecific**, histiocytes without emperipolesis
Emperipolesis is a pathognomic feature.	Histiocytes with less cytoplasm, **twisted nuclei with grooves**; no emperipolesis	**Cytologic atypia** with mitosis	
Histiocytes are **S100+**, CD68+, CD163+, cathepsin D and E +, **CD1a-, Langerin-**	**S100+, CD1a+, Langerin+**	S100+, HMB-45+	S100+/-
	Birbeck granules by electron microscopy		

Path Presenter

KIMURA DISEASE

MORPHOLOGY Extranodal sites

- Deep dermis or subcutaneous tissue shows **lymphoid infiltrates with follicle formation**
- Infiltration of **eosinophils, plasma cells, and mast cells**
- **Eosinophilic microabscesses** within the interfollicular region
- Thin-walled blood vessel proliferation

Lymph Node

- **Distorted architecture** with **hyperplastic follicles**
- **Eosinophilic microabscesses** within the interfollicular region and follicle lysis
- Proteinaceous material deposition in germinal centers (IgE)
- Well-formed mantle zones

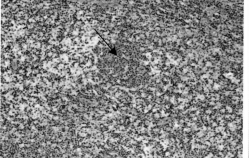

Eosinophilic microabscess

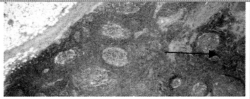

Distorted follicles with interfollicular eosinophils

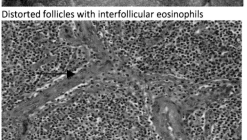

Vascular proliferation

- Necrosis may be present
- Proliferation of vessels in the interfollicular region

OTHER HIGH YIELD POINTS

- Chronic inflammatory disorder with lymphoid **hyperplasia, eosinophilia, and fibrosis commonly** seen in **Young Asian** male with **slow-growing painless subcutaneous masses** in the head and neck (**periauricular** region) and enlarged **regional lymph nodes** .Other sites involved: Salivary glands, oral cavity, axilla, groin.
- Peripheral blood **eosinophilia** and **increased serum IgE** levels with an elevated **ESR**
- Immunophenotype: IgE in germinal centers & background polytypic B & T cells
- Prognosis: Recurrence common

CASTLEMAN DISEASE
UNICENTRIC PLASMA CELL VARIANT OF CASTLEMAN DISEASE
MORPHOLOGY Lymph Node

- **Preserved architecture**
- Follicles with **hyperplastic germinal centers**
- Interfollicular areas with sheets of **polytypic plasmacytosis** and **prominent vasculature**

OTHER HIGH YIELD POINTS

- **Middle-aged adults** with **peripheral lymphadenopathy without B symptoms**
- Immunophenotype: Polytypic light chains, Background B and T lymphocytes in a normal distribution pattern, HHV8 LANA negative.
- Differential diagnosis: HHV8+ multicentric Castleman Disease, Plasmacytoma
- Prognosis: Good prognosis and Treatment: Surgical excision.

UNICENTRIC HYALINE VASCULAR VARIANT OF CASTLEMAN DISEASE
MORPHOLOGY Lymph Node

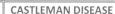

Increased plasma cells in interfollicular areas

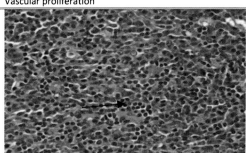

Unicentric Hyaline vascular Castleman disease:Lollipop follicles

- **'Lollipop' follicles**- Enlarged lymph nodes, with **hyalinized blood vessels** radially extending into involuted germinal centers, mantle zone B cells with the **onion-skin appearance**
- Follicles with two germinal centers (**twinning**) or **involuted germinal centers**

OTHER HIGH YIELD POINTS

- Immunophenotype: Background polytypic B and T lymphocytes, follicular dendritic cells: CD21+, CD23+ , plasmacytoid dendritic cells: CD123+, TCL1+
- Differential diagnosis: HIV Lymphadenitis, Kaposi sarcoma, Mantle cell lymphoma.
- Prognosis- Excellent, Treatment-surgical excision of affected LN

MULTICENTRIC CASTLEMAN DISEASE
MORPHOLOGY Lymph Node

- Combination of features of both plasma cell and hyaline vascular variants.
- Lymphocyte depletion, particularly in HIV patients.

OTHER HIGH YIELD POINTS

- **HHV8+** (using LANA1) cells ranging from small lymphocytes to immunoblasts
- Background B and T lymphocytes.
- Prognosis: **Bad prognosis in POEMS syndrome & HIV.**
- Associated neoplasms-Plasmablastic lymphoma, primary effusion lymphoma, Kaposi sarcoma.

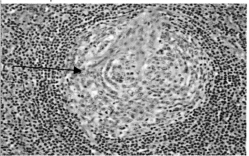

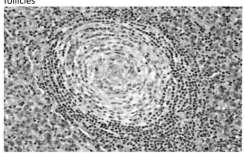

Multicentric Castleman disease

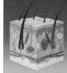
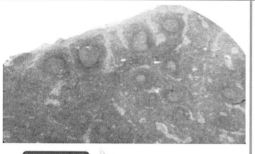

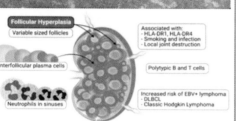

RHEUMATOID ARTHRITIS-RELATED LYMPHADENOPATHY
MORPHOLOGY Lymph Node

- **Follicular hyperplasia** – Variable shapes and sizes
- Interfollicular region with **plasmacytosis**
- **Neutrophils in sinuses**
- IHC: Polytypic B and T cells - normal immunophenotype
- Differential diagnosis:

Rheumatoid Arthritis related lymphadenopathy	Syphilitic Lymphadenitis	Follicular Lymphoma	Reactive Follicular Hyperplasia	Plasmacytoma
Follicular hyperplasia **with Variable shapes and sizes follicles** Interfollicular **region** with plasmacytosis **Neutrophils in sinuses**	Follicular hyperplasia and interfollicular plasmacytosis Hallmark: **vasculitis**, especially in capsule or perinodal area **Warthin-Starry stain** for Spirochetes	Back-to-back neoplastic follicles B cells: **CD10+, Bcl-6+ and Bcl-2+**	Smaller and equally sized follicles	Monoclonal, cytologically **atypical plasma cells** replacing lymph node architecture

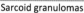

Sarcoid granulomas
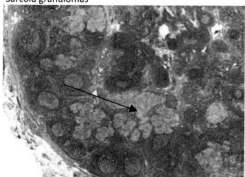

SARCOID LYMPHADENOPATHY
MORPHOLOGY Lymph Node

- Partial or complete involvement, firm cut surface
- **Well-formed, discrete, closely packed, non-necrotizing granulomas containing epithelioid histiocytes**
- **Schaumann bodies (iron and calcium), asteroid bodies (star-like** structures), or **Hamazaki-Wesenburg inclusions** (yellow-brown with lipofuscin) - nonspecific
- Can have foci of fibrosis or fibrinoid necrosis

OTHER HIGH YIELD POINTS

- Diagnosis of exclusion, **R/O infections – AFB, GMS, PAS, Warthin-Starry stains**
- Treatment : Pulmonary sarcoidosis - Glucocorticoids

Nodular paracortical expansion
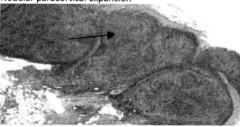

DERMATOPATHIC LYMPHADENOPATHY
MORPHOLOGY Lymph Node

- Lymph node shows **paracortical hyperplasia**, with interdigitating dendritic cells **(IDC)**, Langerhans cells **(LC)**, **macrophages** containing **melanin pigment**, and **T cells**

OTHER HIGH YIELD POINTS

Immunophenotype

- **IDCs, LCs, and macrophages – S100+**
- **Loose clusters of plasmacytoid dendritic cells – CD123+**

Courtesy: Siba El Hussein, MD
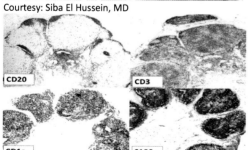

Dermatopathic lymphadenopathy	Mycosis fungoides/ Sézary Syndrome	Langerhans Cell Histiocytosis
Paracortical hyperplasia, **with interdigitating dendritic cells (IDC), Langerhans cells (LC), macrophages containing melanin pigment, and T cells**	Small clusters of lymphocytes with cerebriform nuclei	**Sinusoidal pattern** with **eosinophils and necrosis** Histiocytes with less cytoplasm, **twisted nuclei with grooves**, no emperipolesis
IDCs, LCs, and macrophages – S100+	T-cell gene rearrangements can be helpful with other clues (**CD4:CD8 ratio increased, loss of CD7**)	➤ Langerhans cells: **S100+, CD1a+, Langerin+** ➤ **Birbeck granules** by electron microscopy

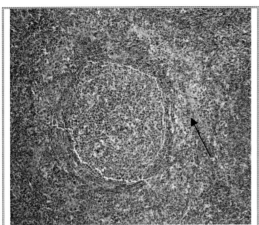

Ring of histiocytes around GC

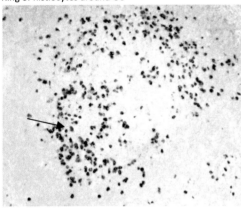

IgG4 stain

IgG4-RELATED DISEASE

Multiorgan fibroinflammatory condition with specific clinicopathologic features

MORPHOLOGY

Extranodal sites	Lymph Node
-Increased lymphocytes and plasma cells, with germinal center formation -Focal storiform fibrosis, **with cartwheel appearance of fibroblasts and inflammatory cells** -Obliterative phlebitis **with lymphocyte and plasma cell infiltration within the vessel wall and lumen (commonly seen in the** orbit) -Destructive inflammation **of the lacrimal and salivary glands and** pancreas	Lymphadenopathy can have **five patterns** with scattered background histiocytes: -Follicular hyperplasia -PTGC -Inflammatory pseudotumor-like fibrosis -- Interfollicular expansion -Multicentric Castleman disease-like

OTHER HIGH YIELD POINTS

Clinical Presentation	Asymptomatic lymphadenopathy- mediastinal or intra-abdominal **in a majority of patients** with autoimmune pancreatitis **Enlarged pancreas on imaging** Increased serum IgG4 levels (>135 mg/ dL), IgG and IgE, **and peripheral** eosinophilia
Immuno - phenotype	Polytypic plasma cells, background B and T cells
Diagnostic criteria	IgG4: IgG plasma cell ratio- > 40% (diagnosis requires clinical, serological, and pathological evaluation) Usually, in the setting of >50 IgG4 cells/HPF
Differential diagnoses	Conditions with increased IgG4 cells: **Inflammatory conditions with increased IgG4** (Primary Sclerosing Cholangitis, Rheumatoid Arthritis, ANCA-associated vasculitis, Rosai Dorfman disease. Low-grade lymphoma with B-cells or Ig light chain restriction **(follicular lymphoma, extranodal MZL)** **Inflammatory Pseudotumor** **Carcinoma of Pancreas** **Type II Autoimmune Pancreatitis**
Prognosis	**Recurrences common**, especially when steroids tapered down **Increased risk for NHL or epithelial malignancies**
Treatment	Symptomatic patients – **steroids or Rituximab** (in patients unresponsive to steroids) **Fibrosis involving the orbit or bile duct – Surgical** resection

Histiocytes with phagocytosis of anucleated RBCs and neutrophils

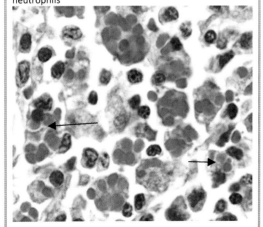

Path Presenter

HEMOPHAGOCYTIC LYMPHOHISTIOCYTOSIS

-**Systemic, non-neoplastic acute condition** with **cytopenias** and **organ infiltration** by histiocytes, frequently with **hemophagocytosis**, usually **fatal if left untreated**
-Defects in cytotoxic T cells or NK cells lead to **increased activation** of **macrophages** and result in **cytokine storm**

MORPHOLOGY

Lymph Node	**Preserved architecture with** bland appearing histiocytes with phagocytosis in the sinuses
Bone Marrow	**Histiocytes with phagocytosis of anucleated RBCs, platelets, and neutrophils** Dysplastic hematopoietic cells, especially erythrocytes
Spleen	Splenomegaly, **red pulp with phagocytic histiocyte**s **Extramedullary hematopoiesis**
Liver	**Kupffer cell hyperplasia with hemophagocytosis**
Skin	Erythematous plaques Increased T cells, histiocytes

OTHER HIGH YIELD POINTS

Prognosis	Better survival with stem cell transplant vs. HLH2004 protocol only
Treatment	•HLH-2004 protocol – 8-week induction with dexamethasone, etoposide, and cyclosporine • Persistent non-familial disease or familial form → stem cell transplant

TABLE: SUMMARY OF REACTIVE LYMPHADENOPATHIES		
Reactive Condition	**Lymph node Morphology**	**Mimics**
Progressive Transformation of Germinal Center • Asymptomatic • Cervical LNs commonly	• Enlarged follicles • Follicular hyperplasia à Follicle lysis • Mantle zones infiltrated by B-cells • Preserved B and T zones	• **NLPHL:** Irregular nodules with LP cells and T-cell rosettes • **FL:** back-to-back packed follicles composed of B-cells (highlighted by CD10, BCl-6, and Bcl-2) • **Reactive:** Smaller follicles. Preserved mantle zone
Kikuchi-Fujimoto disease • Painful posterior cervical LN • Asians • Upper respiratory tract symptoms • Skin papules/erythema	• Paracortical necrosis • Lymphohistiocytic stage (crescentic histiocytes) à Necrotic stage à Phagocytic stage (foamy histiocytes, necrotic debris)	• **SLE lymphadenitis:** hematoxylin bodies, Azzopardi effect, plasma cells • **HSV Lymphadenitis:** Viral inclusions in paracortical lesions
Rosai Dorfman Disease (SHML) • *BRAFV600E* mutation • Young age • B/L cervical lymphadenopathy • Extranodal involvement.	• Sinuses are dilated with histiocytes, plasma cells. • Emperipolesis in the large histiocytes. • Sclerosis and fibrosis	• **Sinus Histiocytosis:** no emperipolesis • **Langerhan's cell histiocytosis:** Nuclear grooves, CD1a +, Langerin +, Birbeck granules on E/M • **Melanoma:** Sinuses are filled with malignant cells. S100, HMB45 +. Mitosis ++
Kimura Disease • Asians • Painless subcutaneous mass	• Eosinophilic microabscesses. Eosinophilia • Hyperplastic follicles • Proteinaceous material (IgE)	• **ALHE:** A vascular tumor in the head-neck region. Plump endothelial cells, however, no LN involvement
Castleman's Disease	**Hyaline Vascular Variant** • Onion skin appearance, involuted germinal centers, hyalinized blood vessels extending into the follicles, twin germinal centers. HHV8 neg **Plasmacytoid Variant** • Preserved architecture. • The Interfollicular area shows sheets of plasma cells (polyclonal). HHV8 negative **Multicentric Castleman's** • Combination of both the features. Associated with plasmacytosis and HHV8 + (LANA1 +)	• **Mantle Cell Lymphoma:** Monoclonal B-cells, CD5, and CyclinD1 + • **Plasmacytoma:** Monoclonal expansion of plasma cells • Hyaline vasculature, follicle lysis is also seen in **HIV and HHV8-associated lymphadenitis**
Rheumatoid arthritis related lymphadenopathy • Associations: Smoking, HLA-DR1, and HLA-DR4	• Follicular hyperplasia • Interfollicular plasmacytosis • Neutrophils are seen in the sinuses	• **Syphilitic lymphadenitis:** Vasculitis is the hallmark. Warthin-Starry stain highlights the bacteria • **Follicular Lymphoma:** neoplastic B-cell follicles (CD10 +, BCl6+, Bcl2+)
Sarcoid Lymphadenopathy • Cervical, peri bronchial LNs. • Raised ESR and ACE levels	• Non-necrotizing granuloma • Fibrotic foci • Non-specific iron, calcium, hemosiderin inclusions	• **Granulomatous lymphadenitis:** needs exclusion by special stains
Dermatopathic Lymphadenopathy • Associated with skin conditions	• Expansion of paracortical areas with dendritic cells, macrophages (melanin pigment within)	• **Pigment in LN:** anthracotic pigment, tattoo dye. Not associated with dendritic cell expansion • **Mycosis Fungoides:** Raised CD4:CD8 ratio, loss of CD7 • **Langerhan's cell histiocytosis:** Nuclear grooves, CD1a +, Langerin +, Birbeck granules on E/M
Hemophagocytic Lymphohistiocytosis • Clinical criteria (5/8 features) • Underlying genetic defect.	• Preserved LN architecture • Histiocytic proliferation in sinus • Hemophagocytosis +	• To be correlated with clinical scenario and exclusion of the common reactive lymphadenopathies.
IgG4-related disease • Painless massive B/L cervical lymphadenopathy	• Distorted LN architecture • Sinuses are dilated, histiocytic proliferation, emperipolesis. Sclerosis and fibrosis • Interfollicular IgG4 plasma cells	

NLPHL, Nodular Lymphocyte-predominant Hodgkin's Lymphoma; FL, Follicular Lymphoma; RLH, Reactive Lymphoid Hyperplasia; SHML, Sinus Histiocytosis with massive lymphadenopathy; AHEH, Angiolymphoid hyperplasia with eosinophilia/ Epithelioid hemangioma

INFECTIOUS LYMPHADENITIS

	CHRONIC GRANULOMATOUS LYMPHADENITIS	SUPPURATIVE LYMPHADENITIS
Clinical presentation	Localized or generalized lymphadenopathy	**Fever, leukocytosis**, lymphadenopathy
Etiology	Infectious agents: **Mycobacteria, fungi, viruses, parasites** Other causes: **Foreign body, autoimmune (e.g., sarcoidosis)**	Most common cause: **Staphylococcus, Streptococcus** Regional lymph nodes draining pyogenic inflammation, e.g., dental abscess, upper respiratory infection, or infected wounds
Morphology	Lymph Node: - **Caseating granulomas** show **central eosinophilic necrosis** with a **rim of epithelioid macrophages, lymphocytes and fibroblasts** - **Non- caseating granulomas** do not show central necrosis. Compose of a collection of epithelioid cells, giant cells, lymphocytes, and histiocytes	Lymph Node: Dilated sinuses, **microabscesses**, fungi, or bacteria with **perilymphadenitis**
Special stains	● Acid-fast bacilli: Ziehl-Neelson, Fite Faraco, Kinyoun ● Fungi: PAS, GMS ● Other bacteria: Gram stain ● Parasites: Giemsa stain	Bacteria: Gram stain Fungi: PAS, GMS
Confirmatory test	PCR	Microbiological Culture, PCR

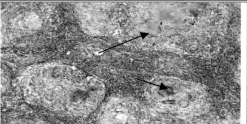

Caseating granulomas with Langhans giant cells

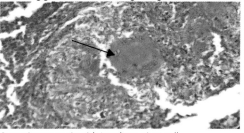

Caseating necrosis with Langhans giant cell

MYCOBACTERIUM TUBERCULOSIS LYMPHADENITIS

Clinical presentation	Lymphadenopathy, **most common cervical**, painless, and progressive **Others: Axillary, inguinal, abdominal (rare)**
Lymph Node	**Single or matted**, the **cut surface may be cheesy-white (caseous)** **Granuloma formation: Necrosis at center** surrounded by **layers of epithelioid cells, and Langhans giant cells** (peripherally arranged nuclei) along with lymphocytes and plasma cells
Special studies	● **Tuberculin skin test** ➤ Positive in most cases of MTB lymphadenitis ➤ False-negative: Immunodeficiency states like HIV ● **Interferon-gamma release assay (IGRA)** ➤ **Highly specific for MTB** ➤ **Negative in patients with previous BCG vaccination, sensitization to non-tuberculous mycobacteria** ➤ **Cannot differentiate between latent and active infection** ● **Direct staining** ➤ Acid-fast bacilli: Ziehl-Neelson, Kinyoun ➤ Fluorochrome stain: Auramine Rhodamine (bacteria appear yellow/orange on a dark background) ● **Culture**: Lowenstein-Jensen medium, automated: BACTEC 460, MGIT 960, MB/ BacT
Treatment	● Adults: 6 months of isoniazid, rifampin, pyrazinamide, and ethambutol ● Children: 2 months of isoniazid, rifampin, and pyrazinamide, plus two months of isoniazid and rifampin

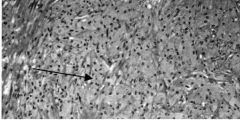

Spindle cells arranged in fascicles

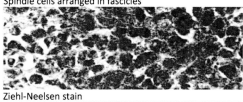

Ziehl-Neelsen stain

MYCOBACTERIAL SPINDLE CELL PSEUDOTUMOR

● Lymph node infection by **Mycobacterium avium intracellulare (MAI)** that causes distinctive tumor-like appearance

Clinical presentation	Lymphadenopathy, **in a background of** immunosuppression, **particularly HIV infection** Other sites: Spleen, skin, bone marrow, lung, and brain
MORPHOLGY lymph node	● **Spindle cells** arranged in **fascicles and storiform** arrays ● Cells have **eosinophilic and granular cytoplasm** ● Clusters of **epithelioid histiocytic cells** with similar cytoplasmic features ● **Acid-fast stain usually shows numerous organisms MAI** within spindled and epithelioid cells
Special studies	SPECIAL STUDIES ● IHC: **CD68 +, lysozyme +, vimentin +, CD31-, CD34-** ● Culture essential for confirmation: Traditional culture media: Löwenstein-Jensen, Liquid media such as BACTEC (growth takes two weeks) ,PCR methods also useful for diagnosis and classification

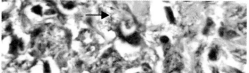

Sheets of large histiocytes with foamy cytoplasm
Courtesy: Olaleke Folaranmi, MD @olalekefolaranmi

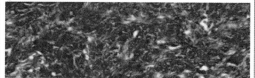

Ziehl-Neelsen stain Courtesy: Olaleke Folaranmi, MD
@olalekefolaranmi

PAS stain, Courtesy: Olaleke Folaranmi, MD
@olalekefolaranmi

ATYPICAL MYCOBACTERIUM TUBERCULOSIS LYMPHADENITIS

Lymph Node Morphology

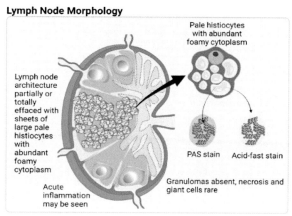

MORPHOLOGY Lymph Node

- Lymph node **architecture partially or totally effaced** with **sheets of large pale histiocytes** with **abundant foamy cytoplasm**
- Granulomas absent, necrosis & giant cells rare.
- Acute inflammation may be seen

CAT SCRATCH DISEASE

Lymph Node Morphology

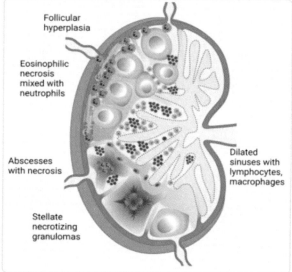

Stellate microabscesses Courtesy:@MComptonMD

MORPHOLOGY Lymph Node:

- Early lesions show **follicular hyperplasia**, with **tingible body macrophages** in germinal centers
- Subcapsular sinuses may show **eosinophilic necrosis mixed with neutrophils**
- **Sinuses appear dilated with lymphocytes, histiocytes and immunoblasts**
- Lymph nodes can show abscesses with Necrosis.
- **Late stages show classic stellate necrotizing granulomas**

OTHER HIGH YIELD POINTS

- **Warthin Starry stain identifies organisms**, best seen at an **early stage** of disease. **IHC: Monoclonal anti-Bartonella antibodies**
- PCR, Serologic testing: Cross-reactivity with B.quintana

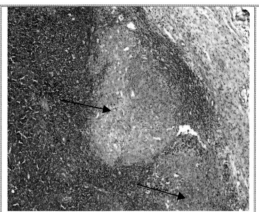

Nodules composed of variable sized and shaped blood vessels.
Bacillary Angiomatosis Courtesy:@MComptonMD

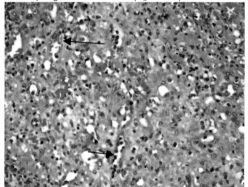

Blood vessels lined by prominent endothelial cells and surrounded by deeply eosinophilic material
Bacillary Angiomatosis Courtesy:@MComptonMD

BACILLARY ANGIOMATOSIS

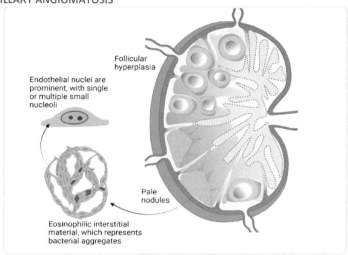

MORPHOLOGY Lymph Node:
- Early lesions show **follicular hyperplasia**
- Nodules composed of **blood vessels of variable size & shape**, can be confluent
- Blood vessels show a **range of differentiation** from round, large, irregular, or ectatic to small solid clusters with pinpoint lumina
- **Endothelial nuclei are prominent, with single or multiple small nucleoli**
- **Mitotic** figures are present; up to **3-5 per HPF**
- Blood vessels can be surrounded by **deeply eosinophilic interstitial material, which represents bacterial aggregates**

OTHER HIGH YIELD POINTS
- **Warthin Starry stain** identifies organisms, best seen at an early stage of disease Immunohistochemistry: **FVIIIAg(+), ULEX-1(+)** can highlight endothelial cells
- TREATMENT - Erythromycin, Doxycycline

LYMPHOGRANULOMA VENEREUM
MORPHOLOGY Lymph Node:
- **Early lesion: Necrosis and accumulation of neutrophils**
- **Progressive lesion: Histiocytes with small or confluent cytoplasmic vacuoles** Organisms larger at the periphery of the vacuole (**reticulate bodies**) and smaller in center (**elementary bodies**) and **maybe visible with routine H&E stain**
- **Lymphocytes and plasma cells** surround foci of necrosis
- **Clusters** of **monocytoid B cells** may be seen in subcapsular or paratrabecular sinuses
- **Coalescence** of **necrotic foci to form a stellate shape**
- Surrounded by **palisading epithelioid histiocytes** and few giant cells

OTHER HIGH YIELD POINTS
- **Giemsa stain: Light blue bacteria within vacuoles**
- **Warthin-Starry stain: Dark, small, round microorganisms within vacuoles**
- **Brown-Hopps-Gram stain: Red to violet microorganisms**
- **PCR, Serologic** testing

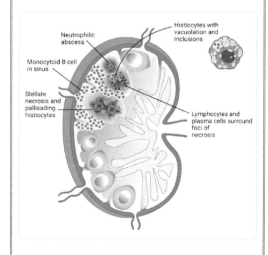

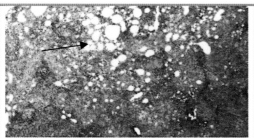
Lipogranuloma in Whipple disease

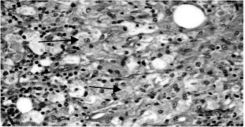
Foamy histiocytes in Whipple disease, PAS positive

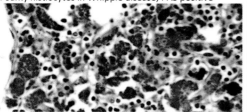

WHIPPLE DISEASE

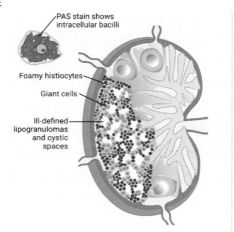

MORPHOLOGY:

Lymph Node	Small intestine
Nodal **architecture obscured by** ill-defined **lipogranulomas** & **cystic spaces** Giant cells may be seen. necrosis usually absent	Submucosal foamy histiocytes containing mucin and PAS + diastase resistant material Gram +, Gomori silver +, Acid-fast − Admixed **inflammatory infiltrate** composed of neutrophils, eosinophils, & lymphocytes **Villous shortening** can be seen

OTHER HIGH YIELD POINTS
- Standard test: PCR using primers common to DNA encoding unique bacterial 16S ribosomal RNA
- Special stain: **PAS**, **IHC: Antibody specific for T. whipplei, histiocytes: CD68+**

Architecture distorted, Germinal centers with tingible body macrophages, Interfollicular immunoblasts

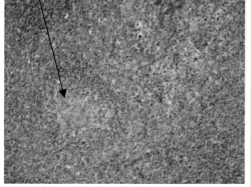

Immunoblasts, small to intermediate sized lymphocytes and plasma cells

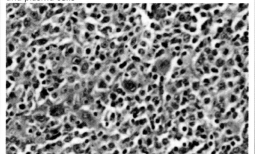

INFECTIOUS MONONUCLEOSIS

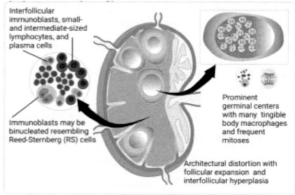

MORPHOLOGY Lymph Node:
- Lymph node **architecture is distorted**, showing predominantly **interfollicular process**, but follicles may also become hyperplastic
- Germinal centers may become prominent with numerous tingible body macrophages and frequent mitoses
- **Interfollicular immunoblasts** (may be binucleated, **resembling RS** cells, making it look like lymphoma), small- and intermediate-sized **lymphocytes, and plasma cells**

OTHER HIGH YIELD POINTS
- **Serologic tests, presence of atypical lymphocytes (Downey cells) in peripheral blood, Monospot test (a.k.a. Heterophile antibody test)**
- EBV-specific antibody tests by immunofluorescence

LN Touch preparation, Histoplasmosis

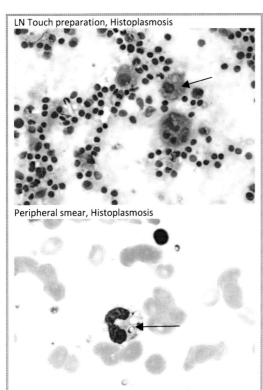

Peripheral smear, Histoplasmosis

HISTOPLASMA LYMPHADENITIS

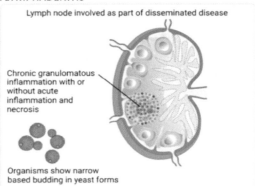

Lymph node involved as part of disseminated disease

Chronic granulomatous inflammation with or without acute inflammation and necrosis

Organisms show narrow based budding in yeast forms

MORPHOLOGY Lymph Node:
- Lymph node involved as part of disseminated disease
- **Chronic granulomatous ± acute inflammation with necrosis**, organisms show **narrow-based budding in yeast forms**

OTHER HIGH YIELD POINTS
- Serologic tests: Complement fixation, ID assay
- Blood culture on Sabouraud's dextrose agar
- EIA for polysaccharide antigen

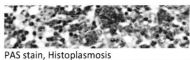

GMS stain, Histoplasmosis   PAS stain, Histoplasmosis

TOXOPLASMA LYMPHADENITIS

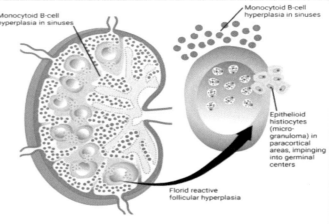

Monocytoid B-cell hyperplasia in sinuses

Monocytoid B-cell hyperplasia in sinuses

Epithelioid histiocytes (micro-granuloma) in paracortical areas, impinging into germinal centers

Florid reactive follicular hyperplasia

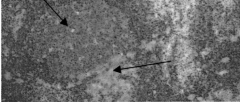

Toxoplasma lymphadenitis

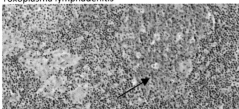

Microgranuloma

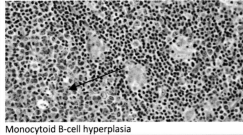

Monocytoid B-cell hyperplasia

MORPHOLOGY Lymph Node:
- Diagnostic triad: **Florid reactive follicular hyperplasia, Monocytoid B-cell hyperplasia in sinuses**, <25 Epithelioid histiocytes (**microgranuloma**) in paracortical areas

OTHER HIGH YIELD POINTS
- **Serologic tests**- IgM screening antibody test positive in 1st three months
- Sabin-Feldman dye test
- Enzyme immunoassays detect positive Toxoplasma-specific antibodies
- **Anti-Toxoplasma immunohistochemistry** detects the presence of parasites Toxoplasma genomes can be detected by **PCR**

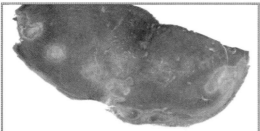

HSV lymphadenitis: punched out appearance Courtesy: Lucas R Massoth, MD

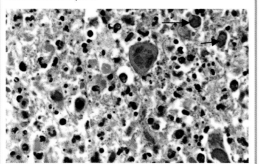

HSV lymphadenitis show multinucleation and intranuclear inclusion. Courtesy: Lucas R Massoth, MD

HERPES SIMPLEX (HSV) LYMPHADENITIS

MORPHOLOGY Lymph Node:

- Imparts **low-power punched-out appearance**
- Interfollicular/paracortical regions focally involved
- **HSV-infected cells show multinucleation & eosinophilic & intranuclear inclusions**() Necrosis, acute and chronic inflammation
- Monocytoid B-cell and follicular hyperplasia

OTHER HIGH YIELD POINTS

- SPECIAL STUDIES -PCR, serology, culture

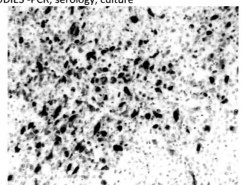

HSV1/2 Immunostain Courtesy: Lucas R Massoth, MD

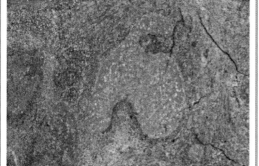

Mixed reactive pattern with mottled appearance

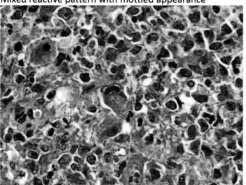

Cytomegalovirus lymphadenitis Courtesy: Teresa Scordino, MD

CYTOMEGALOVIRUS LYMPHADENITIS

MORPHOLOGY Lymph Node:

- Lymph nodes show a **mixed reactive pattern with florid follicular hyperplasia** along with **paracortical and interfollicular hyperplasia**
- Diffuse pattern ± **mottled appearance**
- **Mixed cell population**: Lymphocytes, immunoblasts, and histiocytes
- **Monocytoid B-cell hyperplasia within sinuses**
- The CMV infected lymphocytes, monocytes, and endothelial cells show **nuclear inclusions** (Usually **single, large, brightly eosinophilic nuclear inclusions**, surrounded by clear space -**owl's eye appearance**) and **cytoplasmic inclusions**(smaller, basophilic, and multiple)

OTHER HIGH YIELD POINTS

- Immunohistochemistry for anti CMV antibody
- Antibody titer
- Molecular methods like NASBA, COBAS, AMPLICOR

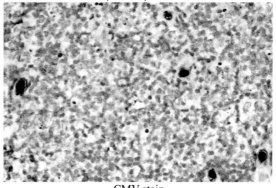

CMV stain

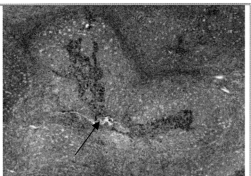
HIV lymphadenitis (Acute phase) -Serpiginous follicles

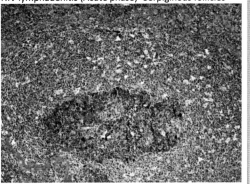

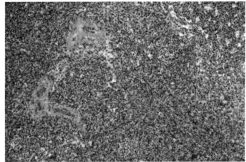
HIV lymphadenitis (Chronic phase)

HIV LYMPHADENITIS
MORPHOLOGY Lymph Node:

- **Pattern A (Florid follicular hyperplasia)**: Serpiginous follicles, followed by follicle lysis, hemorrhage. Sinus are expanded by B-cells and multinucleated giant cells.
- **Pattern B (Mixed pattern)**: Burnt out follicles admixed with hyperplastic follicles. Lymphocyte depletion in interfollicular areas
- **Pattern C (Lymphocyte depletion)**: Poorly defined follicles, subcapsular fibrosis. Lymph node architecture replaced by medullary cords, sinusoids, plasma cells, & histiocytes.

OTHER HIGH YIELD POINTS
- SPECIAL STUDIES
- Serologic testing -Based on the detection **of IgG against HIV antigens in serum**
- **p24 (nucleocapsid protein) becomes positive in a week after detection of viral load**
- **Centers for Disease Control (CDC) criteria for positive serology :**
  - ➢ **Antibodies to gp120 plus antibodies to either gp41 or p24**
  - ➢ Antibodies to gp41 and p24 antigens are 1st detectable serologic marker following HIV infection
  - ➢ **IgG antibodies appear 6-12 weeks following infection in most patients**
  - ➢ Others: gp120 and gp41, envelope proteins
- **Results are reported as positive, negative, or indeterminate**
- Positive 4th generation HIV-1/2 immunoassay should be confirmed by antibody HIV-1/2 differentiation immunoassay
- **RT PCR viral load test: Virus initially detected few days after infection**

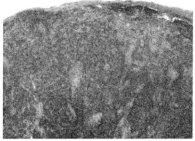
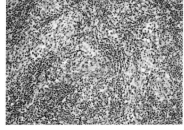
HIV lymphadenitis ("Burnt out" phase)

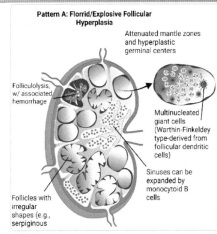
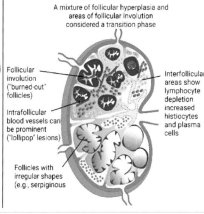
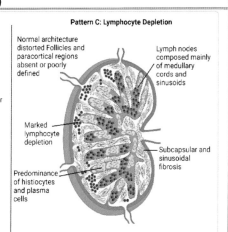

TABLE 2: SUMMARY OF INFECTIOUS CAUSES OF LYMPHADENITIS		
Etiologic Agent	Clinical presentation	Key histological features.
Mycobacterium tuberculosis	<ul><li>Matted lymph nodes</li><li>Fever, weight loss</li><li>May be associated with pulmonary symptoms</li></ul>	<ul><li>Caseous necrosis, necrotizing granulomas</li><li>Langhans giant cells</li><li>Microorganisms highlighted by Zeihl-Neelson stain</li></ul>
Mycobacterium avium intracellulare (MAI)	<ul><li>Immunocompromised state</li></ul>	<ul><li>Epithelioid histiocytic clusters and spindle cells</li><li>Abundant bacteria noted within these cells by ZN stain</li></ul>
Atypical mycobacteria M. scrofulaceum, malmoense, haemophilum	<ul><li>Immunocompromised state</li></ul>	<ul><li>No granulomas</li><li>Lymph node architecture effaced by sheets of histiocytes filled with the bacteria highlighted by ZN stain</li></ul>
Bartonella Henselae	Cat-scratch disease <ul><li>History of cat bite/scratch</li><li>Erythema at the scratch site</li><li>Lymphadenopathy 1-3 weeks later</li></ul>	<ul><li>Follicular hyperplasia</li><li>Abscess</li><li>Stellate necrotizing granuloma</li><li>Microorganisms highlighted by Warthin-Starry stain</li></ul>
	Bacillary angiomatosis <ul><li>Immunocompromised state</li><li>Multiple dome-shaped cutaneous plaques, nodules, regional lymphadenopathy</li></ul>	<ul><li>Follicular hyperplasia</li><li>Ectatic blood vessels with bacterial aggregates around them</li><li>Microorganisms highlighted by Warthin Starry stain</li></ul>
Chlamydia Trachomatis (LGV)	<ul><li>Painless ulcers in the genital area</li><li>Regional lymphadenopathy develops 1-8 weeks later</li></ul>	<ul><li>Neutrophil and vacuolated histiocytes, stellate necrosis</li><li>Reticulate bodies, palisading epithelioid histiocytes</li><li>Microorganisms highlighted by Giemsa, Warthin-Starry stain</li></ul>
Tropheryma whipplei	<ul><li>Mesenteric lymphadenopathy with systemic presentation – arthralgia, diarrhea, steatorrhea</li></ul>	<ul><li>Lymph Node: Effaced architecture replaced by lipogranulomas</li><li>Intestine: Submucosal foamy histiocytes</li><li>Microorganisms highlighted by PAS stain</li></ul>
Treponema pallidum	<ul><li>1^0: Chancre, regional lymphadenopathy</li><li>2^0: Maculopapular rash, generalized lymphadenopathy</li><li>3^0: Gumma, CNS, and CVS manifestations</li></ul>	<ul><li>Non-caseating granulomas</li><li>Parafollicular expansion of immunoblasts, sheets of plasma cells</li><li>Follicular hyperplasia</li><li>Microorganisms highlighted by silver stain</li></ul>
Epstein-Barr virus	<ul><li>Usually affects tonsils</li><li>Hence, pharyngitis and cervical lymphadenopathy</li></ul>	<ul><li>Follicular hyperplasia</li><li>Prominent immunoblasts and are often mistaken as RS-like cells</li><li>Misinterpreted as CHL</li><li>Diagnosis by serology, monospot test, and EBER-ISH</li></ul>
Histoplasma capsulatum	<ul><li>Epidemiology: Ohio and Mississippi regions</li><li>Immunocompromised state</li></ul>	<ul><li>Granulomas, acute inflammation, necrosis</li><li>Intracellular budding yeast forms</li></ul>
Cryptococcus neoformans	<ul><li>CNS and respiratory tract involvement</li><li>Regional lymphadenopathy</li></ul>	<ul><li>Non-caseating granulomas</li><li>Yeast forms with a thick capsule</li><li>Gelatinous fluid-filled spaces, fibrosis noted</li><li>Fungus highlighted by India ink preparation</li></ul>
Toxoplasma gondii	<ul><li>Immunocompromised state</li><li>Posterior cervical lymphadenopathy is typical</li></ul>	<ul><li>Florid reactive follicular hyperplasia</li><li>Sinuses show monocytoid B-cell hyperplasia</li><li>Epithelioid histiocytes in paracortical areas</li><li>Confirmed by serology</li></ul>
Coccidiodes immitis Coccidiodes posadasii	<ul><li>Soil exposure, immunocompromised state, pneumonia, regional lymphadenopathy</li></ul>	<ul><li>Fungus demonstrated as round spherules with endospores within</li><li>Are highlighted by GMS stain</li></ul>
HSV 1/ 2	<ul><li>Skin lesions</li><li>Localized regional lymphadenopathy</li></ul>	<ul><li>HSV infected cells (multinucleation, margination, molding) are seen in paracortical areas. Inflammation and necrosis +/-</li></ul>
Cytomegalovirus	<ul><li>Fever, pharyngitis, lymphadenopathy</li><li>Systemic illness in immunocompromised state</li></ul>	<ul><li>Florid follicular hyperplasia. Viral inclusions (nuclear & cytoplasmic) in endothelial cells and monocytes</li></ul>
HIV	<ul><li>Fever, weight loss, diarrhea</li><li>High-risk behavior</li><li>Opportunistic infections</li><li>Generalized lymphadenopathy</li></ul>	<ul><li>Pattern A (Florid follicular hyperplasia): Serpiginous follicles, followed by follicle lysis, hemorrhage. Sinus are expanded by B-cells and multinucleated giant cells</li><li>Pattern B (Mixed pattern): Burnt out follicles admixed with hyperplastic follicles. Lymphocyte depletion in interfollicular areas</li><li>Pattern C (Lymphocyte depletion): Poorly defined follicles, subcapsular fibrosis. Lymph node architecture replaced by medullary cords, sinusoids, plasma cells, and histocytes</li></ul>

MATURE B-CELL LYMPHOMA

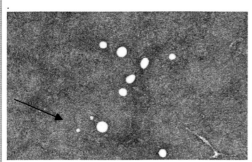

Diffuse architectural effacement, prominent paler proliferation centers (pseudo- follicles), proliferation of small lymphocytes

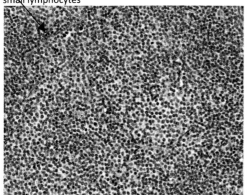

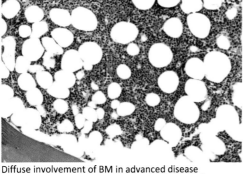

Diffuse involvement of BM in advanced disease

CHRONIC LYMPHOCYTIC LEUKEMIA/ SMALL LYMPHOCYTIC LYMPHOMA (CLL/SLL)

MORPHOLOGY Lymph Node:

- **Diffuse architectural effacement** by proliferation of **small lymphocytes** with variably prominent **paler proliferation centers** composed of prolymphocytes and paraimmunoblasts

Peripheral smear:

- Lymphocytosis composed of small mature lymphocytes with numerous smudge cells

Bone Marrow :

- **Interstitial, nodular, mixed (nodular and interstitial), or diffuse** involvement
- Para-trabecular aggregates are not typical
- Most cases have >30% CLL cells in the bone marrow aspirate

OTHER HIGH YIELD POINTS

- Adults leukemia/lymphoma presenting with lymphadenopathy, splenomegaly, and lymphocytosis
- **Absolute lymphocyte count >5000/ul diagnostic of CLL**
- Immunophenotype: **Positive for CD19, CD20 (dim), CD22, sIg (dim), CD79a, CD5, CD23, LEF1 (specific for CLL), CD200 and Negative for CD10, FMC7, BCL6**
- Cytogenetics: **del 13q14 (most common), trisomy 12, del 11q, and del 17p**
- Prognosis: Transformation of CLL into high-grade lymphoma (proliferation centers broader than a 20x field or confluent), Ki67 >40%, or >2.4 mitoses in the proliferation centers)
- Richter syndrome (transformation to large cell lymphoma): DLBCL type and classic Hodgkin lymphoma type
- Adverse prognostic factors: CD38 and/or ZAP70 expression implying unmutated IgVH status, del 11q, del 13p, high beta-2 microglobulin (>4), higher initial lymphocyte count (>30,000), lymphocyte doubling time <1 year
- Good prognostic factor: Mutated IgVH, del 13q14

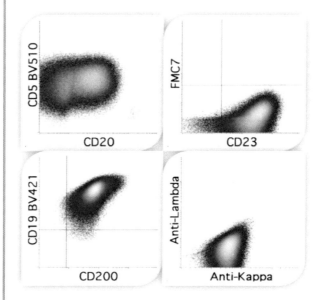

Sheets of neoplastic cells are CD20 positive.

Immunophenotype shows abnormal B-cell population for dim CD20, CD5, CD23, CD19, CD 200 and dim kappa light chain. These cells are negative for FMC7 and lambda.

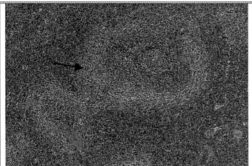
Neoplastic cells surround germinal centers

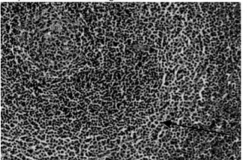
Peripheral (marginal) paler zone of larger cells

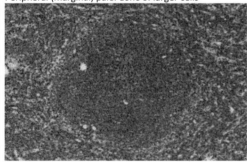
Tumor cells are positive for CD20

SPLENIC MARGINAL ZONE LYMPHOMA (SMZL)

- Involves spleen (mainly white pulp with infiltration into red pulp), splenic hilar lymph nodes (no other nodes), liver (sinusoids), bone marrow (nodular pattern) and peripheral blood (villous lymphocytes)

MORPHOLOGY Spleen

- Neoplastic cells surround and replace the splenic white pulp germinal centers, efface the follicle mantle, and merge with a peripheral (marginal) zone of larger cells, and can also infiltrate the red pulp

MORPHOLOGY Splenic hilar Lymph Node

- Nodular proliferation with preservation of the dilated sinuses
- Lymphoma surrounds and replaces germinal centers, but the two cell types, small lymphocytes, and marginal zone cells, are often more intimately admixed, without the formation of a distinct paler so-called marginal zone

OTHER HIGH YIELD POINTS

- Positive for CD20, CD79a, sIg (IgM and IgD), Ki67 (targetoid pattern)
- Negative for CD5, CD10, CD23, CD43, annexin A1, CD103, cyclin D1
- DIFFERENTIAL DIAGNOSIS

CLL/SLL	Hairy cell leukemia	Mantle cell lymphoma	Follicular lymphoma	Lympho plasmacytic lymphoma
Positive for CD5, CD23, LEF1, CD200	The nodular pattern on bone marrow biopsy excludes HCL {Positive for AnnexinA1 etc.}	Positive for CD5, cyclin D1, SOX11, t(11,14)	Positive for CD10, BCL6, BCL2	MYD88 mutation

- GENETICS-Show Ig genes rearrangement, mutation of NOTCH2, and KLF 2 (associated with del 7q) and Lack translocation typical of other lymphoma like t(14;18), t(11;14); t(11;18) and t(1;14)
- Indolent lymphoma that responds to splenectomy and/or rituximab
- Hepatitis C virus positive cases respond to antiviral treatment using interferon-gamma, with or without ribavirin
- Adverse prognostic factors: NOTCH2, KLF2, p53 mutation and large tumor mass

HAIRY CELL LEUKEMIA (HCL)

MORPHOLOGY Spleen
- Infiltrates in the red pulp, white pulp atrophic
- Blood lakes (red blood cells surrounded by hairy cells)

OTHER HIGH YIELD POINTS

- Indolent neoplasm of small mature lymphoid cells with hairy projections involving peripheral blood, bone marrow, liver (sinusoids) and splenic red pulp (blood lakes)
- Bone marrow fibrosis with a dry tap on aspiration and fried egg morphology on biopsy
- Positive for CD20, CD22, CD11c, CD103, CD25 (bright), CD123, TBX21, annexin A1 (most specific), FMC7, CD200 and cyclinD1 (dim, nuclear)
- Negative for CD5, CD23, and CD10
- BRAF V600E mutation and TRAP-positive on cytochemistry
- Treatment: interferon alfa or nucleosides; for relapse: rituximab, anti-CD22 agents or BRAF inhibitor

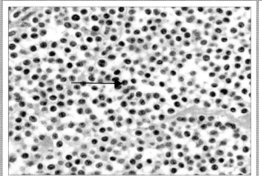
Small lymphoid cells with fried egg appearance

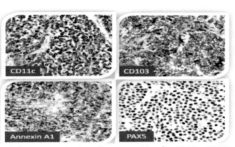

IHC shows neoplastic cells are positive for CD11c,CD103, Annexin A1 and PAX5

Characteristic	HCL (classic)	SMZL
Nucleus	Oval, sometimes "coffee bean"	Round
Cell surface	Circumferential projections	Noncircumferential polar projections
BM infiltration pattern	Diffuse and/or interstitial	Nodular and/or intrasinusoidal
Splenic infiltration pattern	Red pulp, with effacement of white pulp	White pulp
CD123, BRAF V600E, AnnexinA1	Positive	Negative

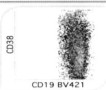

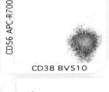
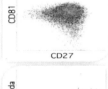

Flow cytometry analysis shows Lymphocytes (blue) positive for CD20,CD19, variable CD38, kappa light restriction and Plasma cells (pink) positive for CD38,CD19,CD20, CD27 and CD81.

LYMPHOPLASMACYTIC LYMPHOMA (LPL)
MORPHOLOGY Lymph Node
- **Normal architecture is retained**
- **Sinuses are dilated and filled with PAS-positive material**
- **Follicular colonization** of monotonous proliferation of small lymphocytes, plasma cells, plasmacytoid lymphocytes
- **Dutcher bodies (intranuclear pseudo-inclusions), mast cells, hemosiderin** can be seen

OTHER HIGH YIELD POINTS
- **Indolent** neoplasm of small B-lymphocytes, plasmacytoid lymphocytes, plasma cells
- Associated with **Hepatitis C and cryoglobulinemia** and presents with IgM paraproteinemia and hyperviscosity syndrome
- **Positive for sIg (IgM > IgG >>> IgA), B-cell antigens: CD19, CD20, CD22, CD79a**
- **Negative for CD5, CD103, CD10, CD23**
- **Plasma cell is positive for CD138, CD19, CD45, PAX5, & Negative for MUM1.**
- **MYD88 L265P mutations (most common)**, CXCR4 truncating frameshift mutations, ARID1A mutations
- Adverse prognostic factors: advanced patient age, cytopenia, high B2-microglobulin levels, serum paraprotein >7 g/dL, del 6q, absent MYD88 mutations (low response to ibrutinib)

HEAVY CHAIN DISEASES (HCD)

Characteristics of Heavy chain diseases

HCD	SITES	ASSOCIATED DISEASES	Morphology	PHENOTYPE
ALPHA IgA	GIT, Respiratory system diseases	Parasitic / bacterial intestinal diseases	-Heavy infiltration of lamina propria of bowel by plasma cells and small lymphocytes -Lymphoepithelial lesions -Progression to diffuse large B-cell lymphoma	Pan B-cell Ag+ CD138+ CD5- CD10- CD20-
GAMMA IgG	Bone marrow, spleen, extranodal sites	Autoimmune Diseases	-Lymph node shows polymorphous infiltration by lymphocytes. Plasmacytoid lymphocytes, plasma cells, immunoblasts, and histiocytes -Lymphocytosis with small lymphocytes, resemble CLL/SLL on Peripheral blood	CD19+ CD20+ CD38+ CD138+ CD5- CD10-
MU IgM	Bone marrow	HSM, pulmonary infection, SLE, systemic amyloidosis	Bone marrow shows vacuolated plasma cells and small round lymphocytes	CD19+ CD20+ CD38+ Kappa CD5+ rare

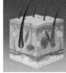

FOLLICULAR LYMPHOMA

MORPHOLOGY Lymph Node

- **Nodular lymphoid proliferation** that typically overruns the lymph node capsule
- **Back-to-back or fused follicles with attenuated mantles, loss of polarity, absence of tingible body macrophages and diminished mitosis**
- Two cell types in varying proportions: small, cleaved cells (**centrocytes**) and large noncleaved cells (**centroblasts**)
- Grading is based on the proportion of large noncleaved cells (centroblasts) in 40x fields of 10 randomly selected neoplastic follicles

OTHER HIGH YIELD POINTS

- Isolated lymphadenopathy without constitutional symptoms, involving bone marrow in 30% of cases at presentation
- **Positive for surface Ig (IgM, IgG), B-cell markers, germinal center markers: LMO2, GCET1, HGAL (GCET2), BCL2, BCL6, CD10**
- **BCL2 expression in follicles: Hallmark of FL and will aid to differentiate reactive follicles vs. FL.** Although BCL2 overexpression is the hallmark of FL, absent BCL2 does not rule out FL.
- In a normal lymph node, BCL2 is expressed in T-cells, primary follicles, and mantle zone
- CD21, CD23 highlight FDC within the follicles
- Grade 3B-cells usually are CD10 negative, BCL2 negative but BCL6 positive
- Ki67 in grade 1-2 is <20%, and in grade 3 is >20%

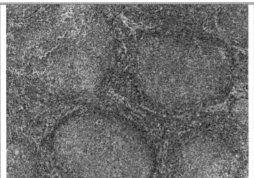

Nodular lymphoid proliferation with back-to-back arrangement

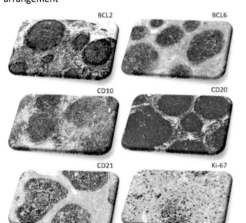

IHC shows positivity for CD20, CD10, Bcl2 and Bcl6. CD21 highlights follicular dendritic meshwork.

Fig 5: Grading of FL based on number of Centroblasts	
Number of Centroblasts per HPF (40x, 0.159 mm^2)	
Grade 1-2 (low grade)	0 – 15
Grade 1	0 – 5
Grade 2	6 – 15
Grade 3 (high grade)	>15
Grade 3A	Centrocytes present
Grade 3B	No centrocytes present

- **Variants of FL**

Diffuse variant FL	-Diffuse involvement with microfollicles seen in background -Inguinal region LN involved -CD10, CD23 Positive, BCL2 weak/- -Absent t (14;18) (q32; q21) IGH/BCL2 - Shows del 1p36, containing gene TNFRSF14
Testicular FL	-High-grade FL with good prognosis -Children >>> adults - lack BCL2 translocation
In situ follicular neoplasia	-Intact nodal architecture with widely scattered involved follicles -Architecturally reactive appearing germinal centers with cytologic features of FL (infiltrate composed exclusively of centrocytes, demonstrated by strong immunostaining for CD10 and BCL2
Duodenal type FL	-Multiple small polyps in the second part of the duodenum detected incidentally on endoscopy -Neoplastic follicles (composed of centrocytes) in the mucosa/submucosa -Low rate of lymph node dissemination with an excellent prognosis -Positive for CD20, CD10, and BCL2; CD21 restricted to the periphery of the follicle -Negative for activation-induced cytidine deaminase

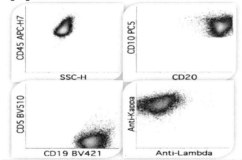

Flow cytometry analysis shows abnormal lymphoid population positive for CD45, CD20, CD19, CD10 with kappa light chain restriction and negative for CD5.

Path presenter

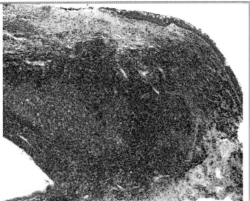

Lymphoepithelial lesions composed of small to medium sized lymphoid cells in conjunctival/ocular MALT lymphoma

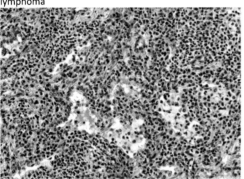

Lymphoepithelial lesions in MALT lymphoma Lung

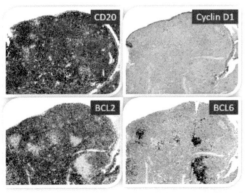

IHC shows neoplastic cells are positive for CD20, Bcl2 and negative for cyclin D1 and Bcl6.

Path presenter

EXTRANODAL MALT LYMPHOMA
MORPHOLOGY Lymph Node
- **Small to medium-sized neoplastic cells** form large **confluent areas in the marginal zone** and can replace germinal centers
- Mantle zone preserved.
- **Lymphoepithelial lesions** are formed in epithelial tissues

OTHER HIGH YIELD POINTS
- Associated with chronic antigenic stimulation: infection or autoimmunity; most commonly involve **stomach**
- **Positive for IgM heavy chains, B-cell markers with light chain restriction, IRTA1, MNDA. Negative for CD5, CD10, CD23, BCL6**
- **Good prognosis**
- **H. pylori antibiotic therapy leads to remission in gastric MALT lymphoma**
- **t (11;18) (q21;q21): resistant to H. pylori eradication therapy**
- Translocations (related to upregulation of NFkB: t (1;14), t (11;18), t (14;18), t (3;14)

Table 3: Genetic alterations in MALT lymphomas

- IG heavy and light chain gene rearrangements are seen with somatic hypermutation of variable regions.
- Biased usage of certain IGHV genes

Translocations (related to upregulation of NF kappa B)

Translocation	Chimeric protein	Locations
t (11;18)	IAP2/MALT1	Pulmonary and gastric tumors
t (3;14)	FOXP1/IGH	Thyroid, ocular adnexa, orbit, and skin
t (14;18)	IGH/MALT1	Ocular adnexa, orbit, and salivary gland
t (1;14)	BCL10/IGH	Intestine, lung, salivary gland

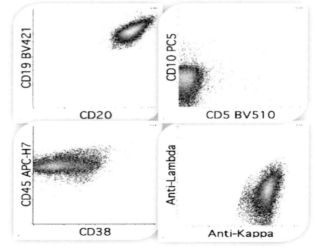

Flow cytometry analysis shows abnormal lymphoid population with bright CD45, CD20, CD19 and kappa light chain restriction. These cells are negative for CD10, CD5, CD38 and lambda.

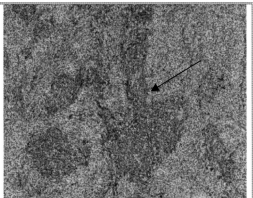

Proliferation of neoplastic cells around the follicles and in interfollicular areas, Follicular colonization

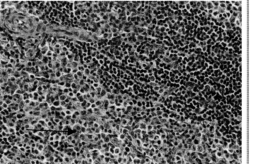

Neoplastic cells- Monocytoid Marginal zone B-cells and Plasma cells

Path presenter

NODAL MARGINAL ZONE LYMPHOMA
MORPHOLOGY Lymph Node
- Proliferation of neoplastic cells around the follicles and in interfollicular area
- **Follicular colonization**: neoplastic cells entering germinal centers noted in a few cases (remnants of follicular dendritic cell (FDC) meshwork noted).
- The neoplastic cell population comprises **Marginal zone B-cells (centrocyte-like, monocytoid), plasma cell cells**, transformed B-cells, and eosinophils.
- Lymphoid cells may show plasmacytoid differentiation.

OTHER HIGH YIELD POINTS
- Morphologically resembles extranodal or splenic type; but **no extranodal or splenic disease**
- Associated with a**utoimmune disease, HCV infections**
- **Positive for pan-B cell markers, CD43, BCL2, MNDA, IRTA1 and Negative for CD5, CD23, cyclin D1, germinal center markers as CD10, BCL6, HGAL, LMO2**
- **Genetics:** Mutations in IGHV 3 & IGHV 4 genes: IGHV 4-34
- MYD88 L265P mutation absent
- Good prognosis in general
- Worse prognosis: advanced age, B symptoms, advanced disease stage

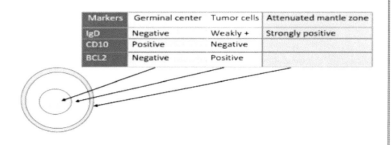

Markers	Germinal center	Tumor cells	Attenuated mantle zone
IgD	Negative	Weakly +	Strongly positive
CD10	Positive	Negative	
BCL2	Negative	Positive	

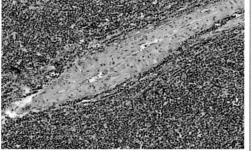

Monomorphic cells in diffuse pattern

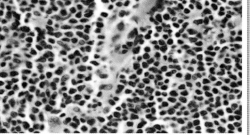

Small to medium sized monomorphic cells with irregular nuclear contours

MANTLE CELL LYMPHOMA
MORPHOLOGY Lymph Node
- **Classical: Monomorphic cells arranged in nodular/diffuse/mantle zone/follicular pattern** (rare)
- **Small to medium lymphoid cells** with **irregular nuclear contours** and dispersed chromatin

Variants of Mantle cell Lymphoma		
Aggressive	**Blastoid**	**Lymphoblast-like cells showing** open chromatin and brisk mitoses
	Pleomorphic	**Mixture of** large and pleomorphic cells showing nuclear irregularity and conspicuous nucleoli
Indolent	**Small cell**	Cells resembling SLL-cells, usually found in **leukemic non-nodal mantle cell lymphoma**
	Marginal zone like	Clusters of monocytoid B-cells, resembling either a marginal zone lymphoma or proliferation center of CLL/SLL

OTHER HIGH YIELD POINTS
- **Aggressive** neoplasm with **CCND1 translocation** in most cases

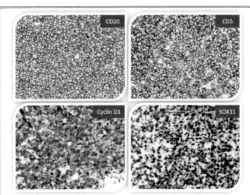

IHC shows neoplastic cells are positive for CD20, CD5, cyclin D1 and SO11

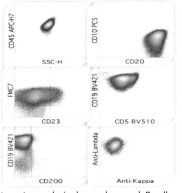

Flow cytometry analysis shows abnormal B-cell population with bright CD20, bright CD19, FMC7, dim CD5 & lambda light chain restriction. These cells are negative for CD10, CD23 and CD200.

- Involves lymph nodes, spleen, and bone marrow, with or without peripheral blood, extranodal sites [Waldeyer's ring, lungs, GIT (as multiple lymphomatoid polyposis)]
- Advanced stage disease with **lymphadenopathy, organomegaly, marrow and peripheral blood involvement** at presentation is common
- IHC- **Positive for surface IgM/IgD (bright), lambda > kappa, cyclin D1, SOX11,** CD5, FMC7, CD43, BCL2 and Negative for CD10, BCL6, CD23
- Proliferative fraction (mitotic count/ **Ki67 index) is extremely important prognostically**
- **t (11;14) (q13; q32); (IGH; CCND1): overexpressing cyclinD1**; abnormal SOX11 expression
- **Incurable, short median survival**
- Adverse prognostic factors: brisk mitoses, Ki67 >30%, blastoid/pleomorphic morphology, leukemia with adenopathy, complex karyotype, TP53 alteration, CDKN2A deletion
- **Leukemic non-nodal mantle cell lymphoma (LNN-MCL):** Small cells resembling CLL cells, involving blood + bone marrow ± spleen, without significant adenopathy; **better prognosis** than classic mantle cell lymphoma

Table 2: Differentiation between classic MCL, LNN-MCL and CLL

	Classic MCL	**LNN-MCL**	**CLL**
Cells	Small – medium	Small	Small
HSM	-	+	+/-
SOX11	+	-	-
CD5	+	+/-	+
CD200	-	+/-	+
CD20	bright	+	dim
Surface light chain	bright	bright	dim
Course	Aggressive	Indolent, rarely progress	Indolent, may progress

- **In-situ mantle cell neoplasia:** Atypical lymphoid cells occupying only the inner mantle zone of a reactive follicle and showing positivity for cyclin D1 with CCND1 rearrangement

DIFFUSE LARGE B-CELL LYMPHOMA, NOT OTHERWISE SPECIFIED (DLBCL, NOS)

MORPHOLOGY Lymph Node

- **Diffuse proliferation of medium or large B lymphoid cells** with nuclei the same size or larger than those of normal macrophages, or more than twice the size of lymphocytes
- **Perinodal** tissue is often infiltrated
- Broad or fine bands of sclerosis may be present
- Morphology:

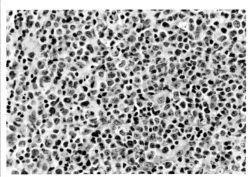

Diffuse proliferation of medium to large B lymphoid cells

Variants:	
Centroblastic	-Most **common** variant -**GCB** type consisting of **centroblasts** which are medium-sized to large lymphoid cells with oval to round, vesicular nuclei with fine chromatin,2- 4 nuclear membrane-bound nucleoli and scant amphophilic or basophilic cytoplasm
Immunoblastic	>90% of the cells are **immunoblasts**, with a single centrally located nucleolus and abundant basophilic cytoplasm
Anaplastic	-**Large cells** with **bizarre pleomorphic** nuclei show **sinusoidal and/or a cohesive growth pattern** and may mimic undifferentiated carcinoma

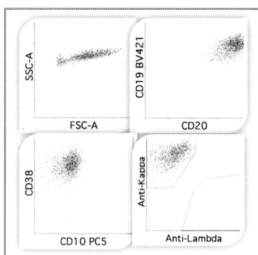

Flow cytometry analysis shows abnormal population with high side and forward scatter, positve for CD19,CD20 and kappa light chain restriction.

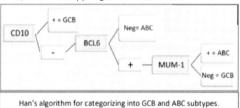

Han's algorithm for categorizing into GCB and ABC subtypes.

Path presenter

Special subtypes	
Primary Breast DLBCL	-ABC subtype and show recurrent MYD88 L265P
Primary Gastric DLBCL	-ABC subtype with recurrent mutations of MYD88
Primary testicular DLBCL	-ABC subtype with high frequency of MYD88 mutations, accompanied by CD79b mutations (in subset of cases) -Testicular DLBCL, NOS, can spread to the CNS and the contralateral testis

OTHER HIGH YIELD POINTS

- Rapidly enlarging, localized, nodal or extranodal mass; with B symptoms in one third patients
- **Positive for CD19, CD20, CD22 and CD45, usually positive for BCL2 with variable expression of CD10, CD5, and BCL6**
- Differential diagnosis includes **extramedullary leukemias, Burkitt lymphoma high-grade B-cell lymphoma with MYC and BCL2 and/or BCL6 rearrangements, and blastoid mantle cell lymphoma**
- CD5+ DLBCL can be distinguished from the blastoid or pleomorphic variant of mantle cell lymphoma by the absence of cyclin D1 and/or SOX11 expression and FISH show t (11;14)
- Morphologically, GCB is more likely to have centroblastic morphology, while ABC often has immunoblastic morphology
- BCL2, t (14;18) rearrangement is common in GCB
- BCL6, t (3; X) rearrangement is more common in the ABC type
- Double expressors (+ IHC for both MYC and BCL2) vs. double hit/ triple hit lymphoma (MYC + BCL2 and/or BCL6 rearrangements)
- Positivity criteria: CD10, BCL6 and IRF4/MUM1 ≥ 30%; BCL2 ≥50%, and MYC ≥ 40%
- Special subtypes: primary breast DLBCL, primary gastric DLBCL, primary testicular DLBCL.

PLASMABLASTIC LYMPHOMA

- Diffuse **proliferation of large neoplastic cells, resembling B immunoblasts or plasmablasts**, that have CD20-negative plasmacytic phenotype
- Occurs in adults in association with immunodeficiency and have a poor prognosis
- Involves extranodal regions of head and neck (oral cavity) and gastrointestinal tract
- **Positive for plasma cell markers (CD38, CD138, VS38c, IRF4/MUM1, PRDM1, XBP1), cytoplasmic Ig (IgG) with light chain restriction, EMA, CD30, CD56 (some cases), high Ki67 >90%, EBER ISH**
- EBER positivity and history of immunodeficiency can aid in differential diagnosis from plasmablastic plasma cell myeloma
- Negative for CD45, B-cell markers, HHV8

GENETICS

- Clonal IGH rearrangement, complex karyotypes, MYC translocation usually with IG gene, seen in EBV positive cases

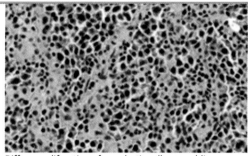

Diffuse proliferation of neoplastic cells resembling immunoblasts to cells with plasmacytic differentiation

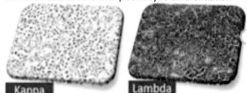
Kappa | Lambda

IHC shows neoplastic cells positive for MUM1, CD138 and lambda restriction. These cells are negative for PAX5 and kappa. CD30 is approx. 20-30%

MUM1

CD138

PAX5

CD30

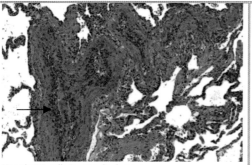

Neoplastic cells in vascular lumen
IHC shows neoplastic cells stain positive with
CD20,PAX5.Ki-67 shows high proliferative index.

INTRAVASCULAR LARGE B-CELL LYMPHOMA

- Aggressive lymphoma involving extranodal sites with the growth of **neoplastic cells within the lumen of vessels, small and intermediate-sized vessels**
- **Fibrin thrombi hemorrhage and necrosis** may be present
- Cytomorphology: Large cells with prominent nucleoli and frequent mitotic figures cells
- Cells may be anaplastic or may be smaller in size
- Sinusoidal involvement in liver, spleen and bone marrow
- **Positive for B-cell antigens**
- CD5 and CD10 can be positive
- Patterns of presentation: classic, hemophagocytic associated and isolated cutaneous
- Complications: CNS relapses and neurolymphomatosis

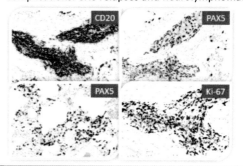

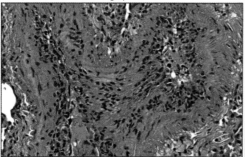

Medium-sized to large cells with round to pleomorphic
nuclei with abundant pale cytoplasm, CD20, CD30 +

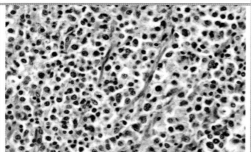

PRIMARY MEDIASTINAL (THYMIC) LARGE B-CELL LYMPHOMA

- Large B-cell lymphoma arising in the anterosuperior mediastinum with distinct clinical, immunophenotypic, genotypic and molecular features mostly affecting young adult females
- Involves anterosuperior mediastinum (thymus) and regional lymph nodes, producing superior vena cava syndrome
- **Diffuse to nodular effacement by medium-sized to large cells** with round to pleomorphic nuclei with abundant pale cytoplasm
- Interstitial fibrosis surrounds nodules of tumor cells
- Positive for **pan B-cell markers, B-cell transcription factors, CD30, IRF4/ MUM1, CD23, MAL1, PDL1/2, CD54, FAS/ CD95, TRAF, REL1, TNFAIP2**
- Variable expressions of CD15, BCL2, BCL6, MYC
- Negative for EBER, CD10, CD5, and sIg
- Mutations in TNFAIP3 (activation of NF-kappa B pathway), SOCS1, STAT6 and PTPN1 (activated JAK/STAT pathway), CIITA (downregulation of MHC class II), BCL6 Poor prognosis: extension into thoracic viscera, pleural/pericardial effusion, and poor performance status

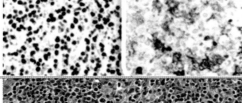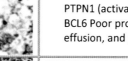

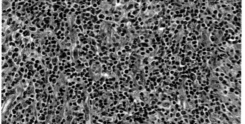

Mucosal infiltration by neoplastic cells

EBV-POSITIVE MUCOCUTANEOUS ULCER

- Ulcerated **lesions with adjacent pseudoepitheliomatous hyperplasia in oral cavities, GIT of elderly or immunosuppressed**
- Reactive lymphadenopathy
- Neoplastic cells have **activated B-cell phenotype (IRF4/MUM1 positive), are positive for EBV markers: LMP-1, EBER; CD30 +, CD15 +** in few cases
- Background scattered lymphocytes are CD8+ T lymphocytes
- Rim of CD3+ T-cells at the junction of the lesion and normal tissue
- Indolent course and responds well to rituximab, local radiation, and chemotherapy

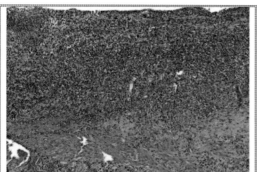

Ulcerated lesion

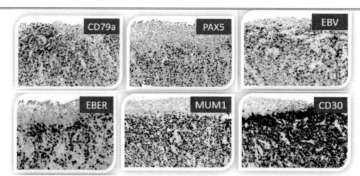

IHC shows neoplastic cells positive for CD79a, PAX5, MUM1, CD30, EBER and EBV

Table: THRLBCL vs NLPHL vs LRCHL			
	THRLBCL	NLPHL	LRCHL
Architecture	Diffuse	Nodular	Nodular/Diffuse
Classic RS cells	-/+	-/+	+
CD45	+	+	−
CD30	−	−	+
CD15	−	−	+/-
CD20	+	+	-/+
CD79a	+	+/-	−
EBV	−	−	+/-
Background lymphocytes	T>>>B	B>>>T	B>T
CD21 FDC	−	+	−
BM inv	+/-	-/+	-/+

T-CELL/HISTIOCYTE RICH LARGE B CELL LYMPHOMA (THRLBCL)
- Involves lymph nodes (diffuse or vaguely nodular), liver (portal tract), spleen (white pulp) and presents as systemic disease

Lymph Node
- Diffuse **or vaguely nodular pattern** replacing most of the normal lymph node parenchyma
- Consist of **dispersed, single large B-cells in the background of small T-cells and variable numbers of bland-looking non-epithelioid histiocytes**
- Large B cells may mimic lymphocyte predominant (LP) cells of NLPHL, centroblasts or maybe more pleomorphic
- Absent follicular dendritic cells meshwork
- On recurrence: the number of atypical cells may increase, resembling DLBCL and rendering an inferior outcome
- Cases lacking histiocytes are currently included in the THRLBCL category with the note about the paucity or absence of histiocytes
- Cases with sheets of neoplastic B-cells should not be included within this category and may be considered a subtype of DLBCL, NOS

OTHER HIGH YIELD POINTS
- Origin: de novo or progression from nodular lymphocyte predominant Hodgkin lymphoma (NLPHL)
- Neoplastic cells are positive for **pan-B markers and BCL6**
- Negative for CD15, CD30, or CD138
- Background consists of CD68+ and CD163+ histiocytes and CD3+ and CD5+ T cells

PRIMARY DIFFUSE LARGE B-CELL LYMPHOMA OF CNS
- DLBCL arises within the brain, spinal cord, leptomeninges or eye
- No association with viruses like EBV, HHV6, HHV8, polyomaviruses SV40 and BK virus
- **Central large areas of geographical necrosis with perivascular lymphoma islands at the periphery**
- Positive for B-cells markers, sIg (IgM and IgD), IRF4/MUM1, BCL6, BCL2, high Ki67 >70%
- Negative for plasma cell markers, **CD10 (positivity should prompt search for systemic DLBCL)**
- Loss of major histocompatibility complex (MHC) class I and/or II expression
- Adverse prognostic factors: del 6q, age >65 years

PRIMARY CUTANEOUS LARGE B-CELL LYMPHOMA, LEG TYPE
- DLBCL arising in cutaneous locations, mostly in the lower legs and predominantly affecting elderly women
- **Non-epidermotropic infiltrate of large B-cells in the dermis**
- **Positive for pan-B-cell markers, BCL2, IRF4/MUM1, FOXP1, MYC, BCL6, IgM and high Ki67**
- MYD88 L265P mutations, CDKN2A loss, and multiple skin tumors are poor prognostic factors
- Treatment: RCHOP (rituximab, cyclophosphamide, doxorubicin, oncovin, prednisone)

Table: EBV Latency patterns	
Latency	**Genes expressed**
0	EBER 1, EBER 2, BART miRNA
I	EBER 1, EBER 2, BART miRNA + EBNA 1
II	EBER 1, EBER 2, BART miRNA + EBNA 1 + LMP1, LMP 2A
III	All genes are expressed, including EBNA 3A, 3B, 3C

LYMPHOMATOID GRANULOMATOSIS
• **EBV+ neoplastic B-cells that are angiocentric and angio-destructive**; commonly affect western adult males
• Large number of reactive CD3+ T-cells
• Most commonly involve lungs, can also involve the brain, kidney, and subcutaneous tissue
• **Positive for B-cell markers, CD30, EBV markers: LMP-1, EBNA2, latency type III**
• **Aggressive behavio**r with grading based on the number of EBV+ cells

DLBCL ASSOCIATED WITH CHRONIC INFLAMMATION
• EBV-associated large B-cell lymphoma arising at sites of long-standing chronic inflammation and most commonly involving body cavities and narrow spaces
• **Diffuse infiltration of large lymphoid cells which simulate immunoblasts and centroblasts**
•Areas of necrosis
• Pyothorax associated lymphoma being the prototype; Males, twin peaks of age • **Positive for B-cell markers, CD30 +/-, EBER, type III EBV latency**
• Genetics: Majority: TP53 mutations, MYC amplification, Del TNFAIP3, Complex karyotype
• Aggressive course and poor prognostic factors: Elevated LDH, ALT

ALK-POSITIVE LARGE B-CELL LYMPHOMA (ALK+ LBCL)
• Aggressive ALK+ LBCL with plasmablastic/ immunoblastic phenotype
Lymph Node
• **Diffuse infiltrate with a sinusoidal growth pattern**
• Cytomorphology: **Large monomorphic immunoblast-like cells** with round nuclei, large central nucleolus, and abundant cytoplasm
• Also, show **plasmablastic or atypical multinucleated giant cell** morphology
• **Positive for ALK (cytoplasmic granular staining), B cell transcription factors (OCT2, BOB1+), EMA, MUM1, plasma cell markers (CD138)**
• Negative for B-cell lineage markers, CD30

EBV-POSITIVE DLBCL (NOS)
• **EBV-positive large B-cell neoplasm** that does not fit into other well defined EBV-positive entities predominantly affecting elderly Asian population
• Aging-associated immune dysregulation plays a role in the development
• Spectrum of morphology varying from polymorphic to monomorphic • **Positive for B-cell markers, IRF4/MUM1, CD30, CD15, EBER, EBV type III or II latency pattern**
• Good prognosis: Younger patients, polymorphic pattern
• Poor prognosis: CD30 positivity, EBNA2 positivity, old age and B symptoms

Table: Grading of Lymphomatoid granulomatosis Based on the number of EBV + cells	
Grade	Features
Grade 1	• Polymorphous cell population • No cytological atypia • Focal necrosis • EBV + cells are < 5/HPF
Grade 2	• Polymorphous background • Occasional large lymphoid cells/immunoblasts • Necrosis is seen • EBV + cells are 5 – 20 /HPF
Grade 3	• Background inflammatory cells • Large, atypical B-cells forming large aggregates • Extensive necrosis • EBV + cells are > 50/HPF, may form sheets

Table : Clinical presentation		
Features	**Pyothorax associated lymphoma**	**DLBCL associated with chronic inflammation at other sites**
Age	20-64 years	40 – 80 years
An associated chronic inflammatory condition	History of spontaneous pneumothorax and TB effusion, history can be **as long as 20 years ago**	Associated with chronic osteomyelitis, metallic implants, surgical mesh implants
Site	Pleural cavity	Joints, bone (femur), periarticular soft tissue
Clinical	Chest pain, respiratory difficulty,raised serum LDH	Pain, lytic lesions on X-ray, raised serum LDH
Morphology	Mass > 10 cm **confined** to the thoracic cavity	Mass lesion at the site

Table: Differentiating features between ALK positive LBCL and ALCL		
	ALK positive LBCL	**ALK + anaplastic large cell lymphoma (ALCL)**
Morphology	Plasmablastic or immunoblastic	Variable, hallmark cells
CD30	-	+ (100%)
CD 20/79a/PAX5	- or weakly +	-
OCT2/BOB1	+	-
CD138	+	-
Granzyme B, Perforin, TIA 1	-	+ (80%)
Translocation	Mostly **t(2;17) CLTC-ALK**	Mostly **t(2;5) NPM-ALK**
ALK positivity	Granular cytoplasmic	Nuclear, nucleolar and cytoplasmic
IgH rearrangement	Monoclonal	Polyclonal
Kappa/lambda ISH	Monotypic	-
TCR rearrangement	Polyclonal	Monoclonal

• Not associated with immunosuppression (HIV, EBV, HHV8)	Molecular t(2;17) (ALK; CLTC) • Does not respond to standard therapy

PRIMARY EFFUSION LYMPHOMA
- **Large B-cell neoplasm strongly associated with the HHV8,** occurring in **immunodeficien**t individuals, and has an extremely **unfavorable prognosis**
- Presents as serous effusions without detectable tumor masses
- Effusion contain large cells with immunoblastic, plasmablastic or anaplastic morphology
- Nuclei are large and round to more irregular in shape, with prominent nucleoli
- Deeply basophilic abundant cytoplasm, with occasional vacuoles
- A perinuclear hof consistent with plasmacytoid differentiation may be seen
- Extracavitary PEL: Rare HHV8-positive lymphomas presenting as solid tumor masses and occurring in lymph nodes or extranodal sites such as GIT, skin, lungs, and CNS
- Positive for CD45, HLA-DR, CD30, CD38, VS38c, CD138, and EMA, HHV8-associated latent protein LANA1 (also called ORF73) (nuclear positivity), EBV (except non-HIV infected population)
- Negative for B-cell markers, BCL6

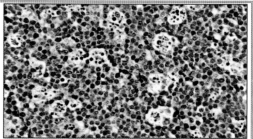

Diffuse monotonous pattern, **Medium-sized cells, Starry sky** pattern due to numerous tingible body macrophages

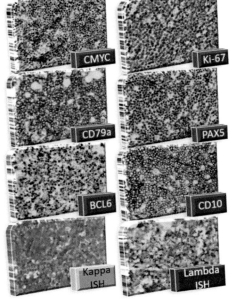

IHC shows positivity for CMYC, CD79a, PAX5, CD10, Bcl6 and lambda restriction. Ki67 (approx. 100 %)

Path presenter

BURKITT LYMPHOMA/LEUKEMIA
- **Aggressive** but curable lymphoma that presents in extranodal sites or as acute leukemia

MORPHOLOGY Lymph Node
- Gross- Masses have a fish-flesh appearance, often associated with hemorrhage and necrosis
- Histologically characterized by diffuse monotonous pattern with **medium-sized B-cells with** round nuclei, finely clumped chromatin, **multiple basophilic medium-sized, paracentrally located nucleoli and basophilic cytoplasm**
- **Numerous mitotic figures**
- Tingible body macrophages impart **starry-sky appearance**
- OTHER HIGH YIELD POINTS
- Three clinicopathological types: Endemic,Sporadic and Immunodeficiency-associated

African (endemic) BL	-Jaw mass in childhood and strong association with EBV
Western (sporadic) BL	Nodal or extranodal (abdominal) of young adults; not associated with EBV Most cases present with abdominal masses, ileocecal region is commonly involved
Immunodeficiency associated with BL	often HIV associated Lymph nodes and bone marrow involved

- Positive for CD19, CD20, CD22, CD10, BCl6, sIg (light chain restriction) and MYC with high Ki67, approximately 100% & Negative for CD5, CD23, BCL2, TdT, CD34
- DIFFERENTIAL DIAGNOSIS:
  - ➢ Lymphoblastic Lymphoma
  - ➢ Blastoid mantle cell lymphoma
  - ➢ Prolymphocytic SLL/CLL
  - ➢ Diffuse large B-cell lymphoma
- Poor prognostic factors: Advanced stage disease, bone marrow, and CNS involvement, unresected tumor >10 cm in diameter, and high serum lactate dehydrogenase level
- **Positive for MYC gene rearrangement as a result of MYC/IgH fusion t (8;14);** also rearranged with IgK (2p12) or Igλ (22q11)

BURKITT-LIKE LYMPHOMA WITH 11Q ABERRATION
- **Resemble Burkitt lymphoma (BL) morphologically and phenotypically but lack MYC rearrangements**

Show chromosome 11q alteration
- Lack 1q gain frequently seen in BL

HIGH-GRADE B-CELL LYMPHOMA (HGBL) (BETWEEN DLBCL, NOS, AND BL)
HGBL with MYC and BCL2 and/or BCL6 rearrangements
- Aggressive lymphoma harboring rearrangement of MYC (8q24) and BCL2 (18q21) and/or BCL6 (3q27); (except for proven follicular lymphomas and B lymphoblastic leukemia/ lymphomas)
- **Double hit lymphomas: MYC + BCL2 or BCL6 translocations**
- **Triple hit lymphomas: MYC + BCL2 + BCL6 translocations**
- Rearrangement of MYC, BCL2, and BCL6 detected by cytogenetic/molecular method like FISH
- Can resemble DLBCL, NOS or BL or intermediate between DLBCL and BL or have blastoid appearance mimicking lymphoblastic lymphoma or blastoid variant of mantle cell lymphoma (negative for TdT and Cyclin D1)

HGBL, NOS
Aggressive lymphomas that lack MYC plus BCL2 and/ or BCL6 rearrangements and do not fall into the category of DLBCL, NOS or BL

PMBL **CHL** 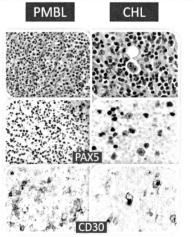 IHC shows CD30 positivity in PMBL type morphology and PAX5 positivity in CHL type morphology	**B-CELL LYMPHOMA, UNCLASSIFIABLE, WITH FEATURES INTERMEDIATE BETWEEN DLBCL AND CLASSIC HODGKIN LYMPHOMA (MEDIASTINAL GRAY ZONE LYMPHOMA PER WHO HAEM5)** • **Lymphomas with overlapping features between CHL and DLBCL**, mainly primary mediastinal (thymic) large B-cell lymphoma (PMBL) • Mediastinal cases are referred as mediastinal gray-zone lymphoma (MGZL) and presents as bulky mediastinal masses leading to superior vena cava syndrome or respiratory distress • Non-mediastinal cases are referred to as gray-zone lymphoma (GZL) • **Cases with CHL on morphology show preservation of the B-cell markers with strong and uniform positivity for CD20 and CD79a** • **Cases with PMBL on morphology show loss of B-cell antigens but positivity for CD30 and CD15** **Aggressive clinical course with poorer outcome** GENETICS Clonal rearrangement of IG genes Gains and amplification of JAK2, **PDL1, PDL2**, REL, MYC Breaks in **CIITA** locus at 16p13.13

T-CELL LYMPHOMAS

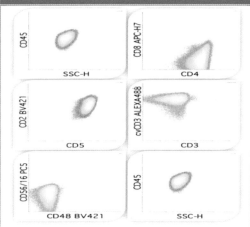 Flow cytometry analysis shows blasts with dim CD45, CD4, CD5, CD2 and cytoplasmic CD3.These blasts are negative for CD8,CD56 and CD48.	**T LYMPHOBLASTIC LEUKEMIA/LYMPHOMA (T-ALL/T-LBL)** Neoplasm with **blasts committed to T-cell lineage,** Involves bone marrow and blood (**T-ALL**) or thymus or nodal or extranodal sites (**T-LBL**) MORPHOLOGY • Lymph Node -Complete effacement, partial effacement and nodular pattern less commonly, Mitotic figures common • Extensive replacement of the thymic parenchyma and infiltration of the surrounding fibroadipose tissue OTHER HIGH YIELD POINTS • Adolescent males • Mediastinal mass • TdT+, cytoCD3+ (lineage specific), CD7+, CD4/CD8 double+ or - • Variable CD2, surface CD3, CD5, CD34, CD10, CD99, CD1a and CD45 • TCR and IGH genes rearranged frequently • Translocations involving chr 7 (TCR) and chr 14 • Activating mutations of NOTCH1 seen in half of the cases • Higher risk disease than B-ALL

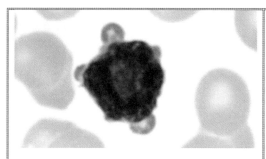

Abnormal T-cell lymphoid population with bright CD45, CD7, CD2, CD5, CD4, CD52, TCL-1 and loss of CD3.

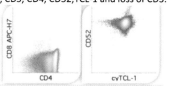

T-CELL PROLYMPHOCYTIC LEUKEMIA (T-PLL)
MORPHOLOGY Lymph nodes
- Diffuse infiltration mainly in the paracortical areas
- Prominent high endothelial venules infiltrated by neoplastic cells

OTHER HIGH YIELD POINTS
- Aggressive leukemia involving blood, bone marrow, liver, spleen
- Positive for T-cell antigens **(CD3, CD2, CD5, CD7), CD52, TCL1**
- CD4+ (most cases), CD8+ (few cases), CD4/CD8 double+ (approximately a quarter of cases)
- Negative for TdT, CD1a
- CD52 (strongly positive): can be used for targeted therapy
- In**v (14) (q11q32)** seen in the majority of cases
- Overexpression of TCL1, used for detecting MRD

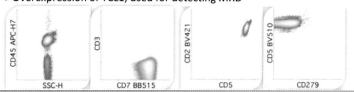

PERIPHERAL T-CELL LYMPHOMA, NOS (PTCL)
Lymph Node Morphology
- Effacement of architecture
- Diffuse and paracortical infiltrates
- Tumor cells are medium to large-sized, with an irregular, pleomorphic, hyperchromatic (sometimes vesicular) nucleus and prominent nucleoli
- Rarely mitotic figures, clear cells, and RS-like cells are seen
- Background of inflammatory cells
- Lymphoepithelioid variant: evidence of epithelioid histiocytes

Path presenter

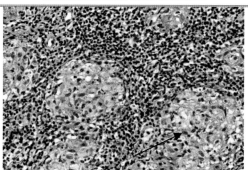

Lymphoepithelioid variant shows epithelioid histiocytes

ADULT T-CELL LEUKEMIA/LYMPHOMA (ATLL)
Morphology
Lymph Node: Early ATLL in the node may resemble Hodgkin lymphoma with **diffuse paracortical infiltration by tumor cells** along with B-cell derived RS-like cells which are **EBV+ and CD30+**

Skin – Epidermal microabscesses, dermal perivascular involvement, and nodules are seen

OTHER HIGH YIELD POINTS
- T-cell neoplasm associated with HTLV-1 infection and endemic in southern Japan, Caribbean and parts of Africa
- Characteristic flower cells (polylobated leukemic cells) seen in peripheral blood
- Clinical variants: acute, lymphomatous, chronic and smoldering
- **Positive: CD4, CD2, CD3, CD5, CD25**
- Negative: CD7, CD8
- Clonal rearrangement of TCR

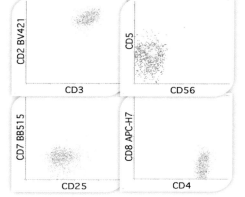

Flow cytometry analysis shows abnormal T cell lymphoid cells positive for CD3, CD2, CD4, dim CD5, dim CD25 and loss of CD7. CD4:CD8 ratio is abnormal.

IHC
Top left: CD2, Top right: CD4, Bottom left: CD7, Bottom right: CD8. CD4>CD8. Loss of CD7.

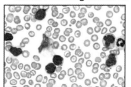
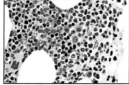
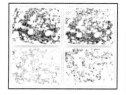

Picture credits: Katelyn Dannheim, MD (@KDannheimMD)

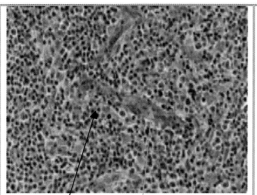
Neoplastic cells cluster around HEV

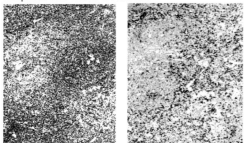
IHC shows positivity for CD3 and PD1.

ANGIOIMMUNOBLASTIC T-CELL LYMPHOMA
Lymph Node Morphology
- Partial or complete nodal involvement with perinodal infiltration
- **HEVs are prominent**
- **Neoplastic cells cluster around HEV**
- Polymorphous inflammatory background: Reactive lymphocytes, histiocytes, plasma cells, eosinophils

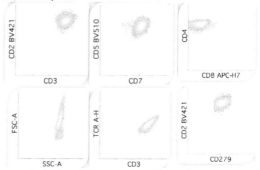

Flow cytometry analysis shows abnormal T-cell population positive for CD3, TCR alpha, CD2, CD5, CD7, CD279 and CD4. The CD4:CD8 ratio is abnormal.

Path Presenter

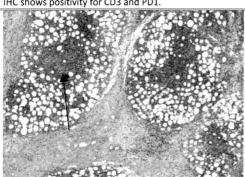
Lymphoma infiltrates the subcutaneous fat

SUBCUTANEOUS PANNICULITIS-LIKE T-CELL LYMPHOMA
- T-cell lymphoma of cytotoxic T-cells (CD8+, cytotoxic markers TIA-1, granzyme B, perforin are positive
- **Lymphoma infiltrates the subcutaneous fat and spares dermis/epidermis, with rimming of fat by tumor cells**
- Cells are of uniform size with irregular hyperchromatic nuclei with a rim of cytoplasm
- Reactive histiocytes
- Karyorrhexis
- Vascular invasion
- Prognosis is good if not associated with hemophagocytosis
- Should be excluded from cutaneous T-cell lymphomas as these have a worse prognosis

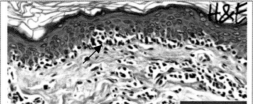
Cutaneous T-cell lymphoma: small to medium sized neoplastic cells with cerebriform nuclei

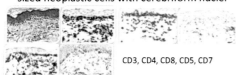
CD3, CD4, CD8, CD5, CD7

MYCOSIS FUNGOIDES
- Epidermotropic primary cutaneous T-cell lymphoma with small to medium sized neoplastic cells having cerebriform nuclei
- Clinically patch, plaque, tumor and erythrodermic stages with dense dermal infiltrate in the tumor stage (epidermotropism may no longer be evident in tumor stage)
- Variants include folliculotropic, pagetoid and granulomatous slack skin variants
- Positive for CD2, CD3, CD5, CD4
- Negative for CD8, CD7 (frequently)
- Cytotoxic CD8+ phenotype has been recognized in cases of pediatric MF
- Expression of CD30 is associated with large cell transformation (defined as >25% large blastic cells)

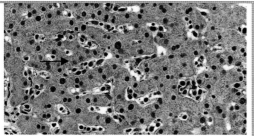

Liver: Sinusoids are infiltrated by tumor cells

HEPATOSPLENIC T-CELL LYMPHOMA
• Aggressive lymphoma of cytotoxic T-cells of gamma delta type commonly involving liver (sinusoids), spleen (red pulp), bone marrow (sinusoidal pattern) and sparing the lymph nodes
• Affects young, immunosuppressed individuals
• Association with isochromosome 7q
• Positive for CD3, TIA-1, granzyme M
• Variable CD56, CD8
• Negative for granzyme B, CD4, CD5, EBV

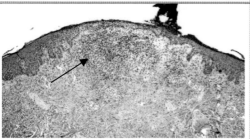

Confluent sheets of tumor cells in the dermis

PRIMARY CUTANEOUS CD30 POSITIVE T-CELL LYMPHOPROLIFERATIVE DISORDER
Lymphomatoid papulosis
• Chronic resolving-relapsing cutaneous disorder with histology mimicking cutaneous T-cell lymphoma and a benign clinical course
• Multiple subtypes with type A being the most common
Primary cutaneous ALCL
• CD30+, ALK-negative primary cutaneous lymphoma composed of large cells
• Exclude MF and systemic ALCL
• Good prognosis

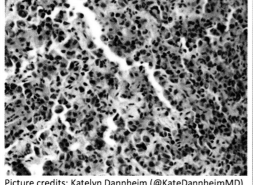

Picture credits: Katelyn Dannheim (@KateDannheimMD)

IHC shows neoplastic cells positive for EMA, CD2 (top row), CD30, AlK1 (middle row), CD43, and MIB1 (bottom row).

Flow cytometry analysis shows an abnormal T-cell population(pink) positive for CD2, CD4, variable CD8, TIA1, Granzyme B, and CD30

Path Presenter

ANAPLASTIC LARGE CELL LYMPHOMA, ALK-POSITIVE
• Hallmark cells: Neoplastic cells with eccentric, horseshoe-shaped nuclei with the eosinophilic region near the nucleus
• t (2;5) (NPM-ALK) fusion most common
• Positive for CD30, ALK, at least some T-cell antigens (CD2, CD4, CD5), cytotoxic markers (TIA-1, granzyme B, perforin), CD25, CD43
• Variable CD45, EMA, CD3, CD8
• Better prognosis than ALK-negative ALCL

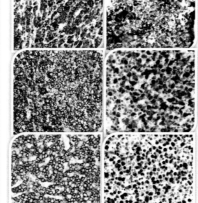
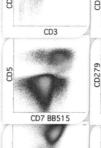
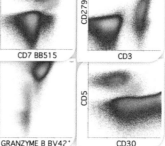

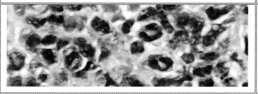

ANAPLASTIC LARGE CELL LYMPHOMA, ALK-NEGATIVE
• Morphologically like ALK + ALCL
• ALK-, CD30+
• DUSP22 rearranged can be MUM1+, negative for cytotoxic markers and good prognosis
• TP63 rearranged are positive for p63 and have a poorer prognosis

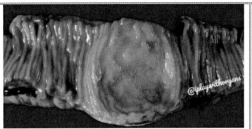
EATL, image credits: Cory Nash

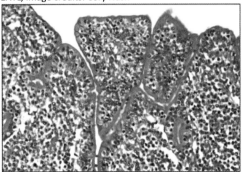
EATL: Medium - large cells with mixed inflammatory cells

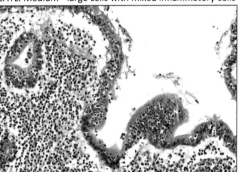
MEITL, monomorphic medium sized cells with epidermotropism

INTESTINAL T-CELL LYMPHOMA

Enteropathy associated T-cell lymphoma
• Occurring commonly in western countries in association with celiac disease (small intestine involved)
• **Medium to large cells with mixed inflammatory cells**
• **Positive for CD3, CD7, CD103, and cytotoxic markers**
• Negative for CD4, CD8, CD56, CD5

Monomorphic epitheliotropic intestinal T-cell lymphoma
• **Monomorphic medium sized lymphoma cells with no inflammatory component, prominent epidermotropism and no association with celiac disease (most common in the small intestine)**
• Occurs in Asian and Hispanic population
• **Positive for CD3, CD8, CD56, TIA1, CD20 (aberrant expression in some cases)**
• Negative for CD5

Indolent T-cell lymphoma of the gastrointestinal tract
• Indolent chronic relapsing disease involving multiple gastrointestinal sites and presenting as mucosal thickening
• Epithelium is not involved
• **Lamina propria is expanded by neoplastic lymphoid cells**
• Positive for CD3, CD8, TIA1, CD2, CD5,
• Negative for CD56, CD7, granzyme B
• Low Ki67

Table: Types of Intestinal T-cell lymphoma	
Type 1 (EATL)	Type 2 (MEITL)
• Enteropathy associated T-cell lymphoma (EATL) • Associated with celiac disease • North Europeans • **Polymorphic population of cells, CD8-, CD56-** • αβ phenotype • Aggressive disease course in adults • Associated with extranodal NK/T-cell lymphoma, nasal type	• Monomorphic epitheliotropic intestinal T-cell lymphoma (MEITL) • Not associated with celiac disease • Asians and Hispanics • **Monomorphic population of cells, CD8+, CD56+** • γδ phenotype • Aggressive disease course in adults • **MATK** is characteristically expressed • Gain of 8q24 (MYC gene) • Mutations in STAT5B, SETD2

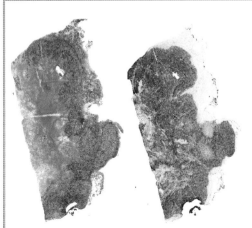
BI-ALCL, CK30 positive

BREAST IMPLANT-ASSOCIATED LARGE CELL LYMPHOMA
Associated with breast implants, morphologic features resemble ALCL but is ALK-negative
Large and pleomorphic tumor cells
Hallmark cells seen in other forms of ALCL can also be identified
Excellent prognosis
Immunophenotype
Positive: CD30 (strong and uniform expression)
Negative: ALK
Incomplete expression of pan-T-cell antigens
Prognosis
Excellent
Most important adverse prognostic factor is the presence of a solid mass of tumor cells, which may indicate a need for systemic therapy

HODGKIN LYMPHOMA

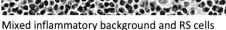

Effaced architecture

CLASSIC HODGKIN LYMPHOMA

- Mixed cellularity CHL(MCCHL): Classic HRS cells in a diffuse mixed inflammatory background
- Nodular sclerosis CHL(NSCHL): Lacunar cells (retracted cytoplasmic membrane) with broad fibroblast poor collagen bands surround at least one nodule
- Lymphocyte-rich CHL(LRCHL): Nodular or diffuse cellular background of small lymphocytes, with an absence of granulocytes and scattered HRS cells
- Lymphocyte-depleted CHL(LDCHL): Predominance of HRS cells and the scarcity of background lymphocytes. Types: Diffuse fibrosis subtype and anaplastic subtype.

OTHER HIGH YIELD POINTS

- Peripheral lymphadenopathy with B symptoms
- Classic Reed Sternberg cells: large cells with bilobed nuclei, prominent eosinophilic viral inclusion-like nucleolus, and abundant basophilic cytoplasm
- IHC: Strong membranous and Golgi zone positivity for CD30 (nearly all cases), CD15 positive (most cases), PAX5 positive (weaker than that of reactive B-cells), weak and variable CD20 positivity
- Type II EBV latency: LMP1 and EBNA1 without EBNA2.
- Prevalence: MCCHL and LDCHL > NSCHL
- PDL1+ T-cell rosettes
- NF-KB is constitutively activated, JAK/STAT signaling pathway
- Treatment: ABVD, BeACOPP, novel agents (CD30 Mab: Brentuximab), immune checkpoint inhibitors (Nevolimumab)

Classic RS cell

NODULAR LYMPHOCYTE PREDOMINANT HODGKIN LYMPHOMA (NLPHL)

- Nodular or vaguely nodular mixed cell proliferation
- Localized peripheral LNs, B symptoms rare
- LP cells (Popcorn cells): Lobed nuclei, with smaller basophilic nucleoli with a rim of pale cytoplasm
- Neoplastic cells positive for CD20, CD45, CD79a, PAX5, OCT2, and BOB1; CD15 and CD30 negative. EBV infection in rare cases
- Clonally rearranged IGH genes and frequent BCL6 rearrangement
- Differential diagnosis: TCRBCL and CHL
- Good prognosis for Stage I and II
- Advanced NLPHL responds better to the R-CHOP used for aggressive B-cell lymphomas

Mixed inflammatory background and RS cells

Path presenter

HISTIOCYTIC AND DENDRITIC CELL NEOPLASMS

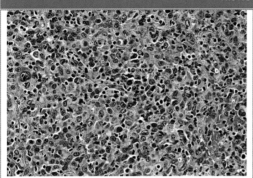

Large neoplastic cells on reactive background

HISTIOCYTIC SARCOMA
MORPHOLOGY Lymph Node
- Diffuse effacement of nodal or extranodal architecture by tumor cells which are large, non-cohesive with abundant eosinophilic cytoplasm and eccentrically placed large nuclei
- Hemophagocytosis, xanthomatous change and sarcomatoid areas may be seen
OTHER HIGH YIELD POINTS
- Wide patient age range, from infancy to old age (predominantly males)
- Associated with malignant mediastinal teratoma or malignant lymphoma
- Fever, weight loss, intestinal obstruction, skin rash/ lesions, pancytopenia, lymphadenopathy, rare systemic
- Positive: CD163, CD68, lysozyme, CD45, 45RO, HLA-DR, CD4
- Isochromosome 12p, BRAF V600E
- Aggressive neoplasm with poor response to therapy

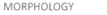

LANGERHANS CELL HISTIOCYTOSIS
MORPHOLOGY
- **Langerhans cells**- Medium-sized oval cells with irregular **grooved nuclei**, inconspicuous nucleoli, and abundant pale, eosinophilic cytoplasm
- Characteristic **background population of eosinophils, neutrophils, small lymphocytes, and osteoclast type giant cells**
- Sinus pattern and paracortex infiltration in lymph nodes, nodular splenic red pulp sclerosing cholangitis,
OTHER HIGH YIELD POINTS
- Childhood, white males > females, smokers (LCH of the lung)
- Transdifferentiation from TALL
- Solitary or multifocal/ multiple sites: bone and adjacent soft tissue (skull, mandible; lytic lesions eroding cortex), skin, liver, spleen, BM
- Positive: **CD1a, langerin, S100, CD68, HLA-DR, PDL1, low CD45 and lysozyme**, variable Ki67
- Electron microscopy shows presence of **tennis racket-shaped Birbeck granules in the cytoplasm**
- **BRAF V600E mutation, MAP2K1**, some with clonal IGH, IGK or TR

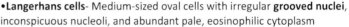

Langerhans cells with irregular,grooved nuclei on background of eosinophils, neutrophils, and small lymphocytes

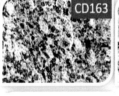 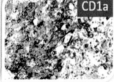

Path presenter

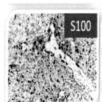 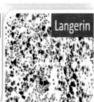 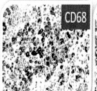 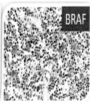

IHC shows neoplastic cells positive for CD163,CD1a,S-100, langerin,CD68 & BRAF

LANGERHANS CELL SARCOMA	tissue, lymph nodes, lung, liver, spleen, bone
Rare, aggressive high-grade neoplasm in adults • Extranodal, multifocal, stage III-IV; skin and underlying soft	• Malignant pleomorphic LC cells with >50 mitoses per 10 HPF • Occasional BRAF V600E mutation
INDETERMINATE DENDRITIC CELL TUMOR • Extraordinarily rare, one or multiple generalized papules, nodules, or plaques on the skin with dermal involvement • Diffuse LCH-like cells with irregular nuclear grooves and typically	abundant eosinophilic cytoplasm, eosinophilic infiltrate usually not present, lack Birbeck granules • S100+, CD1a+, langerin -, variable CD45, CD68, lysozyme and CD4 • Rare BRAF V600E mutation, spontaneous regression or rapid progression

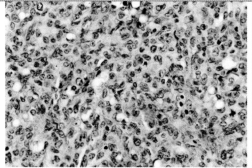

Fascicles of neoplastic cells with nuclear indentations

INTERDIGITATING DENDRITIC CELL SARCOMA
MORPHOLOGY Lymph Node
- Ovoid to spindle cells with nuclear indentations, vesicular chromatin, distinct nucleoli, eosinophilic cytoplasm, and indistinct cell borders forming whorls and storiform pattern
- Tumor infiltrates the paracortex when involving lymph nodes
- Mitotic rate is low
- Multinucleated cells and lymphocytic infiltrate can be seen

OTHER HIGH YIELD POINTS
- Extremely rare neoplasm in adults and children, males > females
- Solitary lymph node lesion or extranodal: skin, soft tissue, hepatosplenomegaly
- ,Birbeck granules not seen

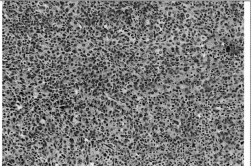

Neoplastic cells forming diffuse sheets and whorls

FOLLICULAR DENDRITIC CELL SARCOMA
- Cervical lymph node, tonsil, GIT, soft tissue, mediastinum, retroperitoneum, omentum
- Slow growing painless mass lesion (>7 cm) or abdominal pain, rare paraneoplasti pemphigus
- Storiform whorls of bland (1-10 mitosis) to pleomorphic (>30 mitoses) cells with cytoplasmic processes and no Birbeck granules, lymphocyte aggregates around blood vessels, epithelioid tumor cells
- Positive: CD21, CD23, CD35, Clusterin, CXCL13, podoplanin, FDCSP, Serglycin, PDL and EBV negative
- Complex karyotype, negative regulation of NF KappaB pathway, BRAF V600E mutation
- Worse prognosis: >6.0 cm tumor size, coagulative necrosis, ≥5 mitosis, marked cytologic atypia, refractory paraneoplastic pemphigus.

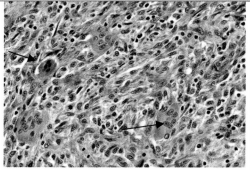

Infiltration by Spindle cells, Touton cells

DISSEMINATED JUVENILE XANTHOGRANULOMA
MORPHOLOGY
- Infiltration by small oval to spindled cells with bland nuclei and vacuolated to pink cytoplasm
- Cells are small without nuclear grooves
- Background inflammatory cells are seen with or without Touton-type giant cells.
- Touton cells less common at non-dermal sites.

OTHER HIGH YIELD POINTS
- Association: NF1; high risk of JMML
- Deep, visceral, and disseminated forms occur by the age of 10 years; half within first year of life
- Skin and soft tissue (commonly, head and neck), upper aerodigestive tract, CNS, eye, liver, lung, LN, BM
- Positive: **Vimentin, CD14, CD68, CD163, Factor XIIIa, fascin, subset S100**
- Negative: CD1a and langerin, BRAF
- All clinical forms are benign, LCH therapy; severe: MAS with cytopenias and liver damage, multiple CNS lesions

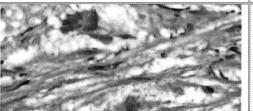

ERDHEIM CHESTER DISEASE
MORPHOLOGY Extranodal sites
- Architectural effacement by sheets of histiocytes with foamy to eosinophilic cytoplasm and small nuclei
- Touton giant cells and fibrosis are seen frequently
- Background polymorphic with infiltrate of plasma cells, neutrophils, and small lymphocytes

OTHER HIGH YIELD POINTS

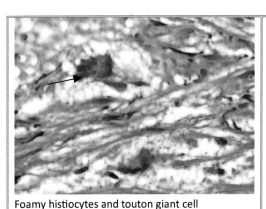

Foamy histiocytes and touton giant cell

- Clonal systemic proliferation of non-Langerhans cell histiocytes, subset with concurrent LCH
- Rare, male preponderance
- Skeletal system, central nervous system, cardiovascular system, kidney, retroperitoneum, and skin involved most commonly
- Coated aorta, diffuse pleural thickening, bilateral symmetrical cortical osteosclerosis of long bones
- Positive: **CD14, CD68, CD163, fascin, Factor XIIIa, BRAF**
- Negative: S100 (rare positive), CD1a and langerin
- Mutations: BRAF V600E (targeted therapy), NRAS, PI3KCA pathway gene
- Severe – cerebellar degeneration, renovascular hypertension, multisystem involvement, increased CRP

BLASTIC PLASMACYTOID DENDRITIC CELL NEOPLASM

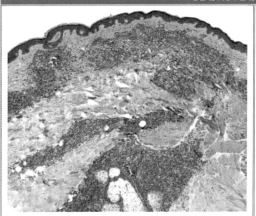

Neoplastic cells infiltration in dermis and subcutaneous fat, epidermis spared.

Path presenter

MORPHOLOGY Skin –Diffuse, monomorphous infiltrate of medium-sized blast cells with irregular nuclear contours, fine chromatin, and one to several small nucleoli and scanty greyish blue cytoplasm
- Mitoses are variable in number, angioinvasion and coagulative necrosis are absent
- Dermis is usually massively involved, with extension to the subcutaneous fat; epidermis and adnexa are spared

Lymph Node –Diffusely involved interfollicular areas & medulla

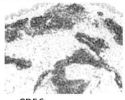

CD123   CD43   CD56

- Absence of lineage associated antigens, together with **positivity for CD4, CD45RA, CD56, and CD123, is considered diagnostic (Mnemonic: 123456)**
- CD303 positivity has the highest diagnostic score within a panel of markers used for BPDCN identification
- Clinical course is aggressive with a short median survival.